Clinical Nursing Procedures

TO ACCOMPANY

FUNDAMENTALS OF NURSING

MARY C. SUNDBERG

Kathleen Hoerth Belland, RN, BSN
Mary Ann Wells, RN, MSEd

Clinical Nursing Procedures

TO ACCOMPANY

FUNDAMENTALS OF NURSING

MARY C. SUNDBERG

Jones and Bartlett Publishers, Inc.
Boston/Monterey

Printed in the United States of America

10 9 8 7 6 5 4 3 2 1

Editorial offices:
Jones and Bartlett Publishers, Inc.
23720 Spectacular Bid
Monterey, CA 93940

Sales and customer service offices:
Jones and Bartlett Publishers, Inc.
20 Park Plaza
Boston, MA 02116

ISBN: 0-86720-400-1

Production: Del Mar Associates
Manuscript Editor: Lillian Rodberg
Interior and Cover Design: Louis Neiheisel
Illustrations: Jack P. Tandy & Associates
Typesetting: Allservice Phototypesetting Company
       of Arizona

Photo Credits
44, 88, 356, 369: Photos by Mark Albertini; 91:
Courtesy Scaletronix, Inc.; 291 (*left*), 292: Courtesy
Stryker Corporation; 291 (*right*): Courtesy Kinetic
Concepts, Inc.

Preface

This book has been written to accompany *Fundamentals of Nursing* by Mary C. Sundberg.

In the table of contents each procedure is keyed to the page of *Fundamentals of Nursing* in which that procedure is applicable. This provides the student with information relevant to laboratory practice and clinical intervention.

PURPOSE

Clinical Nursing Procedures is a manual designed for nursing practice at all levels of nursing care. Both basic and complex skills are included making the manual useful for independent learning situations, and as a primary or supplemental text in a nursing course.

Although the implementation phase of the nursing process is specifically addressed in this manual, it must be utilized within the total nursing process framework. Careful assessment, problem identification, and planning should be included as preliminary steps prior to providing nursing care at any level. Procedures should then be individualized for each patient and documented in the nursing care plan.

ORGANIZATION AND SCOPE

Clinical Nursing Procedures is divided into two sections. The first includes procedures related to basic nursing care; the second deals with procedures related to specific health alterations. Each section is subdivided into units. Specific procedures can be quickly located by referring to the Contents or the comprehensive Index.

Each procedure is divided into seven sections to assist the nurse in understanding the procedure and organizing the patient's care.

- The purpose provides a brief explanation of why the procedure is performed and/or the expected outcome the procedure will have on the patient.
- All requisites are listed for procedures to allow the nurse to organize the procedure prior to implementation. Equipment is listed in general terms to permit health care institutions to substitute requisites according to individual preference.
- Guidelines for each procedure give the nurse additional knowledge related to the procedure. Pathophysiology, anticipated problems, policies, legal implications, and specific assessment parameters are some of the areas identified.
- The nursing action with related rationale section provides a step-by-step approach to implementing the procedures. Illustrations are included to assist in visualizing certain steps of the nursing skill.
- For each procedure, the implementation phase of health teaching is outlined, giving the nurse the opportunity to share the information with both the patient and family. Suggestions for teaching that should be included prior to performing the procedure and suggestions for health maintenance following the procedure are provided.
- The documentation section of each procedure provides a method for utilizing the last step of the nursing process: evaluation. Recording the outcome of nursing interventions offers the opportunity for recording quality care, providing legal protection, and planning reassessment of nursing care.
- References are included with the procedures for further reinforcement of implementation techniques and rationale.

It should be noted that the procedures included in this manual are primarily related to adult patients in the medical-surgical area. Every effort has been made to present the most current information based on scientific principles; however, the nurse must continue to adapt past knowledge to new developments in present and future technologies. Consideration must always be given to hospital and school policies when implementing any procedure outlined in this manual.

The editors and contributing authors hope that this manual will provide a systematic approach to quality nursing care.

Contributors

The following contributing authors are employees of St. Luke's Memorial Hospital in Racine, Wisconsin. All are members of the Nursing Procedure Committee.

Kathleen Hoerth Belland, RN, BSN
In-Service Instructor

Mary Ann Naber Bird, RN
Clinical Nurse, Medical-Surgical

Lucy Antonioni Kohli, RN, BSN
Nurse Epidemiologist

Catherine Shannon Leffler, RN
Clinical Nurse, Nursery

Marianne Key O'Grady, RN, MSN
Clinical Specialist Perinatal Nursing

Linda Johnson Parsons, RN
Clinical Nurse, Critical Care

Sue Hansen Pehlivanian, RN, BSN
Assistant Director of Nursing, Critical Care

Mary Ann Wells, RN, MSEd
Instructor, School of Nursing

Contents

Unit 2 Medication Administration ___ 95

Unit 3 Intravenous Therapy _____ 119

SECTION TWO
PROCEDURES RELATED TO SPECIFIC HEALTH ALTERATIONS
PAGE 175

Unit 4 Cardiopulmonary Procedures _____ 176

Unit 5 Gastrointestinal / Metabolic Procedures _____ 216

Unit 6 Renal/Urological Procedures _____ 250

Unit 7 Musculoskeletal Procedures___285

Unit 8 Sensorineural Procedures___326

Unit 9 Integumentary/Gynecological Procedures _____ 350

SECTION ONE

PROCEDURES RELATED TO SUPPORTIVE NURSING CARE

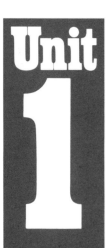

Unit 1

Basic Patient Care

PROCEDURES

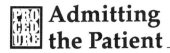 # Admitting the Patient

PURPOSE

1. Assist the patient, family, and/or significant other to feel secure, oriented, and welcome.
2. Make an initial assessment of the patient to identify significant needs.
3. Initiate a plan for nursing care and treatment.

REQUISITES

1. Thermometer
2. Stethoscope
3. Sphygmomanometer
4. Scale
5. Sterile midstream urine specimen kit
6. Nursing history and assessment form

GUIDELINES

1. The patient's condition as well as hospital policy will determine the exact admission procedure.
2. Hospitalization for whatever reason is emotionally stressful for the patient. A warm and understanding nurse can ease the adjustment.
3. Include the family or significant other in admitting the patient.

NURSING ACTION/RATIONALE

1. Assemble all equipment.
2. Identify the patient by name and introduce yourself.
3. Explain the admission procedure and your role as the nurse.
4. Provide privacy.
5. Wash your hands.
6. Place the identification bracelet on the patient's wrist if it is not already in place. Confirm bracelet information with the patient.
7. Orient the patient to the room, the bathroom, and the unit. Explain routines such as times for awakening, retiring, meals, and visiting.
8. Assist, if necessary, in arranging the patient's personal belongings.
9. Request that the patient send home any clothing and articles not needed during hospitalization. In most hospitals, valuables or money can be placed in the hospital safe.

If the patient is incapacitated, prepare a list of his/her belongings and their disposition. Have a second person assist and cosign the list.
10. Inquire whether any medications have been brought to the hospital. If so, request that a family member take them home and explain the procedure for medication administration during hospitalization.
11. Provide the patient with a hospital gown, if appropriate. Assist the patient to dress as necessary.
12. Interview the patient to obtain nursing history. Include:
    a. Chief complaint or reason for admission.
    b. Other current or past health problems.
    c. Current medications and dosages.
    d. Known allergies and the type of reaction.
    e. Comfort status.
    f. Activity, rest, sleep pattern.
    g. Nutrition/fluids pattern.
    h. Urinary and bowel elimination pattern.
    i. Other parameters of physical and psychosocial assessment as appropriate.
13. Obtain baseline vital signs, height, and weight.
14. Obtain a urine specimen if required.
15. Explain to the patient what he/she might anticipate based on his/her condition and the physician's orders.
16. Identify initial nursing diagnoses and, with the patient, formulate short- and long-term goals and a plan for nursing care.
17. Assist the patient to a comfortable position, as appropriate. Place the call signal within reach. Explain and demonstrate the use of the system.
18. Return all equipment to the appropriate area.

PATIENT AND/OR FAMILY TEACHING

1. Explain the admission process to the patient.
2. Reinforce and clarify the physician's explanation of the disease process.
3. Explain any diagnostic testing and therapeutic orders.
4. Instruct the patient to call the nurse with any questions or problems.
5. Explain any activity or diet restrictions.

DOCUMENTATION

1. Disposition of the urine specimen.
2. Initial assessment and nursing history.
3. Nursing diagnoses, goals, and plan of care.
4. Patient's reaction to the hospitalization.

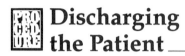 Discharging the Patient

PURPOSE

1. Provide for continuity of care.
2. Assist the patient with the discharge process.

REQUISITES

1. Equipment, supplies, and medication, as appropriate.
2. Written instructions, as appropriate.

GUIDELINES

1. A physician's order is required to discharge a patient from the hospital.
2. The procedure for discharging a patient who wishes to leave the hospital against medical advice varies among health care facilities. Refer to your hospital's policy manual.
3. Inform the patient and family regarding the date of discharge as soon as it is known, so that they can make any necessary arrangements.
4. Planning for a patient's discharge should begin as soon as the patient is admitted. Areas of discharge planning may include activity restrictions, diet modifications, medications, treatments, exercises, follow-up care, community resources, and patient education. Collaboration with other members of the health care team, such as social service and dietary personnel, may be indicated.
5. The patient and family should be involved as much as possible in the discharge planning.
6. Discharge teaching should be done prior to the day of discharge and reinforced on the day of discharge. Written instructions are helpful for the patient to use later as a reference.
7. The return to independence and self-care requires a substantial adjustment for some patients, and comprehensive planning may aid the adjustment.

NURSING ACTION/RATIONALE

1. Assemble all equipment.
2. Identify the patient.
3. Explain the discharge procedure to the patient and family members.
4. Make certain that all equipment, supplies, and medication that the patient is to take home are available.
5. Provide written and oral instructions to the patient regarding prescribed medications, treatments, activity restrictions, dietary modifications, and follow-up care.
6. Ascertain that the patient or a family member has made financial arrangements with the business office regarding the hospital bill.
7. Assist the patient to dress, as necessary.
8. Assist the patient to collect and pack all belongings.
9. Transport the patient by wheelchair to his/her vehicle and assist as needed. Use of a wheelchair conserves the patient's energy. It is the hospital's responsibility to ensure the safety of the patient while on hospital property.
10. Return all equipment in the patient's room to the appropriate area or discard, as indicated.
11. Notify necessary hospital departments of the patient's discharge.
12. Complete the medical record.

PATIENT AND/OR FAMILY TEACHING

1. Explain the discharge procedure to the patient and the family.
2. Reinforce and clarify the physician's discharge instructions.

3. Incorporate the family in discharge planning and teaching and include:
   a. Activity—any restrictions or limitations.
   b. Diet—any special diet modifications.
   c. Medications—names of the medications, when to take them, their action, and any side effects.
   d. Treatments—any procedures to be done at home such as dressing changes or blood pressure monitoring.
   e. Exercises—any special exercises to be done at home.
   f. Follow-up care—doctor's visits, laboratory work, or public health nurse visits, and so on.
   g. Community resource needs—wheelchair or hospital bed rental, financial assistance, support groups, and so on.

4. Have the patient or a family member demonstrate any procedure that will be required at home.
5. Review with the patient the nursing goals or discharge objectives that have been met during hospitalization.

DOCUMENTATION
1. Date and time of discharge, the mode of transportation used, and the name of the person accompanying the patient home.
2. Summary of the patient's hospital course.
3. Assessment of the patient's condition at discharge.
4. The patient's reaction to being discharged.
5. Any special arrangements made.
6. All patient and/or family teaching done and the level of understanding.

Bathing

PURPOSE
1. Cleanse the skin.
2. Promote circulation.
3. Relax muscles.
4. Promote physical, emotional, and mental well-being.
5. Provide an opportunity for patient assessment.

REQUISITES
1. Bath basin
2. Soap
3. Toilet articles
4. Washcloth
5. Towel
6. Bath blanket
7. Clean linen
8. Clean hospital gown

GUIDELINES
1. The type of bath or shower and the patient's role are determined by the patient's condition and the physician's activity orders.
2. A complete bed bath is performed by the nurse. A partial bed bath is performed by the patient with the nurse usually washing the back, legs, and feet. A tub bath or shower is for the more mobile patient. See "Towel Bath" procedure for another type of complete bed bath.
3. Allow as much patient participation as possible.
4. Make every effort to duplicate the patient's usual bathing habits.
5. The patient's skin condition and amount of excretions determine the frequency of bathing.
6. Care must be taken if a patient has intravenous fluids infusing, a cast, or dressings.
7. Use appropriate body mechanics when bathing the patient or assisting the patient to move.

NURSING ACTION/RATIONALE

Bed Bath

1. Assemble all equipment.
2. Explain the bath to the patient.
3. Provide privacy.
4. Raise the bed to the work level. Raise the siderail on the far side of bed.
5. Wash your hands.
6. Remove the top bed linen and replace with a bath blanket.
7. Provide or assist the patient with oral hygiene (see "Oral Hygiene" procedure).
8. Fill the bath basin two-thirds full with warm water at 40.5 to 43 °C (105 to 110 °F). Change the water as necessary during the bath.
9. Remove the patient's gown. If it is the patient's own nightwear, avoid placing it with the soiled hospital linen.
10. Proceed with the bath in the following order: face, neck, arms, hands, chest, abdomen, legs, back, and perineum.
11. Protect the bed by placing a towel under the body part being bathed.
12. Wrap your hand in a washcloth to make a mitt for bathing.
13. Wash, rinse, and thoroughly dry each part before moving on to the next part.
14. Use firm strokes to increase circulation and remove dead skin.
15. Provide support when elevating extremities to wash them.
16. Remove the bath blanket as each part is bathed. Use a towel when additional covering is needed for privacy and warmth.
17. Offer deodorant, lotion, or powder to the patient.
18. Assist the patient to put on clean nightwear.
19. Change the bed linen.
20. Adjust the bed to the lowest level and position the siderails as needed. Place the call signal within reach.
21. Clean and dry the equipment and place it in the bedside cabinet.
22. Place a clean towel and washcloth within reach.
23. Dispose of the soiled linen.

24. Offer hygienic measures:
    a. Clean and trim the patient's nails as needed. Trim fingernails rounded and toenails straight across. Take precautions not to break the skin.
    b. Comb or brush the patient's hair after covering the shoulders with a towel. To remove snarls, begin at the end of the hair and work to the scalp. Peroxide helps in removing blood and emesis from hair.

Tub Bath or Shower

1. Explain the bath or shower to the patient.
2. Assist the patient in putting on a robe and slippers.
3. Accompany the patient to the bath or shower room as necessary.
4. Protect any casts or dressings with plastic and tape or cast protectors.
5. Fill the bathtub or adjust the water temperature for the shower. Position the shower chair, if needed, and lock. Have the patient test the water for the desired temperature.
6. Stress safety precautions to the patient: to use the handrail and not to add hot water while in the tub. Point out the location of the call signal and explain its use.
7. Arrange towels, soap, and personal care items within the patient's reach. Position bath mat.
8. Assist the patient into the tub or shower. If the patient needs assistance with bathing, place a towel across the patient's lap to avoid completely exposing the patient.
9. Place "Occupied" sign on bath or shower room door.
10. Check the patient frequently.
11. Assist the patient out of the tub bath or shower as necessary.
12. Assist the patient with drying and dressing as required.
13. Dispose of all soiled linen after a tub bath or shower. Clean the tub or shower and spray with disinfectant.

PATIENT AND/OR FAMILY TEACHING

1. Explain why the patient's medical or surgical condition may limit activity and self-care.
2. Teach the patient appropriate skin care and personal hygiene techniques.
3. Teach the patient safety measures appropriate for a tub bath or shower.

DOCUMENTATION

1. Type of bath and time taken.
2. Skin condition, if appropriate.
3. Any observations and the patient's response to the bath.

4. All patient teaching done and the patient's level of understanding.

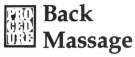 # Back Massage

PURPOSE

1. Promote relaxation.
2. Increase circulation to the area.
3. Assess the skin condition.

REQUISITES

1. Body lotion
2. Towel

GUIDELINES

1. A massage can be given with the bath, before bedtime, or at any other time the patient requests.
2. The greatest relaxation effect of a massage occurs when the rhythm of the massage is coordinated with the patient's breathing.
3. A back massage should take about 5 to 10 minutes.
4. Ascertain any patient allergies or skin sensitivities before you apply lotion to a patient's skin.
5. Avoid massaging over reddened areas unless the redness disappears during the massage.
6. Back massage may be contraindicated in certain immobilized patients susceptible to clotting disorders.

NURSING ACTION/RATIONALE

1. Assemble all equipment.
2. Identify the patient.
3. Explain to the patient that you will be massaging his/her back.
4. Wash your hands.
5. Assist the patient to the prone position. If the patient cannot lie prone, an effective massage can be performed with the patient in the side-lying position.

6. Place a small pillow under the patient's abdomen to maintain correct body alignment.
7. Pour a small amount of lotion onto the palm of your hand. Rub your palms together to warm the lotion, especially if it contains menthol.
8. Massage the back in the sequence shown in Figure 1-1. Massage with your palms and fingers rather than the fingertips, using long firm connecting strokes. Use additional lotion as needed.
   a. *Hand-over-hand.* Massage the back with short quick strokes, alternating hands (Figure 1-1a).

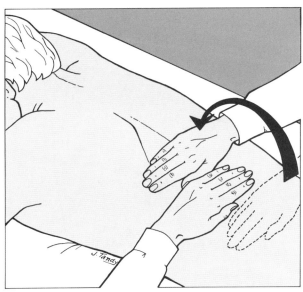

Figure 1-1. Sequence for back massage.
(a) Hand over hand massage.

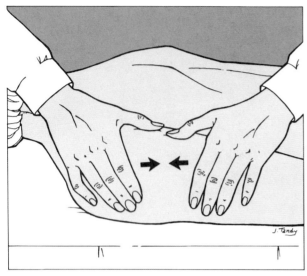

Figure 1-1(b). Kneading.

b. *Kneading.* Squeeze the shoulder muscle with each hand as you slide the hands together (Figure 1-1b).

c. *Friction.* Massage the back with your thumbs, in a circular motion and an upward direction along the spine from the sacrum to the shoulders. Move outward each time until the entire back is covered (Figure 1-1c).

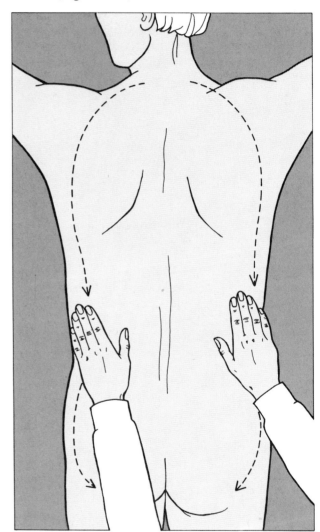

Figure 1-1(c). Friction (shown at left and above).

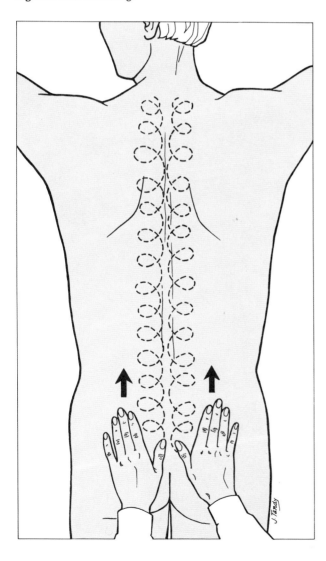

d. *Effleurage.* Massage the back with both hands, using long strokes upward from the sacrum to the shoulders and down again. Use firmer pressure with the upward motion to aid in venous return (Figure 1-1**d**).

e. *Petrissage.* Stroke the back horizontally. Move hands in opposite directions using a kneading motion (Figure 1-1**e**).

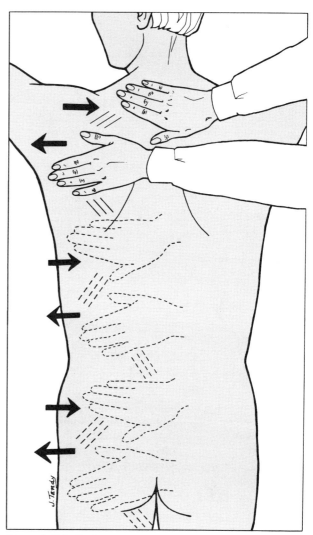

Figure 1-1(e). Petrissage.

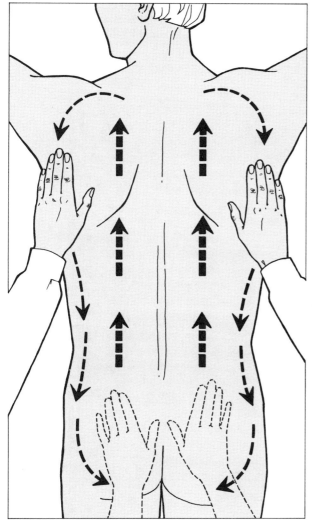

Figure 1-1(d). Effleurage.

f. *Brush-stroking.* Lightly stroke the back with your fingertips to complete the massage (Figure 1-1f).

9. Assist the patient to a comfortable position.

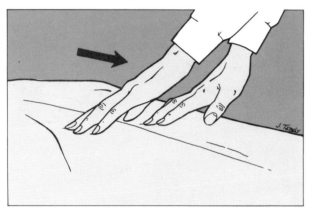

Figure 1-1(f). Brush-stroking.

PATIENT AND/OR FAMILY TEACHING

1. Explain the nature and purpose of the back massage.
2. Encourage the patient to relax and breathe easily during the back massage.
3. Teach the patient actions that can be taken to promote relaxation while confined to bed or hospitalized.
4. Teach back massage to family members for use at home, if appropriate.

DOCUMENTATION

1. The time the back massage was given.
2. An assessment of the patient's skin condition.
3. The patient's response to the back massage.
4. All patient teaching done and the patient's level of understanding.

Towel Bath— Totman Technique

PURPOSE

1. Give a bath that provides the patient with comfort, relaxation, and a minimum of exertion.
2. Maintain or restore healthy, soft skin.

REQUISITES

1. 9 ounce terry cloth towel (36 × 90)
2. 2 quart plastic pitcher
3. 1 ounce of Septi-Soft® concentrate or 3 ounces of Septi-Soft® solution (Vestal Laboratories, St. Louis, MO)
4. Large plastic bag
5. 2000 cc water, 46 to 49 °C (115 to 120 °F)
6. Bath thermometer
7. Bath blanket
8. Bed linen

GUIDELINES

1. A towel bath is especially beneficial to patients who are immobile, have dry skin, or are anxious and agitated. It is quick and relaxing, and it requires no rinsing or drying.

2. Take precautions to keep the patient from becoming chilled. Keep the patient well covered with the bath blanket as you move the towel up. Transfer the towel from front to back quickly.

NURSING ACTION/RATIONALE

1. Assemble all equipment.
2. Identify the patient.
3. Explain the towel bath to the patient.
4. Provide for privacy.
5. Wash your hands.
6. Undress the patient and cover him/her with a top sheet that has been loosened from the foot of the bed. Remove any excess covers.
7. Protect any dressings or casts with plastic and tape.

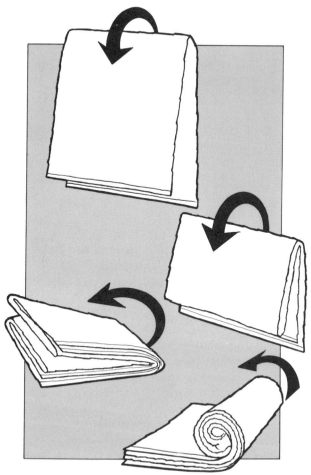

Figure 1-2. Folding and rolling the towel.

8. Fanfold the bath blanket at the foot of the bed.
9. Place the patient in a supine position with legs apart and arms at his/her sides.
10. Prepare the towel.
    a. Fold the towel in half from top to bottom twice. Then fold in half again from side to side. Roll the towel snugly, beginning with the folded edges (Figure 1-2).
    b. Place the rolled towel in the plastic bag with the selvage edges upward.
    c. Fill the plastic pitcher with 2000 cc water warmed to 46 to 49 °C (115 to 120 °F). Add 30 cc Septi-Soft® concentrate or 90 cc Septi-Soft® solution.
    d. Pour the contents of the pitcher into the plastic bag and onto the towel.
    e. Work the solution quickly into the towel. Turn the bag with the open end into the sink and wring out excess solution.
    f. Take the towel in the plastic bag to the patient's room.
11. Bathe the patient:
    a. Fold the top sheet down, exposing the patient's chest. Remove the towel from the bag. Place the towel on the patient's right or left chest with the selvage edges up, and unroll it. Then unfold the towel once, to cover the chest. Fold the top edge down 8 to 12 inches. (This will be used later to wash the face, neck, and ears.) Unfold the remainder of the towel to cover the entire body, remove the top sheet, and tuck the towel around the body (Figure 1-3).

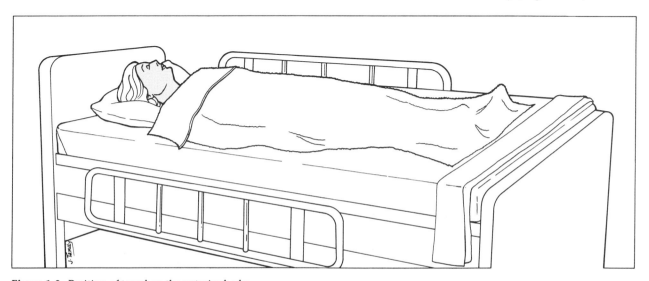

Figure 1-3. Position of towel on the anterior body.

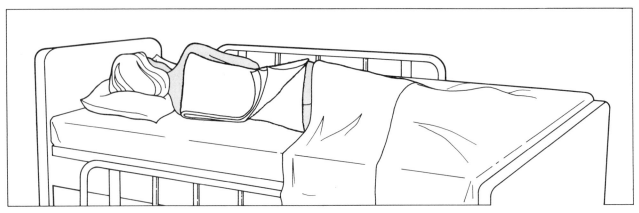

Figure 1-4. Position of towel on the posterior body.

b. Begin the towel bath at the feet. Cleanse the body in an upward direction, massaging gently. Use a clean part of the towel for each section of the body as you progress toward the patient's head. Fanfold the soiled part of the towel toward the head as the bath continues.

c. Unfold the clean bath blanket over the patient as you move upward. Leave several inches of exposed skin between the towel and the bath blanket to allow the skin to air dry.

d. Bathe the face, neck, and ears with the section of the towel folded under the chin.

e. Remove the towel from the patient. Fold into quarters with the soiled side turned inward.

f. Position the patient on his/her side.

g. Place the folded towel on the patient's back with the selvage edges toward the bed and with the four corners over the buttocks (Figure 1-4). Bathe the patient's back beginning at the shoulders. Use the four corners to cleanse the perineal area. Provide additional peri-care if indicated.

h. Remove the towel when bathing is completed.

12. Make the bed, dress the patient, and assist him/her to a comfortable position.

13. Dispose of equipment or return it to the appropriate area.

PATIENT AND/OR FAMILY TEACHING

1. Explain the towel bath to the patient.
2. Instruct the patient to notify the nurse during the bath should chilling occur.
3. Reinforce and clarify the physician's orders for limitation of mobility.
4. Explain any further activity restrictions.
5. Teach the patient appropriate aspects of hygiene.

DOCUMENTATION

1. Time that the bath was given.
2. Temperature of the solution.
3. Patient's skin condition.
4. Patient's reaction to the towel bath.
5. All patient teaching and the patient's level of understanding.

Oral Hygiene

PURPOSE
1. Provide oral care for the teeth, gums, and mouth.
2. Remove offensive odors and food debris.
3. Promote patient comfort.

REQUISITES

Brushing/Flossing
1. Toothbrush
2. Toothpaste
3. Emesis basin
4. Towel
5. Cup
6. Exam gloves
7. Dental floss
8. Dental-floss holder
9. Mirror
10. Lip moisturizer

Denture Care
1. Denture brush
2. Denture cleaner
3. Towel
4. Exam gloves
5. Denture cup
6. Tissue

GUIDELINES
1. Oral hygiene should be offered before breakfast, after each meal, and at bedtime.
2. Oral hygiene is especially important for patients receiving oxygen, for patients with nasogastric tubes, and for patients with no food or fluid intake.
3. Flossing should be done before the brushing procedure and at least once a day in order to prevent plaque formation.
4. For patients with dexterity problems, an electric toothbrush and a floss holder may be helpful (Figure 1-5).
5. If dentures are removed, they should be stored in water in a clearly labeled, covered container placed in a safe location.

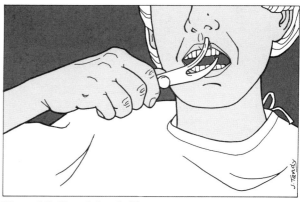

Figure 1-5. Dental-floss holder.

6. Dentures should be cleaned over a basin or sink partially filled with water and padded with a towel to prevent breakage if the dentures are dropped.
7. For complex oral care, refer to the procedure "Special Mouth Care."

NURSING ACTION/RATIONALE
Tooth Brushing and Flossing: Independent Patient
1. Assemble all equipment.
2. Provide privacy.
3. Assist the patient to a high-Fowler's position.
4. Wash your hands.
5. Place a towel across the patient's chest.
6. Arrange oral hygiene equipment within the patient's reach.
7. Assist the patient with flossing and brushing, as necessary.
8. Rinse and return the equipment to the appropriate location.
9. Wash your hands.

Tooth Brushing and Flossing: Dependent Patient
1. Assemble all equipment.
2. Provide privacy.
3. Assist the patient to a semi- to high-Fowler's position, if permitted. If not, turn head to one side.
4. Wash your hands.

5. Place a towel across the patient's chest.
6. Put on the exam gloves.
7. Hold the dental floss in both hands or put it in a floss holder and floss between all teeth, using a clean section of floss for each space (Figure 1-6).

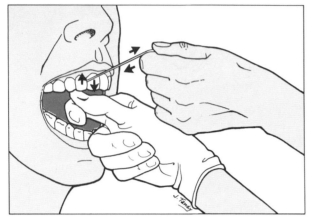

Figure 1-6. Flossing the teeth.

8. Assist the patient with rinsing his/her mouth.
9. Moisten the toothbrush with water and spread toothpaste on the brush.
10. Brush the teeth and gums in a vertical or circular motion, using friction.
11. Assist the patient with rinsing his/her mouth.
12. Wipe the patient's mouth.
13. Apply lip moisturizer, if appropriate.
14. Remove the exam gloves.
15. Assist the patient to a comfortable position.
16. Rinse and return the equipment to the appropriate location.
17. Wash your hands.

Denture Care
1. Assemble all equipment.
2. Provide privacy.
3. Put on the exam gloves.
4. Assist the patient with the denture removal. Using a tissue, remove the top denture by grasping the denture with your thumb and forefinger and pulling downward (Figure 1-7). Remove the bottom denture.
5. Handle the dentures very carefully to avoid breakage. Place the dentures in a dental cup.
6. Line the sink bowl with a towel and fill the sink partially with water.

7. Brush the dentures with a denture brush or toothbrush using denture cleaner. Rinse well.
8. Assist the patient with rinsing his/her mouth.
9. Assist the patient with replacing the dentures and wiping his/her mouth.
10. Remove the exam gloves.
11. Rinse and return all equipment to the appropriate location.
12. Wash your hands.

PATIENT AND/OR FAMILY TEACHING
1. Instruct the patient regarding proper brushing and flossing techniques.
2. Instruct the patient and/or family regarding proper denture care and storage.
3. Explain the importance of oral hygiene care in health maintenance.
4. Stress the importance of regular dental care.

DOCUMENTATION
1. Frequency and method of oral hygiene.
2. Condition of the mouth and gums.
3. Patient's ability to perform oral hygiene, if appropriate.
4. Denture storage location, if appropriate.
5. Any patient and/or family teaching done and the level of understanding.

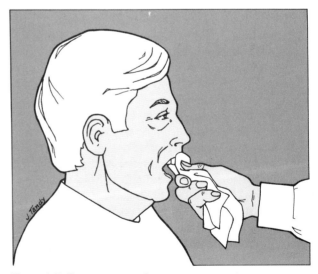

Figure 1-7. Denture removal.

Special Mouth Care

PURPOSE

1. Preserve the integrity and hydration of the oral mucosa and the lips.
2. Prevent dental caries, peridontal disease, and halitosis.
3. Alleviate pain and discomfort, thereby enhancing oral intake.

REQUISITES

Special Mouth Care

1. Toothbrush and/or toothette
2. Toothpaste
3. Cup
4. Emesis basin
5. Dental-floss holder
6. Dental floss
7. Mouthwash (optional)
8. Suction machine
9. Suction catheter
10. Plastic Asepto syringe
11. Exam gloves
12. Towel
13. Lip moisturizer

Special Requisites for Mouth Complications

1. Bleeding
   a. Soft toothbrush or toothette
   b. Tongue blade
   c. 3 × 3 gauze sponges
2. Infections
   a. Prescribed solution
   b. 3 × 3 gauze sponges
   c. Tongue blade
3. Ulcerations
   a. Cotton-tip applicators
   b. 3 × 3 gauze sponges
   c. Tongue blade
   d. Milk of magnesia

GUIDELINES

1. Oral hygiene is a nursing responsibility, but oral care of the patient with oral complications such as infections, ulcerations, or bleeding tendencies is a responsibility shared with the physician.
2. Mouth complications are common in patients receiving chemotherapy and radiation therapy.
3. An oral assessment with a tongue blade and a flashlight should be performed on admission and daily if an oral problem exists.
4. Mouth lesions should be cultured frequently to assess for the presence of microorganisms.
5. Oral care for an unconscious patient should be performed every 2 to 4 hours. For patients with oral bleeding, infections, or ulcerations, oral care frequency and specific treatments should be prescribed by the physician.
6. Care should be taken when performing oral hygiene for patients with thrombocytopenia, infections, or ulcerations. Flossing should be discontinued. Brushing the teeth and cleaning the mouth should be done with a soft toothbrush, a toothette, or a gauze-padded tongue blade.
7. If the patient's mouth is extremely painful, rinsing the mouth with a local anesthetic before performing oral care may be required.
8. Gloves should be worn by the nurse during the special mouth care procedure to protect the patient and to prevent cross infection. Do not put your fingers in the mouth of an unconscious or uncooperative patient.
9. Refer to the procedure "Oral Hygiene" for further guidelines concerning routine oral hygiene.
10. Oral suctioning may be required while performing oral hygiene for an unconscious patient to prevent aspiration. Refer to the procedure "Oropharyngeal/Nasopharyngeal Suctioning" for the appropriate technique.

NURSING ACTION/RATIONALE

1. Assemble all equipment.
2. Identify the patient.
3. Explain the procedure to the patient regardless of mental alertness.
4. Position the patient in the lateral position with the head turned toward the side (Figure 1-8).

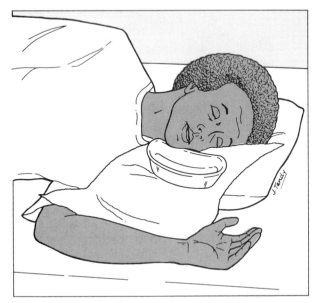

Figure 1-8. The lateral position for special mouth care.

5. Place a towel under the face and over the shoulder of the patient.
6. Provide adequate lighting.
7. Provide privacy.
8. Wash your hands.
9. Put on the exam gloves.
10. Assess the condition of the patient's mouth.
11. Perform flossing and brushing as described in the "Oral Hygiene" procedure.
12. Rinse the mouth carefully with water using an Asepto syringe and oral suction.
13. Dry the patient's mouth.
14. Apply lip moisturizer to prevent cracking and drying.
15. Remove your gloves.
16. Reposition the patient in a comfortable position appropriate for the level of consciousness.
17. Discard, clean, or return all equipment to the appropriate location.
18. Wash your hands.

Special Mouth Care: Bleeding

Refer to the procedure "Oral Hygiene" with the following exceptions:

1. Assess the patient's mouth for the amount of bleeding present and specific areas of bleeding.
2. Do not floss teeth.
3. Brush the teeth and clean the mouth using one of the following methods:
   a. Brush the teeth carefully with a very soft toothbrush or toothette.
   b. Wrap a tongue blade with a 3 × 3 gauze sponge saturated with mouthwash or a prescribed solution. Carefully swab the teeth and mouth.
4. Rinse the mouth with warm tap water.

Special Mouth Care: Infection

Refer to the procedure "Oral Hygiene" with the following exceptions:

1. Assess the patient's mouth for appearance, integrity, and general condition.
2. Obtain a culture, if ordered.
3. Do not floss the teeth if the mouth is irritated or painful.
4. Assist the patient with brushing the teeth and cleaning the mouth, using a soft toothbrush, a toothette, or a gauze-padded tongue blade.
5. Rinse the mouth with water and the prescribed solution, if ordered.

Special Mouth Care: Ulcerations

Refer to the procedure "Oral Hygiene" with the following exceptions:

1. Assess the patient's mouth for appearance, integrity, and general condition.
2. Obtain a culture, if ordered.
3. Do not floss the teeth.
4. Assist the patient with brushing the teeth and cleaning the mouth, using a soft toothbrush, a toothette, or a gauze-padded tongue blade.
5. Rinse the mouth with water.
6. Apply the sediment from milk of magnesia to the ulcerated areas with a cotton-tip applicator. Allow to remain on the ulcerations for 15 minutes.
7. Rinse the mouth with water.

PATIENT AND/OR FAMILY TEACHING

1. Explain the special mouth care procedure to the patient and/or family, including the frequency of oral hygiene.
2. Reinforce and clarify the physician's explanation of the disease process.
3. Instruct the patient to inform the nurse if excessive pain occurs during the procedure.
4. Explain any diet modifications that may be required.
5. Teach the patient and/or family the special mouth care procedure if treatment will be continued following discharge.

DOCUMENTATION

1. Time of the procedure and type of procedure.
2. Any medicated solutions applied.
3. Patient's response to the procedure.
4. Any assessment parameters including the appearance and condition of the mouth.
5. Any cultures obtained and disposition of the specimen.
6. All patient and/or family teaching done and the level of understanding.

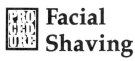 # Facial Shaving

PURPOSE

1. Remove facial hair.

REQUISITES

1. Disposable razor or electric shaver
2. Washcloth and two towels
3. Shaving cream or soap
4. Washbasin
5. Mirror (optional)
6. Pre-shave lotion for electric razors
7. After-shave lotion

GUIDELINES

1. If the patient is alert, question the patient regarding his shaving habits. Follow the patient's routine as closely as possible.
2. Use the patient's own shaving equipment whenever possible.
3. When using the health care facility's electric shaver, the shaver must be cleaned and the shaver head soaked in disinfectant after each patient use.
4. Always use an electric shaver on patients with prolonged coagulation times to prevent uncontrollable bleeding from facial cuts.
5. Never use plugged-in electric shavers on patients who are receiving oxygen therapy because of the danger of combustion. Rechargeable (battery-operated) shavers or safety razors can be used.
6. Consult with the physician before shaving a patient who has had facial surgery or any facial incisions.
7. Patients who are combative, suicidal, or disoriented should have supervision and assistance if able to shave themselves.

NURSING ACTION/RATIONALE

1. Assemble all equipment.
2. Identify the patient.
3. Explain the procedure to the patient.
4. Provide privacy.
5. Provide adequate lighting.
6. Assist the patient to a comfortable upright position, if allowed.
7. Wash your hands.
8. Wash the patient's face with soap and water, and dry thoroughly.
9. Use one of the following methods to shave the patient.

Dry Shave Using an Electric Shaver

a. Apply pre-shave lotion if available.
b. Plug the shaver into the electrical outlet, unless using a rechargeable shaver (see caution in Guideline 5).
c. Turn the shaver on.
d. Use short up-and-down motions, with the grain of the beard, for a shaver with a regular flat or flexible head. Use small circular motions if a circular-head shaver is being used.
e. Shave the cheeks first, then around the mouth, and then the neck.
f. Pull loose skin taut with your free hand, to get a close smooth shave and to avoid pinching the patient's skin.
g. Assist the patient to tilt his head slightly back, if allowed, when shaving the neck.
h. Trim the sideburns with the trimmer if the shaver is equipped with one.
i. Apply after-shave lotion.
j. Assist the patient to a comfortable position.
k. Clean and return all equipment to the appropriate location.

Wet Shave with a Nonelectric Razor

a. Fill the basin with warm water.
b. Apply a warm, wet towel to the face for five minutes to soften the beard.
c. Apply shaving cream or soap with a thick lather to all areas of the beard.
d. Pull the skin taut and shave, using quick firm strokes. Shave each area of the beard in the direction shown (Figure 1-9).
e. Rinse the razor frequently in warm water.
f. Change the razor blade if the razor is pulling at the beard.
g. Wash off excess lather with a cool washcloth and dry.
h. Apply after-shave lotion.
i. Assist the patient to a comfortable position.
j. Discard or return all equipment to the appropriate location.

PATIENT AND/OR FAMILY TEACHING

1. Explain the procedure to the patient before starting.
2. Instruct the patient in safety factors for shaving as they relate to the disease process or medication regimen.
3. Instruct the family members on facial shaving if they will need to provide care after discharge.

DOCUMENTATION

1. Procedure performed.
2. Patient's participation and reaction to the procedure.
3. All patient teaching done and the patient's level of understanding.

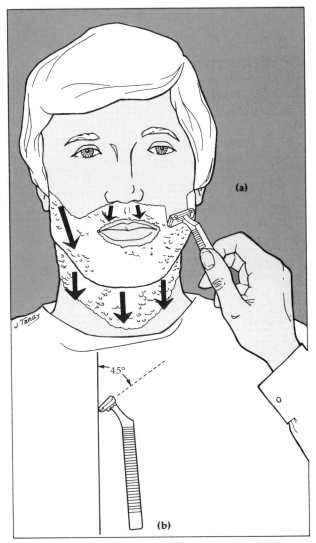

Figure 1-9. Direction of the stroke for shaving the beard **(a)** and angle of razor **(b)**.

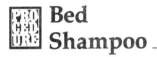 # Bed
Shampoo

PURPOSE

1. Promote cleanliness, comfort, and a positive self-image.
2. Apply a medicated shampoo.

REQUISITES

1. Shampoo drain tray
2. Bed protector
3. Water pitcher
4. Hair dryer
5. Shampoo (medicated, if prescribed by the physician)
6. Comb
7. Bucket
8. Bath towels—3
9. Washcloth
10. Conditioner
11. Clean patient gown
12. Exam gloves (optional)

GUIDELINES

1. A physician's order may be required for a bed shampoo. Refer to your health care institution's policy.
2. If the patient tires easily, the shampoo should not be given at the same time as the bath.

NURSING ACTION/RATIONALE

1. Assemble all equipment.
2. Explain the procedure to the patient.
3. Wash your hands.
4. Place a bath blanket over the patient and fanfold the top linen to the foot of the bed.
5. Assist the patient into a recumbent position close to the side of the bed.
6. Place the bed protector and towel under the patient's head and shoulders.
7. Place the shampoo tray under the patient's head with one end extending over the bucket, which may be placed on a chair to catch the flow of water (Figure 1-10).
8. Provide the patient with a washcloth to cover the eyes.

9. Fill the pitcher with warm water.
10. Pour water onto the patient's hair until it is thoroughly wet.
11. Apply the shampoo and work it into a lather.
12. Massage the patient's scalp with your fingertips.
13. Rinse the hair by pouring additional warm water over it until it is thoroughly rinsed.
14. Re-lather if indicated and rinse thoroughly.
15. Apply conditioner and again rinse thoroughly.
16. Remove the shampoo tray, bed protector, and wet towel.
17. Place a dry towel around the patient's shoulders and position the patient comfortably.
18. Dry the patient's hair with a towel. An electric dryer will facilitate the drying process.
19. Comb and/or brush the patient's hair. Arrange as desired. Allow the patient to participate if possible.
20. Clean all equipment and return to the appropriate area.

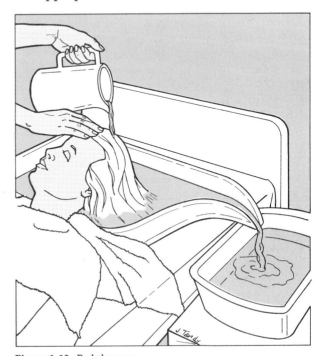

Figure 1-10. Bed shampoo.

PATIENT AND/OR FAMILY TEACHING

1. Explain the procedure to the patient prior to starting.
2. Instruct the patient to inform the nurse if any discomfort is experienced during the procedure.

DOCUMENTATION

1. Time of the procedure.
2. Patient's response to the treatment including any pertinent assessment parameters.
3. Any patient teaching done and the patient's level of understanding.

 # Bedmaking: Unoccupied

PURPOSE

1. Provide a clean change of linen and a comfortable bed for the patient.

REQUISITES

1. Bottom sheet—straight or fitted
2. Top sheet
3. Bedspread
4. Pillowcases—2
5. Blanket
6. Mattress pad, if required
7. Draw sheet, if required
8. Waterproof sheet, if required

GUIDELINES

1. An unoccupied bed is made when the patient is able to get out of bed or is away from the bed for any reason.
2. A post anesthesia bed is required when a patient is recovering from anesthesia. The linen must be placed so that it can be changed readily and the patient transferred easily.
3. Sterile sheets may be required for burn patients.
4. If the patient is incontinent, has profuse drainage, or is being treated with wet compresses, a waterproof draw sheet may be indicated.
5. The bed linen should be changed after the patient's bath or as necessary.
6. Avoid shaking soiled linen or placing soiled linen on the floor to decrease the spread of microorganisms.
7. Use appropriate body mechanics while making the patient's bed.
8. Bedmaking is an opportune time to assess the patient's condition as well as to develop the nurse-patient relationship.

NURSING ACTION/RATIONALE

1. Assemble all linen.
2. Identify the patient.
3. Explain to the patient that you will be making the bed.
4. Wash your hands.
5. Assist the patient out of bed if necessary.
6. Remove any equipment attached to the bed linen and remove any personal items.
7. Adjust the bed to a comfortable height to prevent straining your back. Adjust to a flat position.
8. Change the bed linen.

   Unoccupied Bed
   a. Lower the siderails if appropriate.
   b. Remove the pillows and pillowcases. Set the pillows aside in a clean area.
   c. Loosen and remove the linen, beginning at the head of the bed on one side and moving around the bed to the head of the bed on the other side.

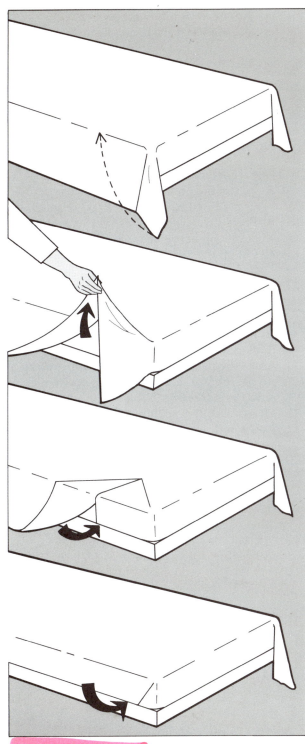

Figure 1-11. Mitered corner.

d. Fold and set aside any linen to be reused.
e. Straighten the mattress.
f. Replace the mattress pad, if necessary.
g. Apply the bottom sheet, using one of the following methods:
   (1) Apply a straight sheet with the seam side down, extending the bottom edge just over the end of the mattress. Miter the top corner on the side where you are standing (Figure 1-11).
   (2) Apply a fitted bottom sheet by placing the fitted corners over the top and bottom mattress corners.
h. Place the draw sheet, if used, on the center of the bed. Tuck in the bottom linen on the side where you are standing.
i. Place the top sheet on the bed, seam side up with the top hem even with the head of the mattress.
j. Place the blanket, if used, on the bed about 8 inches below the top sheet.
k. Place the bedspread over the blanket and even with the top sheet. Fold the top of the bedspread under the blanket.
l. Fold the top sheet over the bedspread.
m. Miter the bottom corner of all three top layers, allowing the top linen to hang over the side of the bed.
n. Move to the opposite side of the bed and repeat the procedure. Pull the linen tight, and smooth out any wrinkles.
o. Fanfold the top linen to the foot of the bed (Figure 1-12).

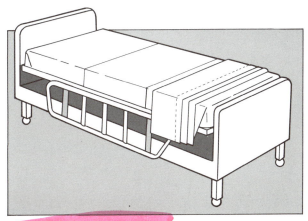

Figure 1-12. Fanfolded top linen.

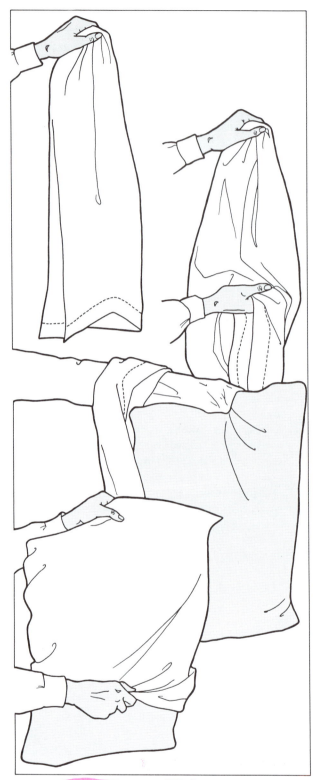

p. Apply clean pillowcases. Grasp the pillowcase at the center of the closed end. Invert the pillowcase over one hand and forearm. Grasp the end of the pillow with the same hand, pulling the pillowcase over the pillow (Figure 1-13).

q. Place the pillow on the bed with the closed end toward the door.

r. Adjust the bed to the low position.

Post Anesthesia Bed

a. Put on the bottom linen as with an unoccupied bed, using a draw sheet.

b. Place a waterproof sheet or disposable pad at the top of the bed instead of the pillow.

c. Put on the top linen as with an unoccupied bed, but do not tuck in the bottom.

d. Fanfold the top linen to the side of the bed away from the door (Figure 1-14).

e. Adjust the height of the bed to the level of the stretcher.

9. Replace the call signal.
10. Assist the patient back to bed if appropriate. Adjust the bed to a comfortable position and raise the siderails.
11. Place the soiled linen in the appropriate area.
12. Wash your hands.

PATIENT AND/OR FAMILY TEACHING

1. Explain the operation of the bed, if appropriate.
2. Instruct the patient to notify the nurse if bed linen becomes wet or soiled.
3. Instruct the patient regarding activity restrictions as appropriate.

Figure 1-13. Applying a pillowcase.

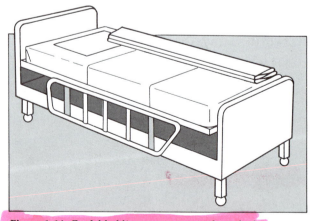

Figure 1-14. Fanfolded linen on post anesthesia bed.

DOCUMENTATION

1. Any observations of soiled linen that indicate need for further patient assessment.
2. Tolerance of activity level while out of bed, if appropriate.
3. Any patient teaching done and the patient's level of understanding.

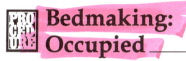

Bedmaking: Occupied

PURPOSE

1. Make the patient's bed comfortable and clean by changing the linen.

REQUISITES

1. Bottom sheet—straight or fitted
2. Top sheet
3. Bedspread
4. Pillowcases—2
5. Blanket
6. Mattress pad, if required
7. Draw sheet, if required
8. Waterproof sheet, if required

GUIDELINES

1. An occupied bed must be made if the patient is unable to get out of bed or complete bed rest is prescribed.
2. If the patient is in traction, the bed must be made so that the traction weights are not disturbed. Assistance will be needed.
3. If the patient cannot be turned, the bottom sheet can be changed from head to foot.
4. Sterile sheets may be required for burn patients.
5. Whenever patients have integumentary, vascular, or orthopedic problems, care must be taken when turning them in bed.
6. If the patient is incontinent, has profuse drainage, or is being treated with wet compresses, a waterproof draw sheet may be indicated.
7. The bed linen should be changed after the patient's bath or as necessary.

8. Avoid shaking soiled linens or placing soiled linens on the floor to decrease the spread of microorganisms.
9. Use appropriate body mechanics when making the patient's bed.
10. Bedmaking is an opportune time to assess the patient's physical condition as well as to develop the nurse-patient relationship.

NURSING ACTION/RATIONALE

1. Assemble all linen.
2. Identify the patient.
3. Explain to the patient that you will be making the bed. Include turning instructions if appropriate.
4. Provide privacy.
5. Wash your hands.
6. Position the patient in a flat supine position if tolerated. Leave the pillows in place.
7. Remove any equipment attached to the bed linen and remove any personal items.
8. Adjust the bed to a comfortable height to prevent straining your back.
9. Remove the blanket and bedspread. Fold and set them aside if they are to be reused. Leave the top sheet on the patient for warmth and privacy. A bath blanket may be used if the top linen has been removed for bathing.
10. Raise the siderail on the far side of the bed.
11. Assist the patient to roll away from you, maintaining proper body alignment.
12. Straighten the mattress, using assistance if necessary.
13. Loosen the top and sides of the bottom linen on the side where you are working. Roll the soiled linen as close to the patient as possible, soiled side inward.

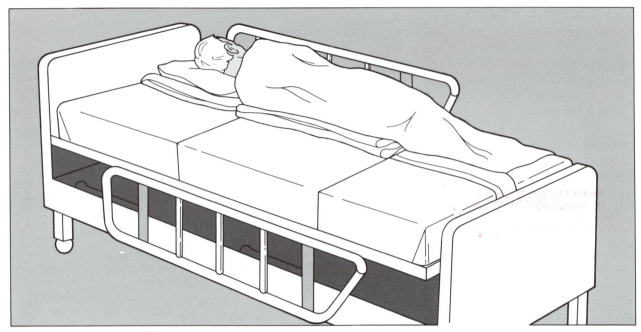

Figure 1-15. Clean linen rolled behind patient.

14. Position half of the clean mattress pad, bottom sheet, and draw sheet on the bed. Tuck in the bottom linen, mitering the top corner or applying the fitted bottom sheet, as described in "Bedmaking: Unoccupied."
15. Roll the clean bottom linen to the middle of the bed with the top side inward. Place it tightly against the patient's back (Figure 1-15).
16. Assist the patient to roll back toward you over all the linens.
17. Raise the siderail to provide patient support and safety.
18. Move to the opposite side of the bed and lower the siderail.
19. Loosen and remove all of the soiled bottom linen. Unroll the clean bottom linen and tuck in linen as described in "Bedmaking: Unoccupied."
20. Return the patient to the supine position. Lower the siderail.
21. Place the clean top sheet over the patient, seam side up. Remove the soiled top sheet or bath blanket from below while maintaining the position of the clean top sheet.
22. Apply the remaining top linen as described in "Bedmaking: Unoccupied," but make a small toe pleat in the top linen at the foot of the bed (Figure 1-16).

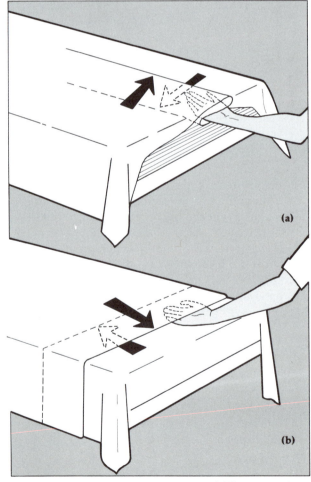

Figure 1-16. Types of toe pleats. **(a)** Vertical. **(b)** Horizontal.

23. Remove the pillows while supporting the patient's head. Change the pillowcases as described in "Bedmaking: Unoccupied." Replace the pillows.
24. Assist the patient to a comfortable position in bed.
25. Replace the call signal. Raise the siderails if appropriate, and return the bed to the desired height. Return the patient's personal articles to the bedside, within reach.
26. Place all soiled linen in the appropriate area.
27. Wash your hands.

PATIENT AND/OR FAMILY TEACHING
1. Explain the turning instructions to the patient.
2. Reinforce and clarify the physician's explanation of the patient's activity restrictions.
3. Relate the activity restrictions to energy conservation and the patient's disease process, if appropriate.
4. Instruct the patient to inform you of any chilling or discomfort during the procedure.
5. Teach the family how to make an occupied bed if the patient will be bedridden at home.
6. Provide information to the patient and/or family regarding the rental of a hospital bed for home use, if appropriate.

DOCUMENTATION
1. Any untoward reactions to the procedure.
2. Activity level achieved.
3. Any assessment done during the procedure.
4. Any patient teaching done and the patient's level of understanding.

Administration of Bedpan or Urinal

PURPOSE

1. Provide facilities for elimination if the patient is unable to use the bathroom or bedside commode.

REQUISITES

1. Bedpan/fracture pan
2. Urinal
3. Toilet tissue
4. Specimen container, if appropriate
5. Towel and washcloth
6. Graduated container, if appropriate

GUIDELINES

1. A female patient on bedrest uses a bedpan or female urinal for urination and a bedpan for defecation (Figure 1-17). A male patient on bedrest uses a urinal for urination and a bedpan for defecation.

2. Metal receptacles can be warmed under warm water before use.

3. Whenever possible, the patient should be encouraged to use the bathroom or the bedside commode for elimination.

4. A bedside commode may be used for a patient who can get out of bed but is unable to get to the bathroom. The procedure for the commode is similar to administering a bedpan, except that the patient is out of bed.

5. Privacy is necessary when using the bedpan/urinal. Many people are unable to evacuate in the presence of a roommate or nurse.

6. Prolonged use of a bedpan or urinal may create constipation or difficulty voiding. There is often a time lag between the urge to evacuate and actual use of the bedpan/urinal if the patient is embarrassed to ask for assistance or the nurse does not respond promptly.

7. It is difficult to relax the sphincters that control urine and feces while lying supine on a bedpan. The patient should be placed in a semi- to high-Fowler's position unless contraindicated.

8. Do not place a bedpan on the bedside table or chair.

9. Skin friction can be prevented by dusting the bedpan with powder before offering it to the patient.

10. A weak patient should not be left on the bedpan or bedside commode for a long time.

11. A separate waste receptacle should be provided for toilet tissue if a specimen is to be collected.

12. If the patient has difficulty voiding, warm water poured over the perineum (measure first if the urine is to be measured), water running from a nearby faucet, or allowing the patient to drink a glass of water may assist the patient to relax. Male patients should be allowed to stand while voiding unless contraindicated.

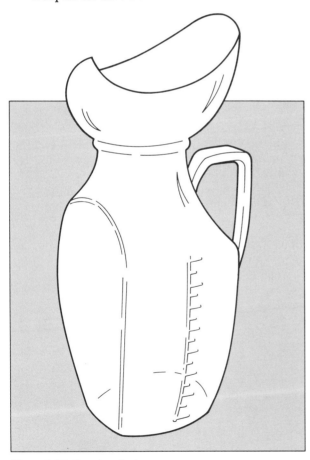

Figure 1-17. Female urinal.

13. A reassuring and supportive attitude on the part of the nurse may decrease the patient's anxiety or embarrassment.
14. A fracture pan is available for very thin patients or for those who are immobile as a result of paralysis, casts, or traction. However, urine is easily spilled from the fracture pan (Figure 1-18). A female urinal that fits against the perineum is also available for immobile patients.
15. Use proper body mechanics whenever assisting a patient to move.

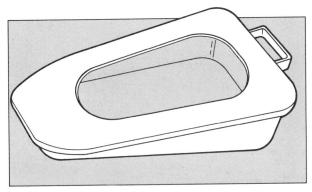

Figure 1-18. Fracture pan.

NURSING ACTION/RATIONALE

1. Assemble all equipment.
2. Explain the procedure to the patient. Explain if a specimen is to be collected.
3. Provide privacy.
4. Wash your hands.
5. Administer the bedpan or urinal.

Bedpan/Fracture Pan (Non-Assistive Patient)

a. Raise the bed to a working level. Raise the siderail on the far side of the bed. Prefold the top bed linen back.
b. Roll the patient toward the far side of the bed.
c. Place the bedpan under the patient's buttocks with the open, pouring side of the pan toward the foot of the bed.
d. Return the patient to the supine position, adjust the bedpan, and replace the top covers.

e. Raise the other siderail. Elevate the head of the bed as allowed or as desired by the patient.
f. Place toilet tissue and the call signal within reach. Instruct the patient to notify the nurse when finished.
g. When the patient has finished, lower the head of the bed as allowed and steady the bedpan while assisting the patient to roll to the opposite side of the bed.
h. Cleanse the patient as necessary with tissue wrapped around your hand, wiping toward the rectum. Use soap and water if necessary.

Bedpan/Fracture Pan (Assistive Patient)

a. Elevate the head of the bed. Pie-fold the top bed linen back.
b. Have the patient spread his/her legs, flex the knees, and lift the buttocks by pressing the heels into the mattress. Assist the patient with one hand under the buttocks. With the other hand, place the bedpan under the patient's buttocks with the open, pouring side of the pan toward the foot of the bed.
c. Raise the siderails if needed for support. Replace the top sheet.
d. Place the toilet tissue and the call signal within reach.
e. When the patient is finished, assist the patient off the bedpan in the same manner in which it was offered.

Urinal

a. Elevate the head of the bed as allowed or as desired by the patient.
b. Instruct the patient to tilt down the closed end of the urinal to avoid spilling.
c. Place the urinal, call signal, and toilet tissue within reach. If the patient is unable to hold the urinal, place it between his legs and position the penis inside. Cover the patient.
d. When the patient has finished, remove the urinal.

6. Assist the patient to a comfortable position.
7. Offer the patient a cleansing towelette or assist with handwashing as desired.
8. Collect any urine or stool specimen as ordered. Label and send the specimen to the laboratory.

9. Empty and discard or clean and return the equipment to the appropriate area.
10. Wash your hands.

PATIENT AND/OR FAMILY TEACHING

1. Explain to the patient how you will be offering and removing the bedpan/urinal.
2. Reinforce and clarify the physician's explanation of the patient's activity restriction.
3. Relate the activity restrictions to energy conservation and the patient's disease process.
4. Instruct the patient to notify the nurse if further assistance is needed or discomfort occurs while using the bedpan.
5. If the patient will be bedridden at home, teach the patient and family how to use the bedpan and/or urinal.
6. Teach proper handwashing and hygiene to the patient and family.
7. Instruct a female patient on intake and output to put toilet tissue in separate receptacle.

DOCUMENTATION

1. Time and type of evacuation.
2. Assessment of the urine or stool.
3. Amount of output.
4. Patient's reaction to the procedure.
5. All patient teaching done and the patient's level of understanding.

 # Providing Drinking Water

PURPOSE

1. Replenish the patient's drinking water.
2. Prevent cross-contamination.

REQUISITES

1. Cart
2. Water pitchers
3. Water-pitcher liners
4. Water
5. Ice
6. Paper cups

GUIDELINES

1. Providing drinking water to a group of patients is a clean procedure. Handwashing should be done between patients.
2. Water-pitcher liners and cups should be changed regularly to prevent the growth of microorganisms. The water pitcher should be replaced every 7 days, or more often if necessary.
3. Every patient, on admission to the hospital, should receive a labeled water pitcher. The label should include the patient's name, room number, date, and "No Ice" alert, if appropriate.
4. Each ice machine should be cleaned regularly with a disinfectant.
5. A water pitcher should never be removed from an isolation room. Ice and fresh water should be taken to the room in a clean water-pitcher liner.
6. The cart for distributing water should be cleansed with disinfectant prior to use.
7. Fresh water should be distributed in the morning, at noon, at night, and at any other time as necessary.

8. A list of patients receiving nothing by mouth should be placed on the cart for reference during the procedure.
9. When distributing drinking water to the patient, pour a small amount of water into the drinking cup and leave the pitcher and cup within the patient's reach.

NURSING ACTION/RATIONALE
Providing Drinking Water: Clean Liner
1. Assemble all equipment.
2. Clean the cart with disinfectant.
3. Wash your hands.
4. Fill the clean water-pitcher liners with ice and water.
5. Distribute the clean, filled liners. Provide clean cups.
   a. Discard the ice in the patient's room and fill the liner with tap water if the patient does not require ice.
   b. Empty the used liner into the sink and discard it in the waste receptacle in the patient's room.
6. Wash your hands between patients.
7. Discard equipment or return it to the appropriate location.
8. Wash your hands.

Providing Drinking Water: Used Liner
1. Assemble all equipment.
2. Clean the cart with disinfectant.
3. Wash your hands.

4. Collect the labeled water pitchers from each room, excluding isolation rooms.
   a. Empty the water from each pitcher in the patient's room. Do not touch the rim or inside of the pitcher.
   b. Place each labeled water pitcher on the cart, making sure that they do not touch each other.
5. Fill each water pitcher with water and ice. Do not touch the ice dispenser or water dispenser with the pitcher.
6. Distribute the labeled water pitchers to the correct patients. Provide clean cups as necessary.
7. Wash your hands between patients if additional care is provided.
8. Discard equipment or return it to the appropriate location.
9. Wash your hands.

PATIENT AND/OR FAMILY TEACHING
1. Reinforce information regarding adequate fluid intake or fluid restrictions, as appropriate.
2. Explain intake and output recording, if appropriate.

DOCUMENTATION
1. Any intake, if appropriate.
2. All patient teaching done and the patient's level of understanding.

Delivering Diet Trays to Patients

PURPOSE
1. Serve meals to patients.

REQUISITES
1. Diet tray, as ordered
2. Oral hygiene equipment, if appropriate
3. Towel and washcloth

GUIDELINES
1. A physician's order is required for diet management.
2. Appetite may be affected by illness. Stress as a result of the hospitalization may cause a decrease in appetite.
3. The patient who is weakened by illness will take a longer time to eat.
4. Most patients prefer to sit up while eating. Allow the patient to sit in a chair or to sit in bed whenever possible. If the patient cannot sit, eating is easier and safer in a lateral position rather than supine.
5. Dependent or confused patients should be assisted with eating and fed, if necessary. The patient's family should be encouraged to participate in assisting the patient at mealtime.
6. The hospital dietician should be consulted for nutrition counseling or any special dietary problems.
7. An awareness of cultural factors related to food and eating habits is important.
8. Treatments should be avoided just before and after meals whenever possible.
9. Typical hospital diets are:
   a. General—regular, well-balanced meal.
   b. Soft—easily chewed and digested foods.
   c. Full liquid—liquids or foods that become liquid at body temperature.
   d. Clear liquid—water, tea, coffee, clear juice, gelatin, or broth.
10. Therapeutic diets may contain reductions in the amount of calories, sodium, cholesterol, sugar, protein, or other substances related to managing the disease process. Therapeutic diets may also require additions of calories, protein, or other substances.
11. Foods should be served at the proper temperature and warm foods reheated, if necessary.
12. Arrangements should be made so that patients who require feeding will have assistance as soon as the tray is served.

NURSING ACTION/RATIONALE
1. Prepare the patient prior to mealtime:
   a. Offer the dependent patient an opportunity for voiding, handwashing, and oral hygiene, as indicated.
   b. Assist the patient to a comfortable position and provide a clean area for the meal tray.
2. Wash your hands.
3. Identify the patient's diet tray according to your health care facility's policy.
4. Assess the tray for correct dietary content. Serve immediately.
5. Identify the patient.
6. Place the tray within the patient's reach. Remove any food covers.
7. Provide a napkin or towel for protection from food spillage.
8. Assist the patient with opening and preparing foods as necessary.
9. Remove the tray after the patient finishes eating.
10. Clean the patient's eating area if spillage has occurred. Change the bed linen and gown, if necessary.
11. Offer the dependent patient an opportunity for oral hygiene and handwashing after eating.
12. Reposition the patient comfortably.
13. Assess the patient's appetite and satisfaction with the meal. Record fluid intake, if appropriate.

PATIENT AND/OR FAMILY TEACHING

1. Discuss the importance of handwashing before meals.
2. Teach the appropriate aspects of nutrition and reinforce dietary counseling.
3. Reinforce and clarify the physician's explanation of the disease process as it relates to the patient's diet.
4. Teach the patient and the family members ways to meet nutritional needs for the patient at home, with economic and cultural adaptations as necessary.

DOCUMENTATION

1. Assessment of the patient's food intake, appetite, and nutritional status.
2. Any fluid intake, if appropriate.
3. All patient teaching done and the patient's level of understanding.

Assisting the Adult Patient to Eat

PURPOSE

1. Assist the patient to obtain nourishment and fluids.

REQUISITES

1. Prescribed diet
2. Large napkin or towel
3. Special cups or utensils as appropriate

GUIDELINES

1. Patients should be assessed on admission and frequently thereafter to determine the type of assistance they may need at mealtime. Any problems identified should be noted on the nursing care plan along with specific corrective approaches.
2. Patients should be encouraged to feed themselves whenever possible and to make decisions concerning the order in which the meal will be eaten.
3. The patient and the environment should be prepared prior to the delivery of the diet tray, as described in the procedure "Delivering Diet Trays to Patients."
4. Whenever possible the patient should be assisted to a sitting position in bed or assisted into a chair. A side-lying position with support pillows can be used for the patient who is unable to sit.
5. Special cups and utensils can usually be obtained from the physical therapy or occupational therapy department to assist the patient to eat more independently.

6. A patient with restricted vision should be told what food is available for the meal and the locations of the food on the tray or plate. The location of the food is usually described in terms of the face of a clock; for example, meat at 12 o'clock, potatoes at 4 o'clock.
7. Patients who have poor vision or difficulty handling objects should never be given very hot food because of the danger of burns if the food is accidently dropped. Hot coffee can be a particular problem.
8. Any personnel assisting the patient at mealtime should try to take a sitting position next to the patient. The manner of assisting should be unhurried, and the conversation should be pleasant and related to a topic of interest to the patient.
9. All attempts should be made to assist the patient with eating as soon as the tray is delivered.
10. If a patient refuses to eat the prescribed diet, discuss food likes and dislikes with the patient. Consult with the dietician if modifications in the diet can be made. Never force a patient to eat.

NURSING ACTION/RATIONALE

1. Prepare the patient and the environment for mealtime:
   a. Remove unpleasant sights from the environment.
   b. Provide good ventilation and adequate lighting.
   c. Assist the patient with urination or defecation as necessary.
   d. Assist the patient with handwashing. Brushing of the teeth or use of a mouthwash can also enhance the patient's appetite.
   e. Position the patient appropriately with consideration of his or her activity limitations.
   f. Provide analgesics if appropriate.
2. Wash your hands.
3. Obtain the patient's tray.
4. Verify the food on the tray with the patient's diet card to ensure that the correct food is on the tray.
5. Identify the patient.
6. Place the tray on the overbed table or other appropriate table.
7. Remove the food covers and prepare the food as necessary for the patient. Depending on the patient's condition, this may include:
   a. Cutting meat.
   b. Opening condiment packages.
   c. Buttering bread.
   d. Pouring tea or coffee.
   e. Opening milk cartons.
8. Place a napkin or a small towel under the patient's chin to prevent soiling of the bedclothing if food is dropped.
9. Assist the patient as necessary. If the patient needs to be fed:
   a. Ask the patient about the order in which he or she would like to eat the meal.
   b. Feed the patient at a comfortable rate for the patient. Allow the patient to chew and swallow the food before offering more.
   c. Allow for rest periods for the patient who tires easily.
   d. Offer fluids as the patient requests or after every three or four mouthfuls of solid food. Special drinking cups with pour spouts can be used for patients in a side-lying position.
10. Remove the tray after the meal. Note fluid intake and proportion of food eaten.
11. Assist the patient with mouth care and washing of hands and face.
12. Change the patient's clothing or bed linen if soiled.
13. Assist the patient with urinating or defecating as necessary.
14. Reposition the patient comfortably.
15. Clean any special feeding aids and return them to the bedside table. Return all other equipment to the appropriate location.

PATIENT AND/OR FAMILY TEACHING

1. Instruct the patient regarding the use of any special feeding devices.
2. Review with the patient any special diet or restriction in diet as ordered.
3. Teach a family member the technique of assisting the patient to eat if this will be required following discharge.

DOCUMENTATION

1. Amount of food consumed by patient during meal.
2. Amount of fluid intake during the meal.
3. An assessment of the patient's ability to feed him- or herself and any necessary changes in the plan of care related to mealtime.

Handwashing Technique

PURPOSE

1. Prevent or minimize the spread of infection.

REQUISITES

1. Antiseptic agent or plain (non-medicated) soap
2. Paper toweling

GUIDELINES

1. Handwashing before and after physical contact with each patient is the single most important means of preventing the spread of infection in the hospital.
2. A variety of antiseptic agents are available for use within a hospital. Although antiseptics and other handwashing soaps do not sterilize the skin, the agents can reduce microbial contamination depending on the following conditions:
   a. Type and amount of contamination.
   b. Type of antiseptic or agent used.
   c. Length of exposure to the antiseptic or agent.
   d. Presence of residual microbial activity.
   e. Handwashing practices followed.
3. Indications for handwashing technique can depend on the type, intensity, and length of personnel-patient contact.
4. Handwashing with an antiseptic agent may be recommended by hospital policy during certain circumstances and in certain areas such as:
   a. Special care units.
   b. Isolation units.
   c. Nursing units where invasive procedures are performed.
   d. Nursing units with patients who have low resistance to infection.
   e. Nursing units with patients infected with multiple-resistant bacteria.
5. Handwashing with plain soap and water is recommended for most situations when there is prolonged physical contact with any non-infected patient. Indirect patient contact usually does not require handwashing.

6. Antiseptics that do not require water may be recommended by hospital policy to eliminate the spread of infection when no large amount of physical soil is involved and sinks are not conveniently located.
7. For effective handwashing, nails should be kept short. The greatest number of organisms is found around and under the fingernails, so added attention should be devoted to cleansing this area.
8. Rings and watches should be removed from the hands and wrists prior to handwashing, since these articles may shelter microorganisms.
9. During routine patient care, a vigorous washing with friction under running water for 15 seconds is recommended. Hospital policy will dictate the duration of the wash, the type of agent to be used, and when hands, wrists, and/or elbows are to be washed. Recommendations depend on the purpose of the washing.
10. Containers or cleansing agents might serve as reservoirs for microorganisms and should be cleaned regularly according to hospital policy. Bar soap, although not recommended, should be stored on a drainable soap tray.
11. Regular use of hand lotion after hospital duty time can help reduce or prevent dermatitis due to handwashing.
12. Hands should be washed after close patient contact even when gloves are worn.
13. Faucets are considered contaminated; when turning off the faucets use a dry paper towel to prevent reinfecting hands and fixtures.
14. Except for a true emergency, hospital personnel should always wash their hands:
    a. Before and after the tour of duty.
    b. Before performing any invasive procedure.
    c. Before and after physical contact with each patient.

d. After handling a source that is likely to be contaminated, such as equipment, dressings, and secretions and excretions from patients.

e. Between patient care sites, if indicated.

f. Whenever your hands become physically soiled.

g. After using the bathroom, blowing your nose, or covering a sneeze.

h. Before eating, drinking, or handling food.

NURSING ACTION/RATIONALE

1. Obtain the paper toweling for drying your hands. If using a dispenser with a handle, pull down the paper but do not tear it off at this time.
2. Turn on the water, adjust the temperature, and allow water to run continuously.
3. Wet your hands. Keep fingers pointing down at all times.
4. Apply a generous amount of soap. Lather all surfaces of the hands and wrists including the backs of the hands, between the fingers, and the areas around the nail edges (Figure 1-19).

5. Wash for 15 seconds or as indicated by hospital policy, using friction.
6. Rinse thoroughly, holding your hands downward. Avoid splashing or allowing your hands to touch the sink. Allow the water to drain off the fingertips (Figure 1-20).
7. Dry your hands thoroughly with the paper toweling.
8. Turn off the faucets, using a dry paper towel (Figure 1-21).
9. Discard the paper toweling into the disposal provided.

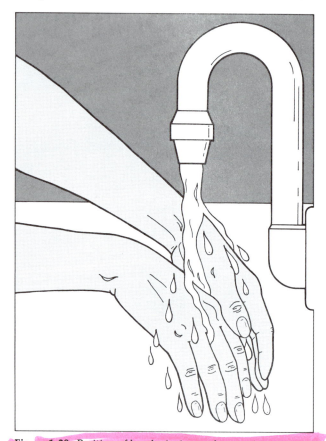

Figure 1-20. Position of hands rinsing under running water.

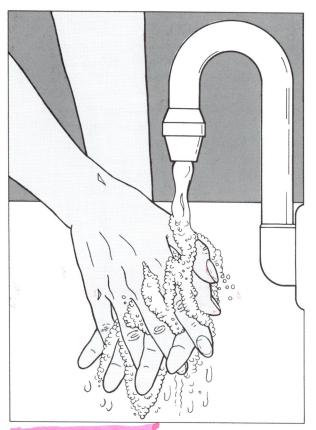

Figure 1-19. Lathered hands.

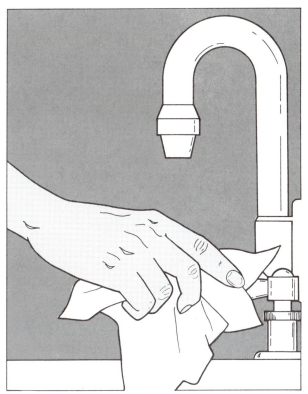

Figure 1-21. Turn off faucets using dry paper toweling.

PATIENT AND/OR FAMILY TEACHING
1. Explain to the patient and/or family the importance of proper handwashing.
2. Demonstrate proper handwashing technique to the patient, and the family if appropriate.
3. Display the hospital instructional handwashing sign in a suitable prominent location, if appropriate.
4. Reinforce the importance of handwashing and good hygiene when discharged.

DOCUMENTATION
1. Any patient teaching done and the patient's level of understanding.

Non-Sterile Gloving Technique

PURPOSE
1. Prevent the transmission of infectious organisms.
2. Provide personal protection.

REQUISITES
1. Non-sterile exam gloves
2. Waste receptacle

GUIDELINES
1. Wearing gloves does not replace handwashing.
2. Non-sterile gloves are worn if infectious transmission could occur by:
   a. Direct patient contact.
   b. Indirect contact with contaminated equipment and/or body secretions.
3. Sterile gloves are always worn when the procedure requires sterile technique. Sterile gloves are applied after the sterile gown and mask, if these items are to be worn.
4. Gloves are worn once and discarded.
5. When indicated, have a supply of gloves readily available for use.

NURSING ACTION/RATIONALE
1. Wash and dry your hands thoroughly.
2. Remove the gloves from the box or the wrapper by the folded wrist edge, one at a time.
3. Place your hand through the opening and pull the glove up to the wrist. Repeat with the second glove.

4. Adjust the gloves so they cover your wrists, or the cuffs of a long-sleeved gown.
5. Complete patient care.
6. Remove the first glove by grasping the outside surface of the glove with the other gloved hand. Pull off, inside out (Figure 1-22a).
7. Remove the second glove by reaching under the remaining glove cuff and pulling the glove off, inside out (Figure 1-22b).
8. Discard the gloves in a waste receptacle.
9. Wash your hands.

PATIENT AND/OR FAMILY TEACHING
1. Explain that the gloves are worn as a precaution to protect the patient and others from infection.
2. Demonstrate to visitors how to put on and how to remove the gloves properly, if appropriate. Provide for a return demonstration.
3. Instruct the patient on the proper disposal of gloves, if appropriate.

DOCUMENTATION
1. Type of gloving used for a particular procedure, when appropriate.
2. All patient and/or family teaching done and the level of understanding.

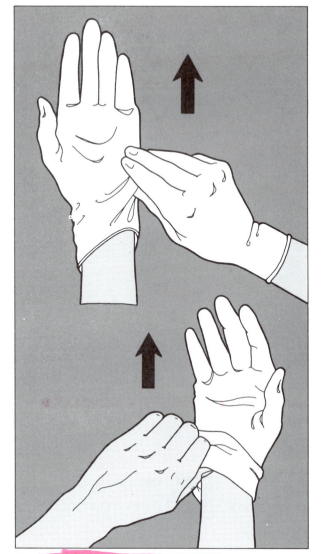

Figure 1-22. Removing non-sterile gloves.

Sterile Gloving Technique

PURPOSE
1. Provide personal protection.
2. Provide asepsis while performing invasive procedures.

REQUISITES
1. Sterile gloves
2. Waste receptacle

GUIDELINES
1. Wearing gloves does not replace handwashing.
2. Non-sterile gloves are worn if infectious transmission could occur by:
   a. Direct patient contact.
   b. Indirect contact with contaminated equipment and/or body secretions.
3. Sterile gloves are always worn when the procedure requires sterile technique. Sterile gloves are applied after the sterile gown and mask if these items are to be worn.
4. Gloves are worn once and discarded.
5. When indicated, have a supply of gloves readily available for use.

NURSING ACTION/RATIONALE
1. Wash and dry your hands thoroughly.
2. Read the directions on the package for instructions regarding opening the sterile glove package.
3. Open the package carefully, touching only the outside of the wrapper.
4. Remove the first glove, touching only the folded edge of the cuff (Figure 1-23a).
5. Avoid touching the wrapper with the glove.
6. Put on the first glove. Do not permit the outside of the glove to come into contact with any non-sterile surface.
7. Hold the wrapper with the ungloved hand and remove the second glove with the gloved hand by placing the fingers under the folded cuffs (Figure 1-23b).
8. Put on the second glove. Again do not permit the outside of either glove to come into contact with any non-sterile surface.
9. Adjust your fingers to fit glove.

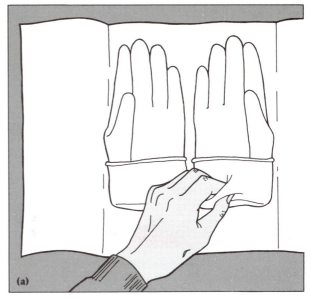

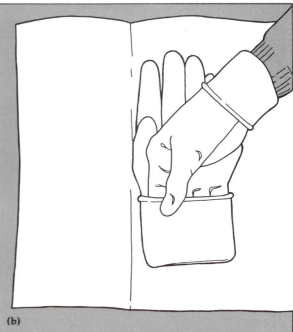

Figure 1-23. Putting on sterile gloves. **(a)** Remove first glove from package. **(b)** Remove second glove from package.

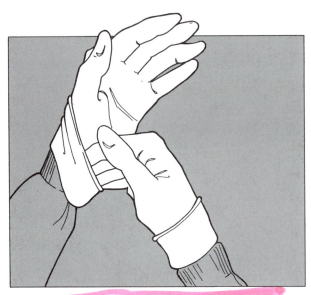

Figure 1-23(c). Pull glove cuff over long-sleeved gown.

10. Pull the glove cuffs over the gown cuffs when wearing long-sleeved gown (Figure 1-23c).
11. Complete patient care.
12. Remove the first glove by holding the outside surface of the glove with the other gloved hand. Pull the glove off, inside out (Figure 1-24a).
13. Remove the second glove by reaching under the remaining glove cuff and pulling the glove off, inside out (Figure 1-24b).
14. Discard the gloves in a waste receptacle.
15. Wash your hands.

PATIENT AND/OR FAMILY TEACHING

1. Explain that the gloves are worn as a precaution to protect the patient and others from infection.

DOCUMENTATION

1. Type of gloving used for a particular procedure, when appropriate.
2. All patient teaching done and the patient's level of understanding.

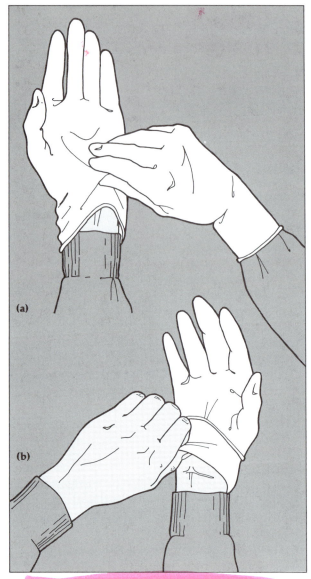

(a)

(b)

Figure 1-24. Taking off sterile gloves. (a) Removing first glove. (b) Removing second glove.

General Draping and Assisting with Physical Examination

PURPOSE
1. Prevent embarrassment and chilling through needless exposure.
2. Assist the person performing the examination.

REQUISITES
1. Bath blanket, sheet, or towel
2. Equipment appropriate to specific exam:
   a. Eye: flashlight, ophthalmoscope, eye chart, and tonometer
   b. Ear: otoscope, ear speculum, and tuning fork
   c. Nose: nasal speculum and flashlight
   d. Throat: tongue depressor and flashlight or headscope
   e. Chest and abdomen: stethoscope
   f. Pelvic: sterile vaginal speculum, sterile gloves, and lubricant
   g. Rectal: exam glove and lubricant
   h. Neurological: percussion hammer and safety pin

GUIDELINES
1. Many patients are anxious before a physical examination. The nurse's sensitivity to these feelings is essential.
2. Tenseness on the patient's part will make the examination more uncomfortable, as well as possibly altering the results.
3. Prevent the patient from becoming chilled during the examination by providing a blanket and avoiding drafts. Make certain that hands and equipment are warmed before touching the patient.
4. Be aware of your non-verbal communication and its effect on the patient.

NURSING ACTION/RATIONALE
1. Assemble any equipment needed.
2. Identify the patient.
3. Explain the examination to be done.
4. Take the patient to the exam room, if the examination is not to be done in the patient's room.
5. Provide adequate lighting.
6. Provide privacy for the patient.
7. Wash your hands.
8. Obtain vital signs, height, and weight if necessary.
9. Remove the patient's gown if necessary.
10. Position the patient and drape as appropriate:
    a. *Chest and axillary region:* Sitting; fold covers to abdomen.
    b. *Abdomen:* Supine; cover the chest with a towel and fold covers to pubic region.
    c. *Back:* Prone; fold covers to sacrum.
    d. *Male genitalia:* Standing.
    e. *Female pelvic area:* Lithotomy; pull gown up to abdomen, drape legs with a sheet.
    f. *Rectal:* Knee-chest or Sim's position; cover upper part of body, drape legs with sheet.
11. Open sterile supplies using aseptic technique.
12. Assist the examiner as required.
13. Explain procedures to the patient and reassure frequently. Instruct the patient to deep breathe during uncomfortable procedures.
14. Assist the patient to a comfortable position after the examination is completed. Assist the patient to his/her room if required.
15. Discard or return all equipment to the appropriate area.

PATIENT AND/OR FAMILY TEACHING
1. Explain the examination to be done.
2. Instruct the patient to deep breathe during uncomfortable parts of the examination.
3. Explain any other diagnostic procedures to be done.
4. Reinforce the physician's explanation of the disease process.

DOCUMENTATION
1. Examinations performed, any observations, and the patient's response.
2. All patient teaching done and the patient's level of understanding.

Blood Pressure Determination

PURPOSE

1. Obtain a measurement of the amount of pressure that blood exerts against the walls of an arterial blood vessel.

REQUISITES

1. Sphygmomanometer
2. Stethoscope

GUIDELINES

1. The appropriate size blood pressure cuff for the individual patient is important:
   a. The width of the bladder, inside the cuff, should be sufficient to wrap at least halfway around the upper arm.
   b. The length of the bladder, inside the cuff, should be sufficient to wrap almost entirely around the arm, but not so long that it would overlap.
2. Any air leaks in the bladder, exhaust valve, and/or tubing will cause erroneous readings.
3. Do not use an extremity that:
   a. Has an intravenous infusing.
   b. Is diseased or injured.
   c. Is paralyzed.
   d. Contains a renal dialysis shunt or fistula.
   e. Is on the same side as a mastectomy.
4. If necessary, the popliteal artery behind the knee may be used for blood pressure determination.
   a. The patient should be in the prone position if possible.
   b. If the patient is unable to lie prone, have him/her lie supine with the knee of the cuffed leg slightly flexed.
   c. The systolic reading in the thigh may be 10 to 40 mm Hg higher than in the arm, but the diastolic reading should be the same.
5. Koratkoff sounds are the tappings and murmurs heard while taking the blood pressure. The Koratkoff sounds are categorized into five different phases according to the distinct changes in sounds heard:
   a. Phase I—A tapping sound is heard which may be followed by an absence of sound (auscultatory gap).
   b. Phase II—A murmur or swishing sound is heard.
   c. Phase III—A crisp clear pulse is heard.
   d. Phase IV—An abrupt muffling of the sound is heard.
   e. Phase V—The first absence of sound occurs.
6. Phase I is considered the systolic reading, phase IV is considered the first diastolic reading, and phase V is the second diastolic reading. Hypertension should be considered in a reading that is above 140/90 mm Hg and hypotension should be considered in a reading below 95/60 mm Hg. The patient's total clinical picture must also be considered.
7. Inflating the cuff 30 mm Hg above the point where arterial pulsations cease is clinically important to prevent the possibility of an oversight of the auscultatory gap. By inflating the cuff arbitrarily to 160 to 180 mm Hg, it is possible to come in at the auscultatory gap and interpret the systolic reading to be much lower than the actual systolic pressure. Routinely inflating the blood pressure cuff to the top of the pressure gauge is poor technique, as this may be very painful and may distort the reading because of pain or induced vasospasm.
8. Drugs such as hormones, vasodilators, and vasoconstrictors may affect the blood pressure.
9. The following situations may create a temporary elevation in blood pressure readings:
   a. Smoking.
   b. Pain.
   c. Emotional stress.
   d. A distended bladder.
   e. A recent meal.
   f. Recent physical exercise.
   g. Cold air or water.

10. If the patient is in shock, with a low cardiac output, and auscultation of the blood pressure with a stethoscope is unsuccessful, the blood pressure can be palpated. Note the point at which arterial pulsations can first be felt during cuff deflation.

11. For consistency, blood pressure readings should be taken in the same arm each time, and with the patient in the same position of sitting, standing, or lying.

12. Patients taking vasodilators, antihypertensives, tranquilizers, or antiarrhythmic drugs, and patients with kidney disease should have their blood pressure taken lying, sitting, *and* standing and each should be recorded. Readings should be taken after the patient has been in the position for 5 minutes.

NURSING ACTION/RATIONALE

1. Assemble the equipment.
2. Identify the patient.
3. Explain the procedure to the patient.
4. Position the patient in a recumbent or sitting position with the arm relaxed on a flat surface at cardiac level. If the arm is below the level of the heart the reading may be erroneously high. Conversely, if the arm is above the level of the heart the reading may be erroneously low.
5. Provide a quiet environment.
6. Push clothing upward and away from the extremity to be used. If clothing is restrictive, remove it.
7. Hold the extremity in a slightly elevated position with the palm up during application and inflation of the cuff, which continues through Step 12. This can be done by supporting the patient's arm between your hip and elbow. If the patient's leg is used, help may be needed to raise the leg while the cuff is applied. Elevation of the extremity decreases the blood volume in the vessels of the forearm; therefore, pressure is decreased. With lower pressure in the forearm, the pressure differential between the forearm and the cuff is increased. This accentuates the Koratkoff sounds so that they can be heard more accurately.

8. Wrap the cuff snugly and smoothly around the extremity with the center of the inflatable bladder directly over the brachial artery and the lower edge of the cuff at least 1 inch above the antecubital space (Figure 1-25).

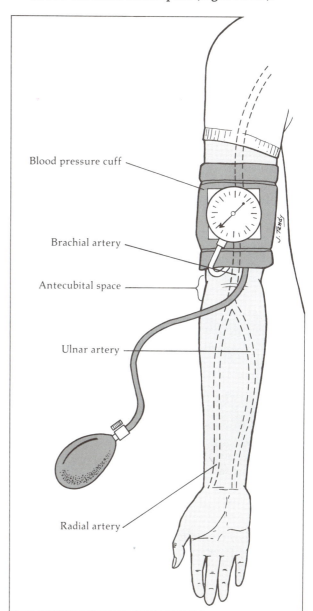

Blood pressure cuff

Brachial artery

Antecubital space

Ulnar artery

Radial artery

Figure 1-25. Proper position for blood pressure cuff.

9. Place the earpieces of the stethoscope in your ears and keep the diaphragm of the stethoscope where it will be readily available.
10. Locate the arterial pulsations of the brachial artery in the antecubital space with the index, second, and third fingertips of your non-dominant hand.
11. Close the central valve of the sphygmomanometer with your dominant hand and inflate the cuff by squeezing the bulb until the arterial pulsations cannot be felt. Continue to inflate the cuff 30 mm Hg beyond this point.
12. Quickly place the stethoscope snugly over the palpated artery of the extremity and lower the extremity to heart level. The stethoscope should be applied firmly but with as little pressure as possible so as not to occlude the artery.
13. Open the control valve and deflate the cuff at a rate not exceeding 2 mm Hg per heartbeat. If deflation is slower, venous congestion develops and increases the diastolic pressure in the extremity. If deflation is too rapid, the exact readings may be missed.
14. Read the gauge when the first faint clear tapping sounds are heard. This reading should be approximately the same as the palpated systolic level.
15. Continue deflating the cuff, reading the gauge when the sounds abruptly soften and muffle and again when the sounds completely disappear.
16. Do not stop during the deflation to reinflate the cuff to take another reading. This causes the forearm to fill with blood and affects the intensity and changes in sound that you will pick up with your stethoscope. If it is necessary to retake the blood pressure reading on the same extremity, wait at least two minutes between readings.
17. Deflate the cuff completely and remove it.
18. Assist the patient to a comfortable position.
19. Return all equipment to the appropriate area.

PATIENT AND/OR FAMILY TEACHING

1. Explain blood pressure and its measurement to the patient.
2. Reinforce and clarify the physician's explanation of the disease process.
3. Explain any additional diagnostic testing or therapeutic orders.
4. Explain the following information to the patient as it is appropriate:
   a. Stress the importance of taking medication as directed to control blood pressure.
   b. Stress the importance of following prescribed dietary restrictions.
   c. Teach the patient the signs and symptoms associated with an elevated or lowered blood pressure.
   d. Teach the patient to avoid such overstimulating items as tobacco and beverages containing caffeine.
   e. Teach the patient to read labeling on over-the-counter drugs carefully for contraindications for patients with hypertension.
   f. Teach the patient to take his/her own blood pressure if required for home monitoring.

DOCUMENTATION

1. Systolic and both diastolic readings (120/80/76). If both diastolic readings are the same, record both as 120/80/80.
2. The position the patient was in and the extremity in which the measurement was taken.
3. All patient teaching and the patient's level of understanding.

Assessing a Temperature

PURPOSE

1. Assess the patient's body temperature.

REQUISITES

1. Thermometer
   a. Electronic thermometer with disposable probe, or
   b. Glass thermometer—oral or rectal
2. Watch or clock
3. Lubricant, if rectal thermometer
4. Disposable tissue

GUIDELINES

1. Body temperature is a measurement of the balance between heat lost and heat produced. It is a useful assessment parameter for a variety of clinical problems including infectious processes and fluid imbalances.
2. Body temperature may be assessed orally, rectally, or at the axilla.
3. Rectal temperature measurement is the most accurate and should be used for any patient who cannot adequately hold an oral thermometer—unless contraindicated because of rectal surgery or disease.
4. Glass thermometers require a specific amount of time to register accurately including:
   a. Oral—8 minutes. (5 min)
   b. Rectal—3 minutes.
   c. Axillary—10 minutes.
5. When using an electronic thermometer, follow the manufacturer's instructions for the time required for temperature measurement.
6. Average normal adult temperatures in various body areas are:
   a. Oral—37°C (98.6°F).
   b. Rectal—37.5°C (99.5°F).
   c. Axillary—36.7°C (98°F).
7. Oral temperatures should not be taken immediately following the ingestion of fluids or following smoking. Wait 15 minutes before assessing the temperature.
8. Electronic thermometers should not be used for patients in isolation precaution. A glass thermometer should be provided.
9. Electronic thermometers should be stored in the recharger when not in use.

NURSING ACTION/RATIONALE

General Preparation

1. Assemble all equipment.
2. Identify the patient.
3. Explain the procedure to the patient.
4. Wash your hands.

Oral: Glass Thermometer

1. Shake down the thermometer below 36°C (95°F).
2. Place the thermometer in the patient's mouth under the tongue in the posterior sublingual pocket (Figure 1-26).

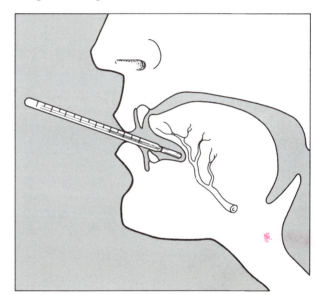

Figure 1-26. Correct oral thermometer placement.

3. Instruct the patient to close his/her mouth.
4. Instruct the patient to leave the thermometer in place for 8 minutes.
5. Remove the thermometer and wipe it with a twisting motion toward the bulb with an alcohol wipe.
6. Read the thermometer at eye level.
7. Wash the thermometer with warm water and soap. Rinse with cold water.
8. Return the thermometer to its appropriate location.
9. Wash your hands.

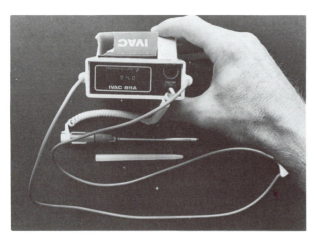

Figure 1-27. Electronic thermometer with probe and cover.

Oral: Electronic Thermometer (Figure 1-27)
1. Remove the oral metal probe from the electric thermometer unit.
2. Insert the metal probe into a plastic disposable cover.
3. Place the covered probe in the patient's mouth in the posterior sublingual pocket.
4. Hold the thermometer in place until the light and auditory signal indicate a final reading.
5. Remove the thermometer and obtain a temperature reading.
6. Discard the plastic probe cover in a waste receptacle.
7. Wash your hands.

Rectal: Glass Thermometer
1. Assist the patient into the lateral (Sim's) position.
2. Provide adequate lighting.
3. Shake down the thermometer below 36°C (95°F).
4. Lubricate the thermometer tip.
5. Insert the thermometer into the rectum approximately 1½ inches.
6. Hold the thermometer in place for 3 minutes.
7. Remove the thermometer and wipe it in a twisting motion toward the bulb with a disposable tissue.
8. Read the thermometer at eye level.
9. Wash the thermometer with warm water and soap. Rinse with cold water.
10. Return the thermometer to its appropriate location.
11. Assist the patient to a comfortable position.
12. Wash your hands.

Rectal: Electronic Thermometer
1. Assist the patient into the lateral (Sim's) position.
2. Provide adequate lighting.
3. Connect the rectal metal probe to the electronic thermometer unit.
4. Insert the metal probe into a plastic disposable cover.
5. Insert the covered probe into the rectum approximately 1½ inches.
6. Hold the temperature probe in place until the light and audible signal indicate a final reading.
7. Remove the temperature probe and obtain a temperature reading.
8. Discard the plastic probe cover in a waste receptacle.
9. Wash your hands.

Axillary: Glass Thermometer
1. Follow the steps in "Oral: Glass Thermometer" with the following exceptions:
   a. Place the thermometer in the center of the axilla with the patient's arm firmly against the side of the chest.
   b. Hold the thermometer in place for 10 minutes.

Axillary: Electronic Thermometer
1. Follow the steps in "Oral: Electronic Thermometer" with the following exceptions:
   a. Place the temperature probe in the center of the axilla with the patient's arm firmly against the side of the chest.
   b. Hold the temperature probe in place until the light and audible signal indicate a final reading.

PATIENT AND/OR FAMILY TEACHING
1. Explain the procedure to the patient.
2. Explain other therapeutic measures prescribed for the patient.
3. Instruct the patient regarding increased fluid intake if temperature is elevated and if fluids are permitted.

DOCUMENTATION

1. Temperature reading.
2. Route of measurement.
3. All patient teaching and the patient's level of understanding.

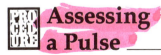 **Assessing a Pulse**

PURPOSE

1. Assess the rate, rhythm, and quality of the patient's heart contractions.

REQUISITES

1. Stethoscope
2. Watch with a second indicator

GUIDELINES

1. The pulse is created by the force of the contraction of the left ventricle of the heart, causing the arterial walls to expand and contract.
2. Common sites for palpating an arterial pulse include the radial artery in the wrist, the carotid artery in the neck, and the femoral artery in the groin. Pulse points are also found in other areas of the body (Figure 1-28).
3. The pulse may also be auscultated on the left chest wall by placing a stethoscope between the fifth and sixth ribs slightly distal to the midclavicular line. In acute care settings, an apical pulse should be taken.
4. The pulse should be assessed for rate, rhythm, quality, and force. To obtain an accurate pulse, the pulse must be assessed for one minute.
5. The average normal adult pulse is between 60 and 100 beats per minute. A pulse rate over 100 is tachycardia. A pulse rate under 60 is bradycardia.
6. Pulse irregularities or arrhythmias may be caused by a variety of clinical problems including cardiovascular disease, respiratory disease, metabolic disorders, and infections.

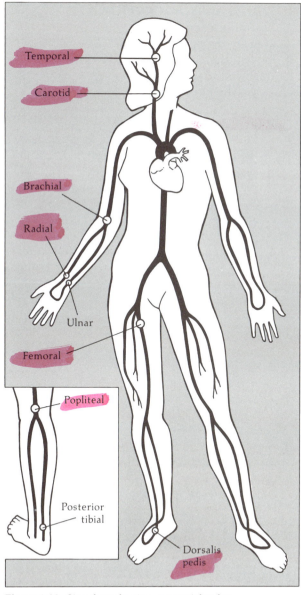

Figure 1-28. Sites for palpating an arterial pulse.

7. Bradycardia may occur normally in the well-conditioned athlete.
8. Any unusual change in heart rate, rhythm, or quality should be reported to the physician.
9. An apical pulse should always be assessed for patients with cardiovascular disease and prior to the administration of cardiac medications. An apical pulse should also be assessed for any critically ill patient.
10. If a pulse deficit is present, an apical-radial pulse should be taken simultaneously by two persons.

NURSING ACTION/RATIONALE

1. Assemble all equipment.
2. Identify the patient.
3. Explain the procedure to the patient.
4. Wash your hands.
5. Assess the pulse.

Radial Pulse

   a. Place the patient's arm on a flat surface at the level of the heart with the palmar surface down.
   b. Place three fingers of your dominant hand against the radial artery (Figure 1-29).
   c. Press gently against the radial artery and palpate the pulse.
   d. Assess and count the pulse for 60 seconds, using the second indicator on your watch.

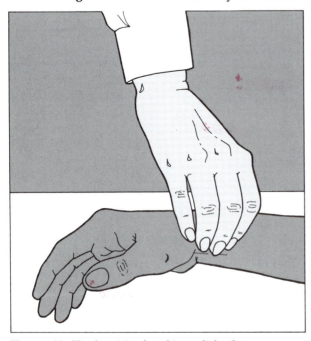

Figure 1-29. Hand position for taking radial pulse.

Apical Pulse

   a. Assist the patient to a recumbent or a sitting position.
   b. Expose the left side of the chest. Drape as required.
   c. Place the stethoscope over the apex of the heart slightly distal to the midclavicular line in the fifth intercostal space (Figure 1-30).
   d. Auscultate and count the pulse for 60 seconds, using the second indicator on your watch.
   e. Assist the patient to a comfortable position.

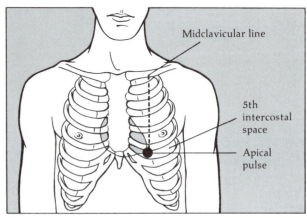

Midclavicular line

5th intercostal space

Apical pulse

Figure 1-30. Apical pulse site.

Apical-Radial Pulse

   a. Follow the procedure for assessing an apical pulse with the following exceptions:
   (1) Place the watch within view of both persons performing the procedure.
   (2) Decide on a starting time on the watch.
   (3) Assess the apical and radial pulses simultaneously for one full minute with one person counting the apical and the other person counting the radial.
6. Wash your hands.
7. Return the stethoscope to the appropriate location.

PATIENT AND/OR FAMILY TEACHING

1. Explain the procedure and its purpose to the patient.
2. Explain other therapeutic measures, if appropriate.
3. Instruct the patient to notify the nurse if experiencing chest pain.
4. Instruct the patient and/or family how to assess the pulse rate if required following discharge.

DOCUMENTATION

1. Location, rate, rhythm, and quality of the pulse.

2. Any physician notification, if appropriate.
3. Any chest pain experienced.
4. Any adjustments in medication administration, if appropriate.
5. All patient teaching done and the patient's level of understanding.

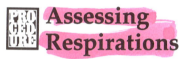 Assessing Respirations

PURPOSE

1. Assess the rate, rhythm, depth, and quality of the patient's respirations.
2. Evaluate the patient's respiratory status.

REQUISITES

1. Stethoscope
2. Watch with second indicator

GUIDELINES

1. Respirations are normally effortless, regular, noiseless, and involuntary.
2. Respiratory rate, rhythm, depth, and quality may change in a variety of clinical problems including respiratory and cardiovascular diseases, metabolic disorders, fluid and acid-base disturbances, trauma, medication overdoses, infectious processes, and neurological disorders.
3. The normal average respiratory rate for an adult is 16 to 20 respirations per minute.
4. An obstructed airway should be suspected if respirations become stertorous (noisy).
5. A complete respiratory assessment, including auscultation of breath sounds, should be performed if a patient is experiencing difficulty breathing.
6. Oxygen and/or respiratory care therapy may be ordered by the physician as an adjunctive treatment for patients experiencing respiratory changes.

7. Any unusual change in the rate, rhythm, depth, or quality of respiration should be reported to the physician.
8. Respirations should be assessed after taking the pulse, while your fingers are still in place over the radial artery. Assessment of respirations will be most accurate when the patient is unaware that you are counting them.

NURSING ACTION/RATIONALE

1. Assemble all equipment.
2. Identify the patient.
3. Wash your hands.
4. Assess and count respirations for 60 seconds, using the second indicator on your watch. Keep your fingers in place over the radial artery to make the patient less aware that you are assessing respirations.
5. Auscultate breath sounds, if appropriate.
6. Wash your hands.
7. Return the stethoscope to the appropriate location.

PATIENT AND/OR FAMILY TEACHING

1. Explain related therapeutic measures such as oxygen or respiratory care treatments, if appropriate.
2. Instruct the patient to notify the nurse if experiencing any difficulty breathing.

DOCUMENTATION

1. The rate, rhythm, depth, and quality of respiration.
2. Any physician notification, if appropriate.

3. Any dyspnea experienced.
4. The patient's position in bed, if appropriate.
5. Any oxygen or respiratory care treatments.
6. All patient teaching done and the patient's level of understanding.

Intake and Output Measurement

PURPOSE

1. Provide an accurate record of the patient's fluid intake and output.

REQUISITES

1. Graduated container
2. Urine collection container
3. Intake and output record
4. Sign: "Intake and Output"

GUIDELINES

1. Fluid balance may be disturbed by a variety of disease processes and drug therapies, making assessment of fluid intake and output essential.
2. Fluid intake includes oral fluids, gavage feedings, and parenteral fluids. Also included are certain instillations of fluids into the body.
3. Fluid output includes urine, liquid stool, blood, emesis, drainage from wounds, and drainage from tubes such as nasogastric, catheters, and drains.
4. Drainage on absorbent pads such as dressings and peri-pads can be assessed accurately by weighing the dressing before and after it is applied to the patient.
5. Chest tube drainage should be included in the total output but should never be emptied. See "Nursing Management of Chest Tubes."
6. For the procedure for emptying a Foley drainage bag, refer to "Care and Maintenance of an Indwelling Catheter."

7. A reference with the liquid-measure equivalents for relevant menu items should be posted at the patient's bedside.
8. An "Intake and Output" sign should be displayed in a convenient location.
9. A patient's 24-hour total of fluid intake and output, along with a daily weight, can be used to determine an accurate assessment of the patient's fluid status.

NURSING ACTION/RATIONALE

1. Assemble all equipment.
2. Prepare an "Intake and Output Record" with the patient's identification data (Figure 1-31).
3. Identify the patient.
4. Place the "Intake and Output Record" in an appropriate, prominent location in the patient's room.
5. Explain the intake and output procedure to the patient.
6. Provide the patient with a urine collection container if the patient does not have an indwelling catheter.
7. Place a graduated container in the patient's bathroom.
8. Post the "Intake and Output" sign in an appropriate, prominent location.
9. Measure and record or instruct the patient to measure and record all intake and output.

INTAKE AND OUTPUT RECORD

THIS RECORD IS IMPORTANT!

INSTRUCTIONS: All fluid taken by mouth MUST be recorded and all urine MUST be measured. The patient must use the bedpan or urinal even if on bathroom privileges. The patient may be helpful by filling in this information or reminding nursing personnel to do so. All fluids taken with and between meals are included. Only record amount of liquid actually consumed.

Date: _____ 1 oz. = 30 cc

UNIT SERVICE		DIETARY SERVICE	
• SMALL PAPER CUP	150 cc	CARTON OF MILK	240 cc
• LARGE PAPER CUP	400 cc	STANDARD JUICE GLASS	120 cc
• PITCHER SET CUP	240 cc	TEA OR COFFEE CUP	200 cc
• WATER PITCHER	800 cc	AV. SERVING SOUP	180 cc
ONE TEASPOON ICE CHIPS	10 cc	SMALL CREAMER	10 cc
• WITHOUT ICE			

DIETARY SERVICE	
AV. SERVING JELL-O	120 cc
AV. SERVING ICE CREAM	105 cc
AV. SERVING SHERBET	105 cc
SODA-CAN	360 cc

	0700 – 1500 (7-3)	1500 – 2300 (3-11)	2300 – 0700 (11-7)	24 HR. TOTAL
ORAL AND PARENTERAL INTAKE				
ORAL FLUID				
TOTAL ORAL INTAKE				
# PARENTERAL FLUID				
TOTAL PARENTERAL INTAKE				
OUTPUT				
URINE				
STOOL (COLOR CONSISTENCY)				
DRAINAGE – GASTRO-INTESTINAL				
DRAINAGE – BILIARY				
DRAINAGE – OTHER				
EMESIS				
TOTAL OUTPUT				

(10-82)

ST. LUKE'S HOSPITAL, RACINE, WISCONSIN   612001

Figure 1-31. Sample Intake and Output Record.

PATIENT AND/OR FAMILY TEACHING

1. Explain the intake and output procedure to the patient and/or family.
   a. Emphasize the purpose and importance of accurate measurement and recording of all intake and output.
   b. Explain the "Intake and Output Record" if the patient is recording his/her own measurements.
   c. Explain the use of the urine collection container and the graduated container.
   d. Instruct the patient to notify the nurse if assistance is needed for collecting, measuring, or recording urine output.
   e. Explain the equivalency reference for hospital menu items that will be recorded as intake.
2. Reinforce and clarify the physician's explanation of the disease process.

DOCUMENTATION

1. All fluid intake and output.
2. Characteristics of the output including color, consistency, and odor.
3. Patency of any drainage systems.
4. Assessment parameters including skin turgor, diaphoresis, alertness, or other symptoms related to fluid balance.
5. Any patient teaching done and the patient's level of understanding.

Application of Elastic Stockings

PURPOSE

1. Promote venous return from the lower extremities.
2. Provide correct application and removal for the patient.

REQUISITES

1. Elastic stockings—correct size for patient
2. Size chart
3. Tape measure

GUIDELINES

1. Elastic stockings are generally ordered for patients who are immobile or for those with vascular disorders. They are also ordered for patients following surgical procedures.
2. Elastic stockings may require a physician's order. Refer to your health care facility's policy manual.
3. Elastic stockings are supplied in a variety of lengths, colors, and sizes. Stockings should be fitted correctly for each patient. Knee-length stockings should end 1 inch below the knee. Thigh-length stockings should end 2 inches below the groin.
4. The tops of elastic stockings should not be folded over, since additional constriction could occur.
5. Elastic stockings should be removed for 20 minutes three times a day to allow for assessment of the leg area. Assessment should include inspection for redness, palpation for tenderness or increased temperature, and testing for Homans' sign.
6. A second pair of elastic stockings should be available to allow for washing at least every other day or when soiled.
7. Elastic stockings should be applied with the patient in a supine position.

NURSING ACTION/RATIONALE

1. Assemble all equipment.
2. Identify the patient.
3. Explain the procedure to the patient.
4. Provide privacy.
5. Assist the patient to a supine position in bed.
6. Wash your hands.
7. Measure the patient's legs.

Knee-Length Stockings

a. Measure the circumference of the calf.
b. Measure the lower leg from the heel to the back of the knee (Figure 1-32).

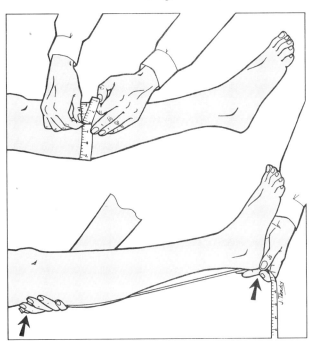

Figure 1-32. Measuring for knee-length stockings.

Thigh-Length Stockings

a. Measure the circumference of the calf and upper thigh.
b. Measure the leg from the heel to the gluteal furrow (Figure 1-33).

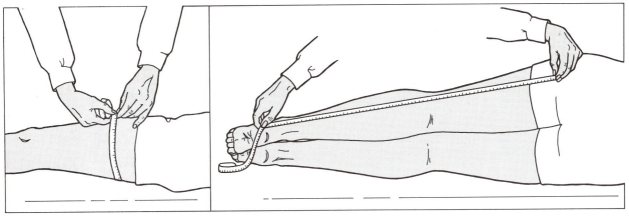

Figure 1-33. Measuring for thigh-length stockings.

8. Compare the patient's measurements with the size chart and select the appropriate size stockings for the patient.
9. Assess the color and sensation of each extremity.
10. Assess each leg for pain in the calf (positive Homans' sign) by dorsiflexing the foot with the knee slightly bent.
11. Insert one hand into the top of the stocking (Figure 1-34a).

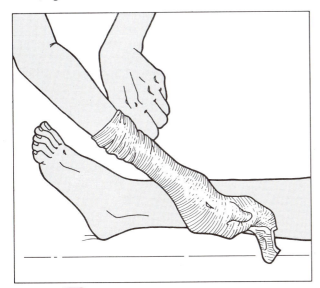

Figure 1-34(a). Inserting one hand into the stocking.

12. Grasp the heel of the stocking and turn the stocking inside out, as far as the heel.
13. Apply the stocking to the foot by stretching the stocking open at the heel and fitting the foot into the toe and heel pockets (Figure 1-34b).

14. Grasp the top of the stocking and pull it over the foot, gathering it at the ankle. Carefully pull it up (Figure 1-34c).

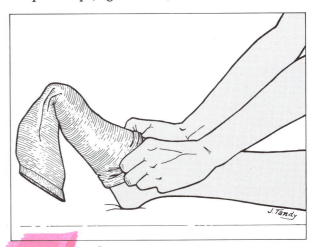

Figure 1-34(b). Applying the stocking to the foot.

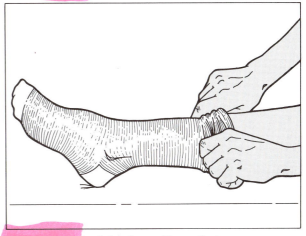

Figure 1-34(c). Applying the stocking to the leg.

15. Apply the other stocking using the same technique.
16. Assess the stockings for proper fit. There should be no wrinkles in the material.
17. Assess the patient for any discomfort from the stockings.
18. Assist the patient to a comfortable position.
19. Return all equipment to the appropriate location.

PATIENT AND/OR FAMILY TEACHING
1. Explain the procedure and its purpose to the patient.
2. Instruct the patient to wear slippers to avoid slipping.
3. Instruct the patient to notify the nurse if any discomfort is experienced.

4. Instruct the patient and/or family **regarding the application and removal of the stockings** if use will be continued following **discharge**.

DOCUMENTATION
1. Time of application and type of elastic stocking applied.
2. Assessment of leg(s) including color, sensations, and Homans' sign.
3. All patient and/or family teaching done and the patient's level of understanding.

Application of Bandages and Binders

PURPOSE
1. Apply pressure to stop bleeding.
2. Assist in absorption of tissue fluids.
3. Limit movement or provide for immobilization of an injured part.
4. Protect open wounds from contamination.
5. Provide support and aid in venous circulation.
6. Provide comfort or security.

REQUISITES
1. Bandage or binder
2. Safety pins or clips
3. Padding
4. Adhesive tape

GUIDELINES
1. The types of bandages and binders available are made from different materials in various sizes depending on the part of the body to be covered and the purpose.

Bandages
a. Tubular elastic—a net-meshed fabric used to secure dressings. It is lightweight and allows ventilation and easy assessment of the wound. It is also available as a shirt and pants.
b. Stockinette—a stretchable cotton or synthetic knit bandage. It is used underneath casts and to cover the head.
c. Tubular support—combinations of stockinette and rubber or elastic yarn. It is available in various widths and lengths and is frequently used to support joints.
d. Cotton gauze—loosely woven bandage. It is used to wrap a wound or secure a dressing while allowing ventilation. It can be impregnated with medication.
e. Elastic roller—woven bandage of cotton or synthetic and rubber or elastic yarn. It is used to provide support, promote circulation, or minimize swelling. Refer to the procedure, "Application of an Elastic Roller Bandage."
f. Adhesive bandage—small patches in many sizes and shapes useful for dressing simple, small wounds.

Binders

a. T-binder—designed in two forms (Figure 1-35). The single T-binder is for the female patient; the double T-binder is for the male patient. This type of binder is used to hold perineal or rectal dressings in place. Secure the waist strap with one pin. Bring the T-strap between the patient's legs and secure it with a second pin. The patient may prefer to apply this binder without assistance. T-binders soil easily, so they should be changed frequently.

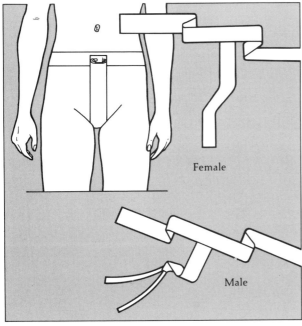

Figure 1-35. Female and male T-binders.

b. Scultetus binder—a many-tailed cloth with interlocking, overlapping bands used to enclose the abdomen with girdlelike support after surgery (Figure 1-36). Beginning at the bottom of the binder, alternate left- and right-side straps with a slight upward slant over the abdomen, covering half of the preceding strap. Secure the final strap with a safety pin.

c. Abdominal binder—a rectangular piece of cotton or synthetic cloth (Figure 1-37). It is used to support the abdomen following surgery. The abdominal binder encircles the waist, overlapping in the center where it is secured with clips or pins.

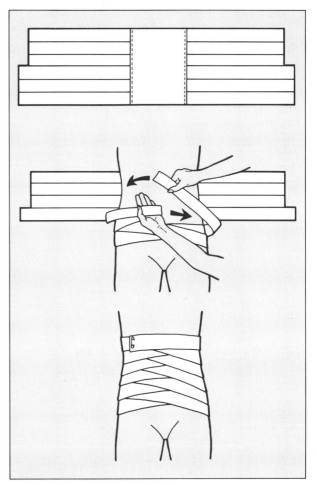

Figure 1-36. Scultetus binder.

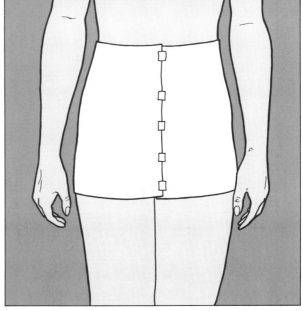

Figure 1-37. Abdominal binder.

d. Breast binder—a sleeveless cloth jacket that is used to hold breast dressings, support the breasts for comfort, or compress the breasts to aid in suppression of lactation following childbirth (Figure 1-38). To provide the most support, apply the binder while the patient is lying supine.

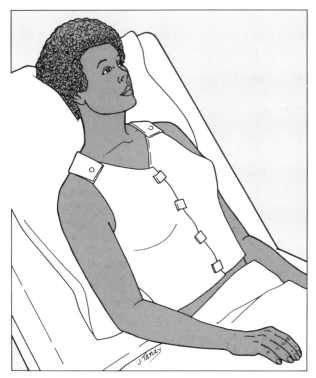

Figure 1-38. Breast binder.

e. Triangular bandage or sling—used to support and immobilize an upper extremity (Figure 1-39). Place the open triangle on the patient's chest with the point toward the affected elbow. Flex the arm at the elbow. One tail is placed around the neck on the unaffected side. The other tail is brought up over the affected arm. The two tails are tied in a square knot off-center behind the neck. Secure the point of the triangle to the sling with a safety pin.

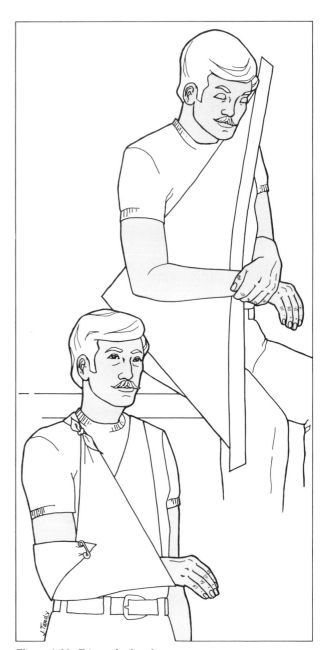

Figure 1-39. Triangular bandage.

2. Bandages and binders should be tight enough to serve their purpose, but not so tight as to impair respirations or circulation to the area.
3. Never begin or end a bandage directly over a wound or bony prominence.
4. Patients who are allergic to rubber may not be able to wear a tubular support or elastic roller bandage that contains rubber.
5. Binders may need to be reapplied frequently. Since they are not attached to the skin, they may slip out of place.

NURSING ACTION/RATIONALE
1. Assemble all equipment.
2. Identify the patient.
3. Explain the procedure to the patient.
4. Provide adequate lighting.
5. Provide privacy.
6. Wash your hands.
7. If an extremity is to be wrapped, place it in a horizontal position for at least 15 minutes to promote normal circulation. Place the body part in good body alignment and position of function.
8. Cleanse the area to be covered. Allow it to dry.
9. Apply a small amount of powder to the skin, unless there is an open wound. This will keep the skin dry and will decrease friction.
10. Place gauze between any adjoining skin surfaces. Pad any bony prominences.
11. Apply bandages from the distal to the proximal part of the body in the direction of venous return. Elevate the extremity while wrapping.
12. Apply bandages and binders securely with even pressure. This will prevent friction and irritation of the involved part and the surrounding area.
13. Leave fingers or toes visible whenever possible for assessing circulation in the extremity.
14. Place pins, clips, and knots used for securing away from any tender, inflamed areas so as not to create unnecessary pressure.
15. Assist the patient to a comfortable position.
16. Discard equipment or return it to the appropriate area.

17. Assess the bandage or binders regularly for correct placement. Assess visible fingers and toes for coolness, cyanosis, tingling, or numbness.
18. Change the bandage or binder regularly. Assess the skin under the bandage or binder for pressure areas, redness, or swelling. Microorganisms will grow in a moist, warm, and unclean environment. Change the bandage or binder on a draining wound frequently to keep it as dry and clean as possible.

PATIENT AND/OR FAMILY TEACHING
1. Explain to the patient how you will apply the bandage or binder.
2. Reinforce and clarify the physician's explanation of the disease process.
3. Explain any additional therapeutic orders.
4. Explain any activity restrictions.
5. Instruct the patient to notify the nurse if any tingling or numbness in the affected body part is experienced.
6. Teach the patient and/or a family member to apply the bandage or binder if it should be required after discharge.

DOCUMENTATION
1. Assessment of the affected body part before and after bandaging including color, motion, and sensation.
2. Type of bandage or binder applied.
3. The patient's reaction to the procedure.
4. Assessment of the underlying skin integrity during bandage changes.
5. All teaching done and the patient's level of understanding.

Application of an Elastic Roller Bandage

PURPOSE

1. Prevent venous stasis or thrombolytic disease or limit its extension if already present.
2. Secure surgical dressings or prevent tension on sutures.
3. Provide support, minimize swelling, and prevent further injury following musculoskeletal trauma.

REQUISITES

1. Elastic roller bandage in appropriate width and length
2. Securing clips or tape

GUIDELINES

1. When bandaging an extremity, wrap from distal to proximal, following the direction of venous circulation.
2. An elastic roller bandage that has been applied too tightly will decrease circulation to that part of the body, resulting in damage to the tissue.
3. If the extremity is wrapped in an improper, non-aligned position, a deformity could result.
4. If an open wound is present on the area to be wrapped, apply the bandage over a sterile dressing.
5. A small amount of powder applied to unbroken skin under the bandage will keep the area dry and reduce friction.
6. To prevent venous stasis in the heel, do not leave the heel exposed when bandaging the foot and leg.
7. If the bandage is to be worn for more than 48 to 72 hours, order two sets for changing purposes. Wash the bandage every two to three days.
8. To decrease the possibility of dislodging blood clots in a patient with thrombolytic disease, never rub or massage the legs when bathing or drying.

NURSING ACTION/RATIONALE

1. Explain the application of the elastic roller bandage to the patient.
2. Provide privacy.
3. Wash your hands.
4. Wash and completely dry the area to be bandaged.
5. Place the extremity or the part of the body to be wrapped at rest in a normal anatomical position.
6. Unroll the bandage by placing the outer surface of the roll next to the patient's skin (Figure 1-40). Begin rolling at the distal portion of the extremity. Leave a small portion of the extremity exposed to check for circulation.
7. Anchor the bandage by securing with one or two complete overlaps.

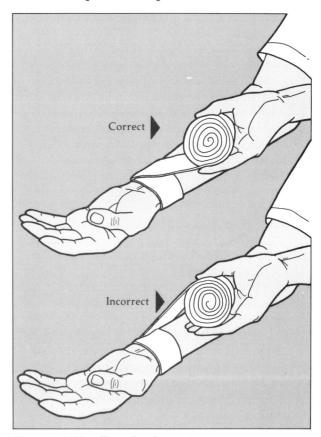

Figure 1-40. Unrolling a bandage.

8. Use one or more of the following methods when applying the bandage:
   a. Spiral wrap is used for cylindrically shaped parts (finger, arm, leg, chest, abdomen). Each turn partially overlaps the previous turn by one-third to two-thirds the width of the bandage (Figure 1-41).

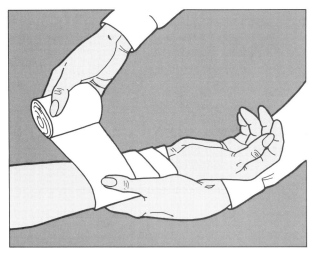

Figure 1-41. Spiral wrap.

   b. Reverse spiral wrap is used for cone-shaped parts (thigh, forearm). Partially overlap each turn but reverse the angle of the turn halfway through each turn (Figure 1-42).

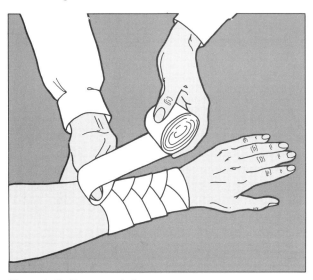

Figure 1-42. Reverse spiral wrap.

   c. Figure-eight wrap is used for joints (elbow, wrist, knee, ankle). Cross each turn over the preceding one, alternately ascending and descending (Figure 1-43).

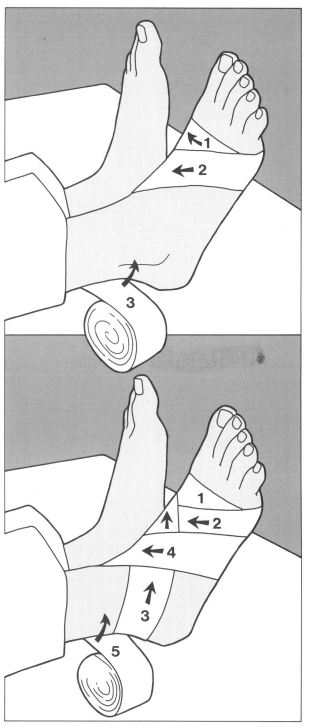

Figure 1-43. Figure-eight wrap.

9. Apply the bandage with firm, even tension and pressure.
10. Tape or clip the bandage in place.
11. Assess the area bandaged for signs of gaps, slippage, unevenness, or constriction. Rewrap if necessary.
12. Assist the patient to a comfortable position.
13. Remove the bandage twice daily unless contraindicated. At this time, wash and dry the skin, assess alignment and circulation, and check for signs of irritation and tenderness.

PATIENT AND/OR FAMILY TEACHING
1. Explain the purpose for the elastic roller bandage.
2. Explain activity restrictions.
3. Reinforce and clarify the physician's explanation of the disease process, surgery, or injury.
4. Teach the patient to assess capillary return in the nail beds by applying pressure and releasing.

5. Instruct the patient to inform the nurse of any signs of impaired circulation: numbness, tingling, cyanosis, or swelling.
6. Teach the patient to apply the elastic roller bandage if it is to be used at home.

DOCUMENTATION
1. Size of bandage, location, and method of wrapping used.
2. Any observations and the patient's response.
3. All patient teaching done and the patient's level of understanding.

 ## Restraints

PURPOSE
1. Maximize patient safety and minimize patient injury.
2. Prevent the patient from injuring others.

REQUISITES
1. Restraints
2. Washcloths, if appropriate

GUIDELINES
1. The use of restraints generally requires a physician's order.
2. Selection of the type of restraint should be based on using the minimum restraint possible to protect the patient and/or staff.
3. A patient should be restrained only after all other methods of control have failed.
4. Vest, waist, and wrist restraints should always be secured to the upper portion of the bedframe so that the head of the bed may be elevated without pulling on the restraints. Do not attach restraints to the siderails.

5. When a patient becomes confused or disoriented with no prior history, a careful assessment should be done to determine possible causes. Consideration should be given to recent medication changes, physical condition, and psychological stress.
6. It is important to select the proper size restraints for the patient to avoid skin irritation or impaired circulation. Padding leather wrist and ankle restraints with a clean washcloth will prevent unnecessary skin irritation.
7. Restraints should be removed as frequently as possible, including all times when nursing staff is present or when family members are available to observe the patient.
8. Restraints should never replace frequent, careful observations.
9. Frequent position changes are necessary for patients in wrist and ankle restraints to prevent the complications of inactivity.
10. If only one wrist and one ankle are restrained, the restraints must be placed on opposite extremities.

NURSING ACTION/RATIONALE

1. Assemble all equipment.
2. Identify the patient.
3. Explain the procedure to the patient, including why the restraints are being applied.
4. Assist the patient to a comfortable position, in good body alignment for restraint application.
5. Apply the type of restraint ordered.

Vest Restraint

a. Assist the patient into the vest restraint with the opening in the front.
b. Cross the straps in the front and secure the straps to the upper portion of the bedframe or around the back of a chair (Figure 1-44).

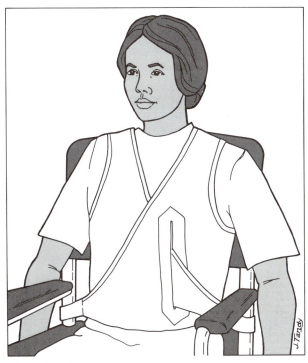

Figure 1-44. Vest restraint.

Waist Restraint

a. Assist the patient into the waist restraint with the opening in the back.
b. Cross the ties, placing one through the opening of the other, and secure the straps to the upper portion of the bedframe or around the back of a chair (Figure 1-45).

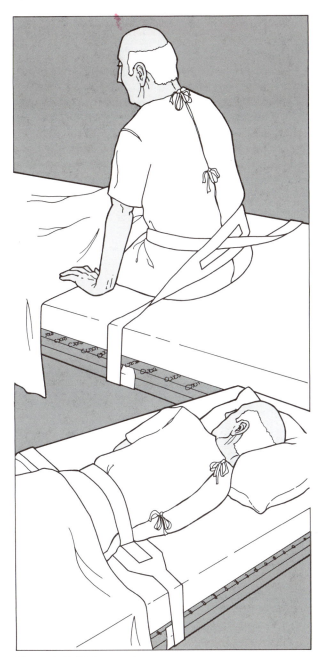

Figure 1-45. Waist restraint.

Wrist and Ankle Restraints: Cloth

a. Apply the cloth wrist or ankle restraints around the extremity.

b. Thread one tie through the opening in the other or secure with a square knot. The restraints should be applied firmly but not too tightly.

c. Fasten the ties of wrist restraints to the bedframe below elbow level. Fasten the ties of ankle restraints to the bedframe below knee level (Figure 1-46).

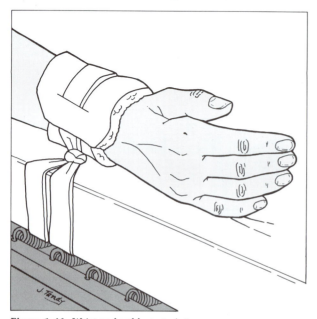

Figure 1-46. Wrist and ankle restraints.

Wrist and Ankle Restraints: Leather

a. Apply the leather wrist or ankle restraints according to manufacturer's instructions. Do not apply too tightly. Place a washcloth under each restraint for additional comfort if appropriate.

b. Fasten the straps to the bedframe and lock in place.

c. Identify the location of the key on the nursing care plan.

6. Raise the siderails and adjust the bed to the low position to further protect the patient.

7. Place the call signal within the patient's reach.

8. Assess the patient frequently for orientation status and skin condition in restraint areas. Evaluate the need for continued use of restraints.

9. Assist the patient with all activities of daily living as appropriate. Offer fluids frequently unless contraindicated.

PATIENT AND/OR FAMILY TEACHING

1. Explain the procedure to the patient and the family. Explain that the restraints are for the patient's protection or for the safety of others.

2. When appropriate, demonstrate removing and reapplying the restraints to the family so they may remove them while they supervise the patient.

3. Encourage the family to assist in reorienting the patient, if appropriate.

DOCUMENTATION

1. Time of application and type of restraints applied.

2. Location of the restraints.

3. Reason for applying the restraints.

4. The patient's reaction to the procedure.

5. Location of the key, if appropriate.

6. Any pertinent assessment parameters such as orientation status, behavior, and skin condition in the restraint areas.

7. All patient and/or family teaching done and the level of understanding.

Sitz Bath

PURPOSE
1. Promote comfort and healing in the perineal area.

REQUISITES
1. Sitz chair, tub, or disposable sitz bath
2. Solution thermometer
3. Bath towels—2
4. Bath blanket
5. Clean gown
6. Perineal dressing, if appropriate
7. Waste receptacle

GUIDELINES
1. A physician's order should be obtained prior to administering a sitz bath.
2. Sitz baths may be given by placing the patient in a sitz chair, a bathtub, or a disposable sitz bath (Figure 1-47).

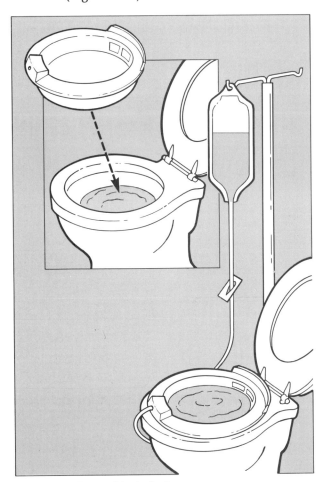

Figure 1-47. Disposable sitz bath.

3. If the patient is in isolation, a disposable sitz bath should be prepared for use in the patient's room.
4. Sitz bath water temperature should be 40.5 to 46°C (105 to 115°F) unless otherwise specified. The treatment usually lasts 15 to 20 minutes.

NURSING ACTION/RATIONALE
1. Assemble all equipment.
2. Verify the physician's order.
3. Identify the patient.
4. Explain the procedure to the patient.
5. Wash your hands.
6. Assist the patient to the sitz chair or tub.
7. Fill the sitz bath with warm water. Assess the water temperature with a solution thermometer.
8. Provide privacy.
9. Assist the patient into a hospital gown. Remove any perineal dressings and place them in the waste receptacle.
10. Place a towel on the back and bottom of the sitz chair if a portable sitz chair is used. Place a towel in the bottom of a tub or disposable sitz bath.
11. Assist the patient into the sitz chair or tub. Stabilize the portable sitz chair.
12. Cover the patient's shoulders with a bath blanket to provide warmth.
13. Place a call signal within the patient's reach.
14. Instruct the patient regarding the length of the sitz bath.
15. Reassess the patient at least once during the sitz bath. Remain with the patient if he or she complains of weakness.
16. Assist the patient out of the bath. Dry the perineal area if assistance is necessary. Assess the perineal area and replace any dressings if appropriate.
17. Assist the patient into a dry gown and back to bed.
18. Clean all equipment and return to the appropriate location. Discard the soiled linen and dressings in the appropriate area.

PATIENT AND/OR FAMILY TEACHING

1. Explain the procedure and its purpose.
2. Instruct the patient to notify the nurse if assistance is required during the bath.
3. Reinforce and clarify the physician's explanation of the disease process.
4. Instruct the patient and/or family regarding performing the procedure at home if prescribed following discharge.

DOCUMENTATION

1. Time and duration of the procedure.
2. The patient's reaction to the procedure.
3. Any assessment parameters including the condition of the perineum.
4. Any patient teaching done and the patient's level of understanding.

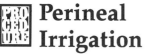 Perineal Irrigation

PURPOSE

1. Cleanse the perineum.

REQUISITES

1. Peribottle or disposable container
2. Warm water 38.0 to 40.5°C (100 to 105°F)
3. Toilet tissue
4. Bedpan (if the patient is on bedrest)
5. Exam gloves
6. Waste receptacle

GUIDELINES

1. Unless contraindicated, perineal care should be given to all patients following vaginal or rectal surgery, obstetrical patients, patients with vaginal infections, and female patients on bedrest, after voiding.
2. Consult with the physician prior to performing this procedure on any postoperative patient who has an unhealed perineal incision. A sterile container, sterile solution, and sterile cotton balls may be indicated to replace the requisites listed.

NURSING ACTION/RATIONALE

1. Assemble equipment.
2. Identify the patient.
3. Explain the procedure and purpose to the patient.
4. Provide privacy.
5. Remove peri-pad or perineal dressings and discard appropriately.

6. Assist the patient to a dorsal-recumbent position on the bedpan with legs separated. Drape the patient with a blanket (Figure 1-48). Ambulatory patients can sit on the toilet, leaning back with legs separated.

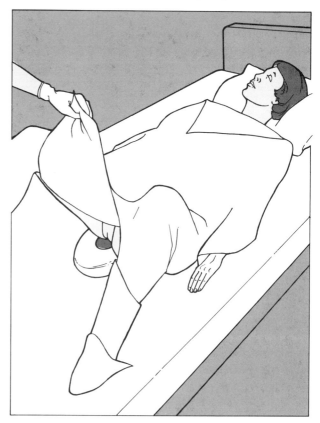

Figure 1-48. Position on bedpan for perineal irrigation.

7. Wash your hands.
8. Apply exam gloves.
9. Fill the peribottle or disposable container with warm water.
10. Pour the water over the perineum. Water should flow from the genitalia to the rectum.
11. Dry the perineum with toilet tissue, using gentle downward strokes. Discard tissue after each wipe.
12. Assess the perineum for signs of healing, drainage, or inflammation.
13. Remove the bedpan and apply a clean peri-pad or dressings as appropriate.
14. Remove gloves.
15. Assist the patient to a comfortable position.
16. Discard equipment or return to the appropriate area, as indicated.

PATIENT AND/OR FAMILY TEACHING
1. Explain the procedure and rationale to the patient before starting.
2. Instruct the patient in the steps for performing the procedure, if the patient's condition warrants self-care. A satisfactory return demonstration is evidence of the patient's understanding.

DOCUMENTATION
1. Procedure performed.
2. Assessment of the perineum as indicated.
3. All patient teaching done and the patient's level of understanding.

 # Hot Water Bottle

PURPOSE
1. Relieve pain, muscle spasm, inflammation, or congestion.
2. Provide warmth.

REQUISITES
1. Hot water bottle
2. Solution thermometer
3. Cloth covering

GUIDELINES
1. Hot water bottle temperatures for adults should range from 46 to 51.5°C (115 to 125°F).
2. Hot water bottle temperatures may have to be adjusted and must be used carefully for patients with a circulatory impairment or a decreased level of consciousness.
3. Never use a hot water bottle on an unconscious patient or on a paralyzed area of the body.

NURSING ACTION/RATIONALE
1. Assemble all equipment.
2. Test the hot water bottle for leaks.
3. Preheat the bottle by filling it with hot water, fastening the top, and inverting it several times, then emptying.
4. Adjust the tap water to the desired temperature by assessing with a thermometer.
5. Fill the hot water bottle one-third to one-half full and expel all air to assure flexibility.
6. Fasten the top of the hot water bottle securely and dry the bottle.
7. Insert the hot water bottle into the cloth cover.
8. Identify the patient.
9. Explain the procedure to the patient.
10. Apply the hot water bottle to the affected area.
11. Assess the patient frequently for signs of skin redness or discomfort.
12. Remove the hot water bottle after 20 minutes. Reapply after refilling as required.
13. Return all equipment to the appropriate area.

PATIENT AND/OR FAMILY TEACHING
1. Instruct the patient to notify the nurse if any sensation of burning or numbness occurs or if the hot water bottle becomes cool.
2. Explain to the patient and visitors that only nursing personnel are to refill the bottles.

DOCUMENTATION
1. Time, temperature, and area of application.
2. All patient assessments including condition of the area of application, if appropriate.
3. All patient teaching done and the patient's level of understanding.

Circulating Water Pad

PURPOSE
1. Apply heat or cold locally for therapeutic effect.

REQUISITES
1. Circulating water pad in appropriate size (Figure 1-49)
2. Distilled water
3. Protective cover

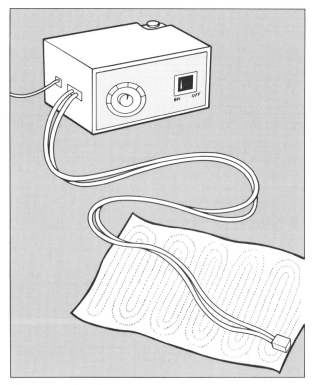

Figure 1-49. Circulating water pad.

GUIDELINES
1. Select the size pad to cover only the area being treated.
2. The circulating water pad and hose should be used at a level below that of its motor to reduce the workload of the motor.
3. Do not secure the pad with pins, which could puncture the pad and cause leakage.
4. If the hose or pad becomes kinked it will not function properly.
5. As with any electrical device, safety precautions must be taken.
6. The affected area must be assessed carefully for signs of hyper- or hypothermia.
7. If oxygen is in use, keep the motor at least 3 feet away from the direct flow of the oxygen.
8. Do not apply the circulating water pad over elastic bandages, surgical hose, or in any area where circulation is impaired, unless specifically ordered.

NURSING ACTION/RATIONALE
1. Assemble all equipment according to manufacturer's directions.
2. Fill the machine unit with distilled water to the indicated level.
3. Tilt the unit from side to side to allow any air bubbles to escape. An air lock would put stress on the motor.
4. Connect the hoses from the pad to the machine unit. Fasten securely to avoid leakage.
5. Set the desired temperature.
6. Identify the patient.

7. Explain the treatment to the patient.
8. Provide privacy.
9. Wash your hands.
10. Position the patient so that the affected area is accessible.
11. Turn the machine unit on.
12. Cover the pad with a protective cover and place on or around the affected area. Secure loosely with ties to prevent restriction of water circulation through the pad.
13. Assist the patient to a comfortable position.
14. Continue heat or cold therapy as prescribed.
15. Check the water level and add additional water as needed.
16. Inspect the affected area frequently for untoward reactions to heat or cold.
17. Return all equipment to the appropriate area.

PATIENT AND/OR FAMILY TEACHING

1. Explain the purpose of the circulating water pad to the patient.
2. Instruct the patient not to change the location of the motor unit.
3. Instruct the patient to call the nurse if the affected area becomes uncomfortable.
4. Reinforce and clarify the physician's explanation of the disease process.
5. Explain any additional therapeutic orders.

DOCUMENTATION

1. Temperature of the unit when treatment was initiated.
2. Time that treatment was initiated and discontinued.
3. Observations of affected area and any therapeutic effect.
4. Patient's reaction to the procedure.
5. All patient teaching done and the patient's level of understanding.

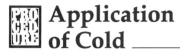

Application of Cold

PURPOSE
1. Apply a hypothermic agent to the body for therapeutic purposes.

REQUISITES
1. Ice bag, ice collar, ice glove, or disposable ice pack
2. Protective covering
3. Ice, if appropriate
4. Patient thermometer

GUIDELINES
1. A physician's order may be required for the application of cold. Refer to your health care facility's policy.
2. Cold therapy is used to relieve pain and/or inflammation, prevent edema, reduce body temperature, and control bleeding by promoting vasoconstriction.
3. An exam glove filled with ice is often used to apply cold to small areas of the body. The flexible glove conforms to the shape of the body as the ice melts.
4. When using disposable ice packs, follow the manufacturer's specific instructions for use.
5. For patients in isolation, use disposable ice packs whenever possible.
6. Cold therapy should not be applied to an already edematous area since the vasoconstricting effect retards the reabsorption of fluid.
7. Cold therapy should be discontinued if pain and edema increase, sensation decreases, mottling occurs, or extreme redness of the skin appears.
8. For best results, cold packs should be left in place for 1 hour, then removed for a period of time to allow the tissue to warm.

NURSING ACTION/RATIONALE
1. Assemble all equipment.
2. Wash your hands.
3. Fill the ice bag, glove, or collar with ice chips according to the patient's needs.
4. Expel the air and fasten the top securely.
5. Dry the outside and test it for leaks.
6. Insert it into a protective cover.
7. Explain the procedure to the patient.
8. Provide privacy.
9. Expose the area to be treated and position the patient, if necessary.
10. Apply the cold packs to the area. Tie loosely in place, if necessary.
11. Assess the skin condition every 20 minutes for blanching, pain, and numbness. Assess the patient's temperature, if appropriate.
12. Remove the cold packs when the treatment is completed.
13. Assess the skin condition in the treated area. Assess the patient's temperature, if appropriate.
14. Assist the patient to a comfortable position.
15. Discard equipment or return it to the appropriate location, as applicable.

PATIENT AND/OR FAMILY TEACHING
1. Explain the procedure and its purpose to the patient.
2. Instruct the patient to notify the nurse if any pain or numbness is experienced.
3. Instruct the patient and family that only the nursing staff is to apply the ice.

DOCUMENTATION
1. Time and type of application.
2. All assessment parameters including the effectiveness of the treatment, the patient's temperature, any reactions, and action taken.
3. Time of removal.
4. All patient teaching done and the patient's level of understanding.

Warm or Cold Soaks

PURPOSE

1. Relieve pain, inflammation, and congestion.
2. Localize infection.
3. Increase drainage.
4. Facilitate debridement.
5. Relax muscles, tendons, and ligaments.

REQUISITES

1. Basin
2. Bath blanket
3. Bath towels—2
4. Solution as prescribed
5. Solution thermometer
6. Dressing, if indicated

GUIDELINES

1. Unless specifically ordered, solution for a warm soak should be 40.5 to 43°C (105 to 110°F) and solution for a cold soak should be 15°C (59°F). An incorrect temperature could burn or chill the patient.
2. When an open wound is to be soaked, sterile technique should be employed. However, if a large area of the body is to be soaked, a compromise may be necessary. When following sterile technique, all requisites listed should be sterile.

NURSING ACTION/RATIONALE

1. Assemble all equipment.
2. Identify the patient.
3. Explain the procedure to the patient.
4. Dress the patient in a hospital gown if there is a possibility of wetting clothing during the soak.
5. Position the patient comfortably in bed or in a chair if appropriate.
6. Provide privacy.
7. Wash your hands.
8. Fill the basin with the prescribed solution heated or cooled to the appropriate temperature.
9. Remove any dressings. If the dressing adheres, allow it to loosen in the soak.

10. Place waterproof material under the basin. Place the affected part in the basin in a comfortable position and in proper body alignment. Place a folded bath towel over the edge of the basin for comfort.
11. Cover the basin with a bath blanket to retain the temperature.
12. Remove the affected part from the basin when adding warming or cooling solution during the treatment. If the original solution contains medication, do not dilute.
13. Continue the soak for 15 to 20 minutes or the prescribed time.
14. Remove the affected part from the solution. Place it on a towel and pat dry. If aseptic technique is necessary, use a sterile towel.
15. Apply a dressing if indicated.
16. Assist the patient to a comfortable position.
17. Discard equipment and linen or return to the appropriate area.

PATIENT AND/OR FAMILY TEACHING

1. Explain the procedure and its purpose to the patient.
2. Instruct the patient to call the nurse if any discomfort occurs from positioning or water temperature during the treatment.
3. Reinforce and clarify the physician's explanation of the disease process.
4. Explain any additional therapy that has been ordered.
5. Explain any activity restrictions.
6. Instruct the patient regarding continuing the soaks at home, if ordered.

DOCUMENTATION

1. Type of solution, solution temperature, and duration of the soak.
2. Any observations and the patient's reaction.
3. All patient teaching done and the patient's level of understanding.

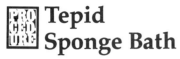 **Tepid
Sponge Bath** _____

PURPOSE
1. Reduce a fever by inducing hypothermia.

REQUISITES
1. Hot water bottle with cover
2. Ice bags with covers—4
3. Washbasin
4. Bath blanket
5. Washcloths—5
6. Bath towels—2
7. Solution thermometer
8. 70% isopropyl alcohol
9. Bed protector

GUIDELINES
1. Tepid sponge bath utilizes the principle of evaporation to increase heat loss through the skin, thus reducing the body's temperature.
2. Alcohol, added to water, evaporates more rapidly than water alone, since alcohol evaporates at a lower temperature than water.
3. If any evidence of shock or chilling occurs during the procedure, discontinue the treatment, apply blankets, and notify the physician.
4. Establish adequate air circulation in the room to prevent vomiting that may occur from inhalation of alcohol vapors.
5. Alcohol sponge baths should not be used for infants or small children.

NURSING ACTION/RATIONALE
1. Assemble all equipment.
2. Identify the patient.
3. Explain the procedure to the patient.
4. Wash your hands.
5. Fill the hot water bottle with 49°C (120°F) water. Fill four ice bags.
6. Prepare basin of solution. If alcohol sponge bath is desired, use equal parts of water and 70% isopropyl alcohol.

7. Test the temperature of the solution with a solution thermometer. Tepid water ranges from 20 to 28°C (68 to 82.4°F). Change temperature gradually to prevent chilling and shock. This can be done by adding ice chips to the water during the procedure.
8. Provide privacy and protect the bed linen with a bed protector.
9. Assess the patient's temperature and other vital signs before the treatment and frequently during the procedure.
10. Remove the patient's gown; position the patient supine; fanfold covers and replace with a bath blanket. Expose as much skin surface as possible to increase the cooling effect from evaporation.
11. Apply a cloth-covered ice bag to the patient's head, axillae, and groin areas.
12. Apply a hot water bottle to the patient's feet to make the patient feel more comfortable and reduce the chance of shivering.
13. Wring out two washcloths and place one under each popliteal area.
14. Use remaining washcloths to sponge anterior chest and both arms, using long, even strokes. Continue sponging for 5 minutes. Leave areas exposed to permit evaporation.
15. Sponge the lower extremities. Continue sponging for 5 minutes. Leave areas exposed.
16. Turn the patient and sponge the back for 5 minutes.
17. Remove the ice bag and hot water bottle. Pat the patient dry; avoid rubbing, which may increase the temperature.
18. Replace the patient's gown. Return the patient to a comfortable position.
19. Assess the patient's temperature and other vital signs and the patient's color. Repeat vital sign checks 30 minutes after the treatment or as ordered.
20. Discard equipment and linen or return to the appropriate area.

PATIENT AND/OR FAMILY TEACHING

1. Explain the procedure to the patient before initiating treatment.
2. Instruct the patient to notify the nurse during the procedure if shivering occurs.
3. Explain aspects of thermoregulation.
4. Reinforce the physician's explanation of the disease process.
5. Explain additional therapy, including prescribed medications.

DOCUMENTATION

1. Time and duration of treatment and solution used.
2. Vital signs before, during, and after treatment.
3. Any observations and effects of treatment.
4. All patient teaching done and the patient's level of understanding.

Preoperative Care

PURPOSE

1. Prepare a patient physically and emotionally for surgery.

REQUISITES

1. Hospital gown
2. Tape—1 inch
3. Blood pressure cuff
4. Stethoscope
5. Thermometer
6. Scale
7. Preoperative assessment record
8. Nail polish remover (optional)
9. Denture cup (optional)

GUIDELINES

1. Reports and forms that should be completed and placed on the patient's chart prior to surgery include a physician's history and physical, all routine and ordered lab work, x-rays (if ordered), electrocardiogram (if ordered), and appropriate surgical consent forms.
2. Health care facility policies dictate the specific diagnostic tests that need to be completed prior to a patient's undergoing surgery. The policies should specify how current the diagnostic test results must be. Refer to your hospital's policy manual.
3. Physician's orders should dictate specific preoperative preparation that may be necessary for individual surgical cases.
4. The physician should be notified the night before surgery, or as soon as possible, if any abnormalities are assessed in test results, lab values, vital signs, or other patient assessment parameters.
5. The requirement for a signed consent form for invasive procedures varies among health care facilities. Refer to your hospital's policy manual.
6. The patient should be wearing a clearly imprinted identification band including the patient's name and hospital number before being transferred to surgery.
7. Valuables should be given to a relative or locked in the hospital safe. Disposition of valuables should be documented in the patient's chart.
8. Food and fluids should be withheld after midnight for patients receiving general anesthesia unless otherwise prescribed.
9. A preoperative assessment form that includes parameters of assessment required for the preoperative patient is a helpful tool in preparing the patient and documenting the preparation (Figure 1-50).

PREOPERATIVE ASSESSMENT RECORD

Allergies: _____   Date _____

	YES	NO	NA		VITAL SIGNS	
				B.P.	Temp.	Weight
Addressograph Card on Chart	☐	☐		Pulse	Resp.	
Surgical Permit signed	☐	☐				
Special Permits/Releases signed	☐	☐	☐	Intravenous Started Yes ☐ No ☐		
History & Physical: On Chart	☐	☐		Type of needle _____		
Dictated	☐	☐		Size of needle _____		
Consultation	☐	☐	☐	Solution _____		
Diagnostic Tests Completed						
Chest X-ray	☐	☐	☐	Time of Last Voiding:		
EKG	☐	☐	☐			
Other____	☐	☐	☐	Time of Last Food - Fluids:		
Clean/Bathed & Proper Attire	☐	☐		Date of Latest Lab Reports		
Oral Hygiene	☐	☐		CBC _____		
Identification Bracelet	☐	☐		Urine _____		
Glasses-Contacts Removed	☐	☐		ESP _____		
Dentures-Dental Appliances:				Other _____		
Removed	☐	☐	☐			
Type Left in Place ____				Comments, Abnormal or Significant Findings:		
Other Prothesis Removed	☐	☐	☐			
Type ____						
Wedding Ring: Removed	☐	☐	☐			
Secured	☐	☐	☐			
Other Jewelry Removed	☐	☐	☐			
Lipstick & Nailpolish Removed	☐	☐	☐	Persons Waiting: Yes ☐ No ☐		
Hairpins, Wigs, Hairpieces				Relationship _____		
Removed	☐	☐	☐	In Family Room Yes ☐ No ☐		
Gum-Candy Removed from Mouth	☐	☐	☐			
Pre-op Medication Recorded	☐	☐	☐	Other _____		

CHART SIGNED OUT AND PATIENT IDENTIFIED BY:

ST. LUKE'S HOSPITAL, RACINE, WISCONSIN   0817 610817

Figure 1-50. Sample preoperative assessment record.

NURSING ACTION/RATIONALE

1. Identify the patient. Apply an identification band if not in place.
2. Assess the patient's knowledge of the operation. Ensure that the consent form is signed and completed according to hospital policy.
3. Explain the preoperative preparation procedure. Answer any questions and provide emotional support as necessary.
4. Wash your hands.
5. Assess all vital signs.
6. Weigh the patient.
7. Assist the patient as necessary with bathing and oral hygiene.
8. Assist the patient into a hospital gown. No other clothing should be worn.
9. Remove hairpins, hairpieces, and hair ornaments, if appropriate.
10. Remove nail polish, lipstick, and facial makeup, if appropriate, so that an accurate assessment of the patient can be made during and after surgery.
11. Remove jewelry, if appropriate. Rings and newly pierced earrings may usually be taped with paper tape. Bandaids are recommended for rings with stones to avoid loosening or pulling out the stone during removal. Refer to your hospital's policy manual.
12. Remove all prostheses and contact lenses. If the patient has a permanent prosthesis, document it on the preoperative assessment record and the nurse's notes.
13. Instruct the patient to void.
14. Administer the preoperative medication as ordered. Explain the anticipated effects of the drug.
15. Instruct the patient to remain in bed. Raise both siderails.
16. Place the call signal within reach. Remove all smoking materials from the area, if appropriate.
17. Allow the family to quietly wait with the patient, if appropriate.
18. Complete the preoperative assessment record and prepare the chart according to your health care facility's policy.
19. Assist surgery personnel with identification of the patient. Verify identification with the patient's identification band and the patient's chart.
20. Release the patient and chart to surgery personnel according to your health care facility's policy.
21. Explain surgical protocol to the family, including the approximate length of time in surgery and in the post anesthesia room.
22. Provide an escort for the family members to the family waiting area.

PATIENT AND/OR FAMILY TEACHING

1. Instruct the patient on deep breathing, coughing, and therapeutic exercises that will need to be done postoperatively. Do this as early as possible preoperatively, so the patient has time to practice.
2. Explain the preoperative preparation procedure to the patient and family, and reinstruct and reinforce throughout the procedure as described in "Nursing Action/Rationale."

3. Reinforce the physician's explanation of the problem requiring surgical intervention.
4. Explain to the patient and/or family the approximate length of the surgery and the approximate length of time in the post anesthesia area.
5. Explain any special postoperative-unit visiting restrictions, if appropriate.
6. Explain postoperative treatments to the patient and/or family as appropriate, including the use of oxygen, monitoring equipment, special drainage tubes, incisional dressings, and intravenous therapy.

DOCUMENTATION
1. All parameters of assessment as outlined on the hospital's preoperative assessment record.
2. Notification of the physician regarding any abnormalities in the assessment parameters.

3. All preoperative procedures performed.
4. All types, amounts, and dosages of medications administered and the patient's response to the medication.
5. Assessment of the patient's psychological and emotional response to the impending surgery.
6. All preoperative teaching done and the patient's level of understanding.

 # Postoperative Care

PURPOSE
1. Provide a safe, supportive environment during the postanesthesia period.
2. Prevent postoperative complications.
3. Identify postoperative complications.

REQUISITES
1. Blood pressure cuff
2. Stethoscope
3. Thermometer
4. Emesis basin
5. IV standard
6. Oxygen equipment, available
7. Oral suction equipment, available
8. Other equipment individualized for each patient

GUIDELINES
1. An initial assessment of the patient following transfer from the recovery room is important in providing baseline data upon which to compare the patient's progress or deterioration during the recovery period.
2. The recovery time from the anesthesia depends on the agent used, the amount of anesthesia used, and the patient's individual rate of metabolism.

3. General areas for assessment that apply to all patients who have received anesthesia are:
   a. Respiratory status.
   b. Neurological status.
   c. Cardiovascular function.
   d. Genitourinary function.
   e. Gastrointestinal function.
   f. Wound status.
   g. Comfort level.
4. Respiratory complications are the most common problem following general anesthesia. The patient should be assessed to assure that an adequate exchange of oxygen is occurring. The rate, rhythm, and depth of respirations along with auscultation of breath sounds and the patient's ability to deep breathe and cough should be assessed.
5. An ongoing assessment of the patient's level of consciousness and reflexes is an indicator of the remaining effects of the anesthesia on the neurological system. It is also a guide in determining when the patient can move from complete dependency to some independent functions.

6. An assessment of the circulatory status should include vital signs. An apical rather than a radial pulse should be taken, since cardiac arrhythmias can be more easily detected with an apical pulse. Peripheral circulation should be assessed, since cool extremities for a patient who is warm and flushed are an early indicator of impending shock with compensation.

7. Diuresis is affected by anesthesia and surgery. In addition, the normal sensations of a distended bladder may be dulled by anesthesia. An accurate intake and output record is an important tool in assessing fluid overload or urinary retention. Abdominal palpation will help to detect bladder distention.

8. General anesthesia, abdominal surgery, and narcotics decrease intestinal peristalsis. An assessment of bowel sounds will help to determine when the patient can have oral intake. The abdomen should be palpated for distention or tenderness which are early indicators of intra-abdominal hemorrhage or gastrointestinal dysfunction.

9. The incisional site should be assessed for drainage or bleeding. Any drains from the incision should be assessed for patency.

10. The patient's comfort level should be assessed along with any need for analgesics. An uncomfortable patient is likely to restrict activities, and resulting immobility could cause respiratory or cardiovascular complications.

11. All support equipment such as intravenous lines, drains, tubes, and irrigations should be assessed for patency and proper functioning.

12. The depth, frequency, and duration of assessments will depend on the condition of the patient, the type of surgery performed, and the patient's postoperative progress. Each type of surgery has specific risks, and the postoperative assessment should be individualized for each patient.

13. A flow sheet for documenting all assessment parameters will aid in identifying early abnormal responses and also provides a fast, easy reference of the patient's post anesthesia status.

NURSING ACTION/RATIONALE

1. Assemble all equipment in the patient's room before he or she arrives. A clean post anesthesia bed should be ready.

2. Receive report from the post anesthesia room nurse.

3. Identify the patient.

4. Wash your hands.

5. Assist in transferring the patient from the stretcher to the bed. Place the call signal within reach.

6. Orient the patient to person, place, and time.

7. Attach any equipment that may be necessary, such as oxygen or suction.

8. Obtain a baseline assessment of all assessment parameters as outlined in the guidelines.

9. Reassess the patient a minimum of every 15 minutes until stable, then every 30 minutes for 1 hour, every hour for 4 hours, then every 4 hours for 24 to 48 hours.

10. Instruct the patient and reinforce as necessary, regarding all areas described in "Patient and/or Family Teaching."

11. Assist the patient with coughing and deep breathing each time an assessment is performed.
   a. Position the patient in a sitting position or in a high Fowler's position, if possible.
   b. Splint any incision with your hands or a pillow, if necessary.
   c. Instruct the patient to take a deep breath, inhaling slowly, holding the breath for several seconds, and exhaling through the mouth. Repeat this twice.
   d. Instruct the patient to cough deeply and forcefully during the third exhalation.
   e. Repeat the procedure at least four times in succession and at least every 4 hours or more often if necessary.

12. Reposition the patient every 2 to 4 hours, or as necessary.

13. Increase activity as ordered by the physician.

14. Provide oral hygiene at least every 4 hours or more often if the patient has oxygen or a nasogastric tube.

15. Begin oral intake and diet based on the physician's orders and the patient's progress in the recovery period.
16. Maintain an accurate intake and output record.
17. Maintain safety factors, including siderails on the bed until the patient is completely awake and oriented.
18. Administer analgesics as ordered by the physician, based on an assessment of the patient's comfort level.
19. Interpret assessment data and notify the physician of any postoperative complications.

PATIENT AND/OR FAMILY TEACHING
1. Explain and reinforce frequently all areas of postoperative care and their importance, including:
   a. Frequency of assessments by the nurse.
   b. All equipment being used in the recovery period.
   c. Coughing and deep breathing exercises.
   d. Activity restrictions.
   e. Oral intake restrictions.
   f. Availability of analgesics.
   g. Specific procedures related to the patient's surgical condition.
   h. Visiting restrictions.
2. Instruct the patient to call the nurse for any problem.
3. Explain the anticipated course of treatment.

DOCUMENTATION
1. Time of the patient's transfer from the post anesthesia room.
2. All baseline and continuous assessment data.
3. All procedures performed.
4. All medications administered.
5. Any complications, interventions, and results.
6. An evaluation of the patient's progress.
7. Notification of the physician, if appropriate.
8. All patient teaching done and the patient's level of understanding.

Isolation Precaution Techniques

PURPOSE

1. Prevent or minimize the transmission of infection to employees, patients, and visitors.
2. Provide nursing care for the patient in an isolation precaution setting.

REQUISITES

1. Hospital information display card identifying the type of isolation precaution and an explanation of the precaution
2. Isolation supplies
   a. Gowns
   b. Caps
   c. Masks
   d. Exam gloves
   e. Plastic bags
   f. Antiseptic soap
   g. Isolation labels and/or marker

GUIDELINES

1. Knowing the chain of infection is an important principle in epidemiology. The three components of the chain are the germ, the link, and the host. Isolation precautions are implemented to break the chain and thus prevent infection.
2. Microorganisms may be transmitted to patients, visitors, and personnel by a variety of routes, including direct contact or indirect contact with contaminated inanimate objects, airborne droplets, and vectors such as mosquitos, fleas, or lice.
3. The parameters for infection control established by the Centers for Disease Control should serve as guidelines for hospitals. Individual hospitals must determine what procedures should be followed carefully and what procedures must be modified to meet the needs of their institutions. Refer to *Guidelines for the Prevention and Control of Nosocomial Infections* for a listing of infectious diseases requiring specific isolation precautions.

4. Isolation precaution is usually ordered by the physician but may be initiated by the responsible nurse when there is a suspicion of an infectious disease or any established diagnosis of infectibility. A physician's order for the isolation precaution should be obtained according to hospital policy.
5. Patients requiring isolation precautions should be placed in a private room if available. Precautionary isolation can be modified as circumstances require according to hospital policy.
6. Isolation precautions differ in degree and method. The form of isolation precaution is based on the communicable disease, its mode of transmission, and the susceptibility of the host. The following are suggested isolation precaution categories to control the transmission of microorganisms:
   a. *Blood/body fluid precaution* is necessary when there is a possibility that blood or body fluids are infected. All blood, blood products, and body fluids should be regarded as a potential source of infection transmission and handled accordingly.
   b. *Enteric precaution* is necessary to prevent the spread of infection that can be transmitted through direct or indirect contact with infected feces or articles contaminated with feces.
   c. *Drainage/secretion precaution* is necessary when the infectious diseases included in this category result in the production of infective purulent material, drainage, or secretions, unless the disease is included in another precautionary category that requires stricter precautions.
   d. *Respiratory isolation* is necessary to prevent the transmission of microorganisms by air or droplet from coughing, sneezing, or breathing.
   e. *Tuberculosis (AFB) isolation* is necessary for all patients with current pulmonary tuberculosis who have a positive sputum smear or a chest x-ray film appearance that strongly suggests current active tuberculosis. Laryngeal tuberculosis is included in this category of isolation.

f. *Strict isolation* is necessary to prevent the transmission of all highly communicable diseases that could be spread by multiple routes. A private room with special ventilation is indicated for strict isolation.

g. *Contact isolation* is necessary to prevent transmission of highly transmissible or epidemiologically important infections (or colonization) that do not warrant strict isolation. Included in this category are diseases spread by close or direct contact.

7. Patients in isolation precaution should have their own personal supplies. Personal belongings should be kept to a minimum. Use of disposable supplies and equipment is encouraged.

8. Visitors should be encouraged to come often, since patients in isolation precaution tend to become lonely and have feelings of being set apart from the other patients and the nursing staff.

9. Specimens should be collected in properly sealed and labeled plastic containers. The outside of the container should be cleaned with a disinfectant and placed in a clear plastic bag using the double-bagging technique. (Refer to the procedure "Double-Bagging Technique.") Mark the outer bag "Isolation."

10. Use preprinted bags marked "Isolation" for collecting isolation equipment and linen. Some hospitals use color-coded bags, but all bags used in isolation should be clearly identified.

11. Disposable needles and syringes should be used whenever possible while the patient is in isolation precaution. Syringes and needles should be disposed of without breaking or recapping the unit and placed in a puncture-resistant box. When filled, the disposable boxes should be sealed with tape and labeled for incineration or steam sterilization and grinding according to hospital policy.

12. Isolation precaution signs are available and should be posted in a prominent location outside the patient's room. The sign should indicate the type of isolation precaution as well as the type of preparation necessary prior to entering the room.

13. Refer to the procedures "Non-Sterile Gloving Technique," "Gowning Technique," "Masking Technique," "Double-Bagging Technique," and "Handwashing Technique" for additional isolation precaution techniques.

NURSING ACTION/RATIONALE
Entering the Room

1. Verify the type of isolation precaution.
2. Remove your watch and rings. Roll your sleeves to the elbow, if appropriate.
3. Assemble all equipment, making sure that you have everything you will need to provide care.
4. Wash your hands.
5. Put on a gown and other appropriate barriers as required, including a mask and non-sterile gloves. Refer to the procedures "Gowning Technique," "Masking Technique," and "Non-Sterile Gloving Technique."
6. Enter the room with all necessary supplies.
7. Explain the isolation precaution to the patient, including any patient participation if appropriate.
8. Provide patient care.
9. Assist the patient to a comfortable position.

Leaving the Room

1. Bag all linen and equipment to be removed from the room in appropriate isolation bags.
2. Place isolation bags inside a second, cuffed bag being held outside the room by an assistant. Take care not to contaminate the outside of the second bag. Refer to "Double-Bagging Technique."
3. Instruct your assistant to carefully fold and tie the top of the bag.
4. Remove the gloves. Refer to "Non-Sterile Gloving Technique."
5. Wash your hands.

6. Remove your mask, touching only the ties, and discard in the appropriate receptacle. Refer to "Masking Technique."
7. Wash your hands.
8. Untie your gown, remove it, and discard it in the appropriate receptacle. Refer to "Gowning Technique."
9. Wash your hands. Refer to "Handwashing Technique."
10. Leave the room, using paper toweling as a barrier for door handles.
11. Wash your hands outside the room.
12. Mark all isolation bags.
13. Discard all isolation bags in the appropriate receptacle.
14. Restock isolation precaution supplies, if necessary.

PATIENT AND/OR FAMILY TEACHING

1. Explain the purpose of isolation precautions to the patient and family.
2. Instruct visitors regarding:
   a. The type of isolation and all necessary barriers required prior to entering the room.
   b. Articles that may be taken into the isolation room.
   c. The procedure for leaving the room.
3. Explain all the precautions necessary for infection control including:
   a. Handwashing.
   b. Waste receptacles.
   c. Personal hygiene.
   d. Visitor rules.
   e. Handling secretions.
4. Explain other therapeutic measures.
5. Instruct the patient to notify the nurse if experiencing any anxiety concerning the isolation precaution.

DOCUMENTATION

1. Type of isolation precaution.
2. Patient's reaction to isolation precaution.
3. Any nursing assessments made.
4. All patient and family teaching and the level of understanding.

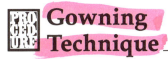

Gowning Technique

PURPOSE
1. Offer a protection barrier to reduce or minimize infectious transmission on clothing.

REQUISITES
1. Cloth or disposable long-sleeved, full-length gown

GUIDELINES
1. Each person should put on a fresh, clean gown every time an isolation room is entered.
2. A gown should be worn only once and discarded in the appropriate receptacle inside the patient's room.
3. The gown should be worn during direct patient care and during indirect contact with items contaminated by excretions or secretions.
4. Do not contaminate your hands by touching the contaminated side of the gown. If this occurs, you must rewash your hands.
5. Uniforms with long sleeves should be rolled up to the elbows prior to gowning.

NURSING ACTION/RATIONALE
Putting on the Gown
1. Wash your hands.
2. Select a gown.
3. Unfold the gown with the opening facing you.
4. Grasp the inside of the gown and slide the gown over your hands and arms. Hold your arms forward and slightly upward (Figure 1-51).

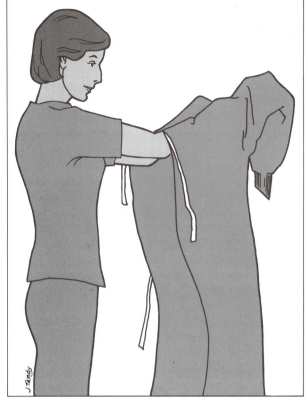

Figure 1-51. Putting on the gown.

5. Adjust the cuffs.
6. Position the gown around your neck and fasten the ties at the neck.
7. Grasp the gown at the waistline in the back, overlapping the edges of the gown as much as possible.
8. Fasten the ties at the waist that have been pulled to the back.

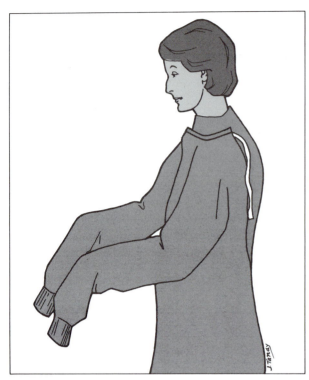

Figure 1-52. Removing the gown.

Removing the Gown

1. Untie the waist tie.
2. Wash your hands.
3. Untie the neck tie.
4. Grasp the neck fastener or the inside of the gown at the shoulder area. Bring the neck of the gown forward and draw it over your arms and hands (Figure 1-52).
5. Hold your arms away from your body and fold the gown so that the contaminated outside of the gown is folded inward and rolled into a bundle.
6. Discard the gown in the appropriate receptacle in the patient's room.
7. Wash your hands.
8. Leave the room.
9. Rewash your hands.

PATIENT AND/OR FAMILY TEACHING

1. Explain that the gowning precaution is being carried out to prevent the transmission of infectious agents.
2. Demonstrate to visitors how to put on and how to remove the gown properly. Provide the opportunity for a return demonstration.
3. Demonstrate to the patient's visitors the appropriate handwashing technique.
4. Instruct the patient's visitors regarding the appropriate disposal of gowns.

DOCUMENTATION

1. All patient and family teaching done and the level of understanding.

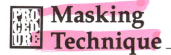 **Masking Technique**

PURPOSE

1. Prevent or minimize the transmission of infection, protecting both the nurse and the patient.

REQUISITES

1. Disposable or cloth face mask.

GUIDELINES

1. When the face mask becomes moist, it becomes ineffective; a new one should be applied.
2. Use a mask only once, since it is considered contaminated and should not be lowered and draped around the neck.
3. The mask should cover the mouth and nose and fit closely.
4. When indicated on the infection precaution display card, the mask must be worn by all persons entering the room. The mask should be put on before entering the room and taken off and discarded before leaving the room.

NURSING ACTION/RATIONALE

Putting on the Mask

1. Wash your hands.
2. Place the mask over your mouth and nose.
3. Fasten both sets of ties securely (Figure 1-53).

Removing the Mask

1. Wash your hands.
2. Untie the mask.
3. Discard the mask in the appropriate receptacle in the patient's room, touching only the ties.
4. Wash your hands.
5. Leave the room.
6. Rewash your hands.

PATIENT AND/OR FAMILY TEACHING

1. Explain that the masking precaution is being taken to protect the patient or personnel from infectious agents that can be transmitted as aerosols or droplets.
2. Demonstrate to visitors how to put on and how to remove the mask properly. Provide for a return demonstration.
3. Demonstrate to visitors the appropriate handwashing technique.
4. Instruct the patient's visitors regarding the appropriate disposal of the mask.

DOCUMENTATION

1. All patient and family teaching done and the level of understanding.

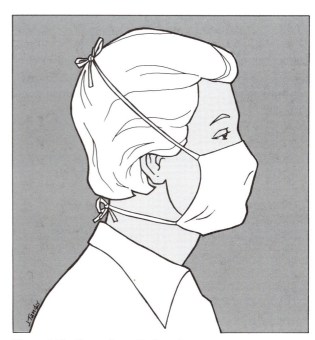

Figure 1-53. Correctly applied mask.

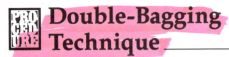

Double-Bagging Technique

PURPOSE
1. Prevent the transmission of infection.
2. Remove contaminated articles and/or linens from the room of a patient in isolation precaution.

REQUISITES
1. Clear plastic bags
2. Plastic, labeled equipment-isolation bags
3. Water-soluble linen bags
4. Identification marker

GUIDELINES
1. Double-bagging technique is used for packaging non-disposable or disposable contaminated articles that are removed from an isolation room such as:
   a. Waste
   b. Linens
   c. Reusable supplies
   d. Laboratory specimens
   e. Patient's personal items
2. All isolation precaution bags must be correctly identified.
3. Reusable supplies such as instruments and basins must be rinsed to remove all gross contamination before bagging and double-bagging.
4. Labeled plastic bags for contaminated items have been specially manufactured to withstand steam and gas sterilization for processing patient care equipment and reusable supplies.
5. Double-bagging is done in the doorway of the patient's room prior to removing the bag from the room.
6. Prevent any wet linens from dissolving the water-soluble bag by wrapping all wet linen in dry, used linens.
7. Have a supply of each type of plastic bag readily available outside the isolation room.

NURSING ACTION/RATIONALE
1. Take the bags used for discarding specific items into the isolation precaution room.
2. Fill all bags and tie them securely.
3. Place the contaminated bag carefully into a second, cuffed bag held outside the room door by an assistant (Figure 1-54).
4. Instruct your assistant to fold the bag cuff up and to tie the outer bag securely.
5. Remove any protective isolation barriers and wash your hands.
6. Label the isolation bags with proper identification.
7. Place each bag in the appropriate area.
8. Wash your hands.

PATIENT AND/OR FAMILY TEACHING
1. Explain the double-bagging procedure to the patient.
2. Instruct visitors that items may not be removed from the room unless appropriately handled.

DOCUMENTATION
1. Disposition of any specimens.
2. All patient and family teaching done and the level of understanding.

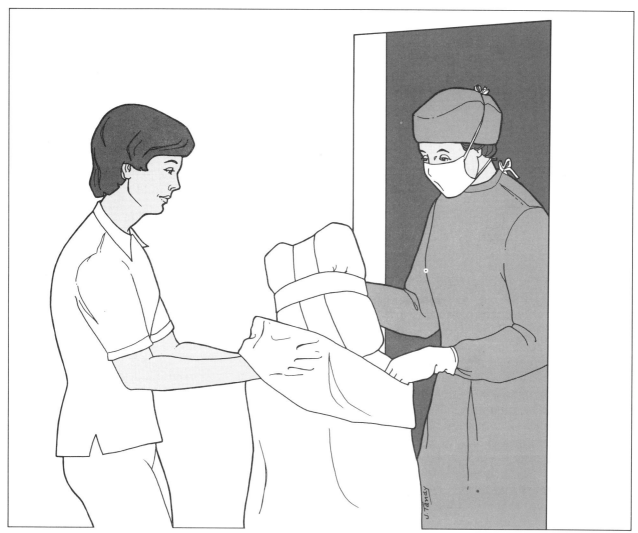

Figure 1-54. Second bag cuffed over hands.

Transporting Technique: Isolation

PURPOSE
1. Provide a barrier to prevent transmission of infection during transport.

REQUISITES
1. Transporting vehicle
2. Isolation supplies
3. Clean patient gown
4. Clean sheet
5. Clean dressings, if appropriate

GUIDELINES
1. Inform the department receiving the patient what type of isolation precaution the patient will need. Instruct the receiving department what precautions need to be followed.
2. The patient should be dressed in a clean gown and fresh dressings should be applied before transport to another department.
3. Personnel must wear isolation barriers appropriate to the type of precaution.
4. Refer to the hospital informational display card for concise information for handling each type of precaution.
5. When wrapping the patient, avoid contaminating the outside of the clean sheet.
6. This procedure may need to be modified and adapted to fit the individual situation.

NURSING ACTION/RATIONALE
1. Notify the receiving department.
2. Before you enter the room, cover the vehicle with a clean sheet.
3. Apply isolation barriers as required.
4. Wheel the vehicle into the room.
5. Identify the patient.
6. Explain the procedure to the patient.
7. Prepare the patient:
   a. Assist the patient into a clean gown.
   b. Apply clean dressings, if appropriate.

8. Assist the patient into or onto the vehicle.
9. Wrap the patient's entire body except the head, with the sheet covering the wheelchair.
10. Apply a mask and/or cap to the patient if appropriate.
11. Wash any exposed part of the vehicle, if appropriate.
12. Remove isolation barriers and wash your hands.
13. Transport the patient to the appropriate area.
14. Rewrap the patient in a clean sheet for the return to the room.
15. Assist the patient from the vehicle.
16. Assist the patient to a comfortable position.
17. Dispose of used linens and barriers in the proper receptacle in the patient's room.
18. Move the vehicle to the entrance of the room.
19. Wash the vehicle.
20. Wash your hands.
21. Move the vehicle out of the room.
22. Rewash your hands.

PATIENT AND/OR FAMILY TEACHING
1. Reinforce the physician's explanation regarding the need to transport the patient.
2. Explain the need for special precautions during transport.

DOCUMENTATION
1. The patient's tolerance of the transport.
2. Precautions taken.
3. All patient teaching done and the patient's level of understanding.

Breakstick Technique or Culturette Method for Aerobic Specimen Collection

PURPOSE

1. Obtain a specimen for culturing to determine the presence of infection due to aerobic bacteria.

REQUISITES

1. Antiseptic swabs
2. Sterile culturette tube or sterile applicator with a culture medium tube
3. Exam gloves
4. Sterile gloves
5. Sterile dressings, as appropriate
6. Waste receptacle

GUIDELINES

1. General signs and symptoms of infection are an elevated temperature, inflammation, an elevated white blood count, and purulent drainage.
2. The breakstick technique is used for culturing aerobes, which are organisms that need oxygen to survive.
3. Some common sites for culturing aerobic bacteria are certain wounds and skin lesions, and the eye, ear, nose, throat, nasopharynx, cervix, and vagina.
4. Always collect specimens for culture before antibiotic therapy is begun.
5. Care must be taken when collecting the specimen to avoid contamination with other organisms. Obtaining cultures is an aseptic procedure.
6. Consult the nurse epidemiologist and the microbiologist regarding infection and specimen collection.
7. Consult with the microbiologist regarding the transport medium to be used for specific specimens.
8. Double-bag all specimens from isolation patients before removing them from the patient's room.

NURSING ACTION/RATIONALE

1. Assemble all equipment.
2. Verify the physician's order.
3. Identify the patient.
4. Explain the procedure to the patient.
5. Provide adequate lighting.
6. Provide privacy.
7. Wash your hands.
8. Position and drape the patient as indicated for the site of the specimen collection.
9. Put on the exam gloves.
10. Remove dressings if appropriate and discard.
11. Remove the exam gloves.
12. Open sterile supplies using aseptic technique.
13. Apply the sterile gloves.
14. Cleanse the skin around the area to be cultured with antiseptic swabs to prevent contaminaton of the specimen by surface bacteria.
15. Obtain the specimen.

Breakstick Technique

a. Remove the cap from the culture tube. Hold the cap in your non-dominant hand, maintaining sterility of the inside of the cap.
b. Using a sterile applicator, swab the exudate from the site.
c. Insert the swab portion of the applicator into the sterile culture tube.
d. Break off the upper portion of the applicator.
e. Replace the cap on the culture tube.

Culturette Method

a. Remove the cap, with the sterile applicator attached, from the culturette tube.
b. Swab the exudate from the site.
c. Replace the swab in the culturette tube, securing the cap.
d. Turn the culturette tube cap-down.
e. Crush the ampule in the bottom of the tube by squeezing it between your index finger and thumb at midpoint.
f. Push the cap down to bring the swab into contact with the medium.

16. Redress the wound with the appropriate dressings, if necessary.
17. Remove the sterile gloves.
18. Label the specimen container.
19. Reposition the patient comfortably.
20. Discard equipment or return it to the appropriate area.
21. Wash your hands.
22. Send the specimen to the laboratory immediately.

PATIENT AND/OR FAMILY TEACHING
1. Explain the procedure and its purpose to the patient.
2. Reinforce and clarify the physician's explanation of the suspected infectious process.
3. Explain any therapeutic orders and additional diagnostic orders.
4. Explain to the patient the purpose and side effects of any antibiotics ordered.

5. Teach the patient the signs of an infection and to report any further signs to the nurse.
6. Instruct the patient regarding handwashing and proper hygiene.

DOCUMENTATION
1. Time, site, and method of specimen collection.
2. Assessment of the site and the specimen collected.
3. The patient's tolerance of the procedure.
4. Disposition of the specimen.
5. All patient teaching done and the patient's level of understanding.

Specimen Collection for Anaerobic Culture

PURPOSE
1. Obtain a specimen for culturing to determine the presence of infection due to anaerobic bacteria.

REQUISITES
1. Antiseptic swabs
2. Sterile gloves
3. Waste receptacle
4. Sterile dressings as appropriate
5. Swab method: anaerobic culture kit, containing
   a. Sterile test tube with cap
   b. Sterile swabs—2
   c. Sterile slides—2 and slide container
6. Syringe method
   a. Sterile 10 cc syringe
   b. Sterile 21-gauge needle
   c. Alcohol wipe
   d. Sterile tube with rubber stopper

GUIDELINES
1. General signs and symptoms of infection are an elevated temperature, inflammation, an elevated white blood count, and purulent drainage.
2. Anaerobic microorganisms require no oxygen to grow. They are found in sterile body fluids or areas with decreased circulation or tissue damage.
3. Some suitable sites for collecting specimens for anaerobic culturing are:
   a. Sinus tracts
   b. Normally sterile body fluids
   c. Uterus
   d. Abscesses or draining wounds
4. Care must be taken when collecting the specimen to avoid contamination with other organisms. Obtaining cultures is an aseptic procedure.
5. Consult the nurse epidemiologist and the microbiologist regarding infection and specimen collection.

6. Always collect specimens for culture before antibiotic therapy is begun.
7. Consult with the microbiologist prior to collecting the specimen to determine the specific culture medium for transporting the specimen.
8. Two methods of collection can be used: syringe method or swab method. The syringe method is used for fluid specimens, such as synovial fluid. The swab method is used for wound drainage.
9. Some health care facilities require the physician to aspirate sterile body fluids using the syringe method, in which case the nurse would assist the physician. Refer to your hospital's policy manual.
10. Double-bag all specimens from isolation patients before removing them from the patient's room.

NURSING ACTION/RATIONALE

1. Assemble all equipment.
2. Verify the physician's order.
3. Identify the patient.
4. Explain the procedure to the patient.
5. Provide adequate lighting.
6. Provide privacy.
7. Position and drape the patient as indicated for the site of the specimen collection.
8. Wash your hands.
9. Apply exam gloves and remove old dressings if necessary. Assess the wound for drainage and/or healing.
10. Remove exam gloves and discard.
11. Wash your hands.
12. Obtain the culture.

Syringe Method

a. Open sterile supplies using aseptic technique.
b. Put on sterile gloves.
c. Cleanse the skin around the area with antiseptic swabs to prevent contamination of the specimen by surface bacteria.
d. Aspirate the specimen with the needle and syringe. Eject all the air from the syringe.
e. Cleanse the rubber stopper of the sterile tube with an alcohol wipe.
f. Inject the specimen into the container.

Swab Method

a. Put on sterile gloves.
b. Follow the procedure "Breakstick Technique or Culturette Method for Specimen Collection."
c. Use the breakstick technique method for obtaining the swab specimen and placing in into the test tube.
d. Use the second swab to swab the drainage area again.
e. Open the sterile slide holder. Roll the swab across each of the two slides in the container.
f. Allow the slides to dry thoroughly, then close the container.
13. Redress the wound site as appropriate using the "Sterile Dressing Change" procedure.
14. Remove the sterile gloves.
15. Label the specimen containers.
16. Reposition the patient comfortably.
17. Discard equipment or return to the appropriate location.
18. Wash your hands.
19. Send the labeled specimens to the laboratory.

PATIENT AND/OR FAMILY TEACHING

1. Explain the procedure and its purpose to the patient.
2. Reinforce and clarify the physician's explanation of the suspected infectious process.
3. Explain any therapeutic orders and additional diagnostic orders.
4. Explain to the patient the purpose and side effects of any antibiotics ordered.
5. Teach the patient the signs of an infection and to report any further signs to the nurse.
6. Instruct the patient regarding handwashing and proper hygiene.

DOCUMENTATION

1. Time, site, and method of specimen collection.
2. Assessment of the wound, if appropriate.
3. Assessment of the specimen.
4. The patient's reaction to the procedure.
5. All patient teaching done and the patient's level of understanding.

Postmortem Care

PURPOSE
1. Prepare the body for family viewing.
2. Prepare the body for transfer to the morgue.

REQUISITES
1. Bath supplies
2. Linen
3. Shroud
4. Bag for personal belongings
5. Identification tags
6. Waste receptacle

GUIDELINES
1. Death, even when expected, can be a very difficult time for the family. Be supportive of the family's need for and method of grieving.
2. The cultural background and religious beliefs of the family affect the meaning of death.
3. Nurses must be aware of their own feelings about death to better support grieving families.
4. Complete identification of the deceased patient is very important.
5. Local laws and hospital policy dictate how the following should be handled:
   a. Removal of equipment from the body.
   b. Autopsy requirements and permission.
   c. Tissue and organ donation and removal.
   d. Identification of the body.
   e. Death certificate.
6. Special identification must be used if the patient was in isolation prior to death. The infectious process will dictate the type of procedure to be used.

NURSING ACTION/RATIONALE
1. Provide privacy for the patient and/or family. Assist the roommate and visitors to leave the room temporarily, if appropriate.
2. Verify that the patient has died and has been pronounced dead by the physician.
3. Notify appropriate persons in the hospital as well as the clergy if requested by the family.
4. Assemble all equipment.
5. Position the body supine in proper body alignment. Close the eyelids. Place a small pillow under the head.
6. Remove and discard all tubes and lines and change all dressings, if appropriate. Remove jewelry and eyeglasses and place with personal belongings. Replace dentures, if possible.
7. Bathe the body.
8. Apply a clean patient gown and clean bed linen if the family will be viewing the body. Leave the head uncovered and have the room arranged neatly.
9. Prepare the family before viewing the body. Offer support and your physical presence, if desired, during their visit. Assist the family with funeral arrangements, if necessary.
10. Identify and assemble the patient's personal belongings for the family.
11. Attach at least two forms of identification to the body. Place one tag on the patient's body (wrist, ankle, or big toe) and the other on the outer covering or shroud, according to specific policy. Leave the wrist identification band in place.
12. Place the body within the shroud.
13. Arrange for transportation to the morgue.
14. Discard equipment or return to the appropriate location.
15. Wash your hands.

PATIENT AND/OR FAMILY TEACHING

1. Explain to the family what the dead body looks like, before viewing.
2. Explain to the family how to make funeral arrangements.
3. Provide information to the family on organ donation and support groups for bereaved persons when appropriate.

DOCUMENTATION

1. Date and time of death.
2. Physician who pronounced the patient dead.
3. Care given to the dead body.
4. Any forms or permits that the family signed.
5. The family or clergy that visited.
6. Disposition of personal belongings.
7. Identification that was attached to the body.
8. Disposition of the body and whether an autopsy is to be performed.
9. All teaching done and the family's reaction.

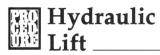 # Hydraulic Lift

PURPOSE

1. Provide a means of lifting and/or transporting a patient with limited mobility.

REQUISITES

1. Hydraulic lift with S hooks and chain
2. Hydraulic lift sling
3. Wheelchair or chair, if indicated

GUIDELINES

1. This procedure describes the Hoyer lift. If your institution uses another type of hydraulic lift, refer to the manufacturer's directions.
2. Do not operate the hydraulic lift alone. Assistance will be needed to guide the patient to another location.
3. Always place some type of protective pad on the sling. Cleanse the sling between patients with antiseptic solution.
4. Never use a torn or damaged sling.
5. The hydraulic lift should always be in good operating condition and should have regular preventive maintenance.
6. The chain attachment to the shoulder area of the sling is shorter than the buttocks chain attachment to allow the patient to maintain a sitting position in the sling.
7. When transferring a patient to a wheelchair, make sure the wheels of the wheelchair are locked.

NURSING ACTION/RATIONALE

1. Assemble all equipment.
2. Wash your hands.
3. Identify the patient.
4. Provide privacy.
5. Explain the procedure to the patient.
6. Replace the top linen with a bath blanket unless the patient is dressed or in a bathrobe.
7. Position the patient in the center of the bed in a supine position.
8. Raise the siderail opposite the work area.
9. Position the patient on his/her side facing the raised siderail.
10. Fold the sling in half lengthwise, placing the smooth surface toward the patient.
11. Position the sling parallel with the patient's back, with the lower edge just below the knees.
12. Assist the patient onto the sling, making sure it is centered.
13. Adjust the head of the bed to the high-Fowler's position.
14. Attach the open S hooks of the chain to the sling hooks. The S hooks should be pointing away from the patient.

15. Position the hydraulic lift so that the open end of the horseshoe base is under the side of the bed.
16. Spread the legs of the horseshoe base.
17. Attach the chains to the ends of the swivel bar, keeping the bar away from the patient's face. Place the patient's arms within the chain attachment (Figure 1-55).

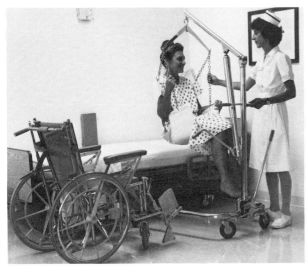

Figure 1-55. Patient positioned in a hydraulic lift.

18. Adjust the release valve to the closed position.
19. Pump the hydraulic handle, using a slow, steady movement, until the patient's buttocks are lifted clear of the bed. It may be necessary to support the patient's head.
20. Lift the patient clear of the bed:
    a. Grasp both feet and swing them over the edge of the bed.
    b. Grasp the steering handles and move the patient away from the bed and to the desired area.

21. Lower the patient gently and slowly into the desired area by opening the release valve.
22. Guide the patient's descent by pushing gently on the patient's knees to gain correct sitting position.
23. Close the release valve as soon as the patient is in position.
24. Detach the chains from the swivel bar.
25. Keep your hands on the swivel bar and move the lift away from the patient.
26. Detach the S hooks and the chains from the sling, and leave the sling under the patient.
27. Assess the patient's body alignment and comfort, the placement of any drainage tubes, and the physical status of the patient. Assess the need for restraints.
28. Return the patient to bed by reversing the procedure.

PATIENT AND/OR FAMILY TEACHING

1. Explain the procedure to the patient step by step before starting. Reinforce the information by explaining the procedure as you proceed.
2. Instruct the patient to keep arms close to the body for safety.

DOCUMENTATION

1. The patient's tolerance of the procedure, including specific assessment parameters such as vital signs, level of consciousness, and color.
2. Any patient teaching done and the patient's level of understanding.

Alternating Pressure Mattress

PURPOSE
1. Prevent skin irritation and breakdown.
2. Relieve pressure to susceptible body areas.

REQUISITES
1. Air mattress
2. Air pump
3. Bed sheet

GUIDELINES
1. Alternating pressure mattresses are used for inactive patients susceptible to skin irritation or breakdown.
2. For maximum effect, only one layer of bed linen should be used between the mattress and the patient.
3. Pins should not be used when an air mattress is in use to prevent puncturing the mattress.
4. Unless contraindicated, frequent repositioning should continue in conjunction with use of the air mattress.
5. Alternative pressure-relieving devices include water mattresses, flotation pads, and eggcrate foam mattresses.

NURSING ACTION/RATIONALE
1. Assemble all equipment.
2. Wash your hands.
3. Explain the procedure to the patient.
4. Provide privacy.
5. Assess the patient's skin condition.
6. Apply a bottom sheet to the patient's mattress. Refer to the procedure "Bedmaking: Unoccupied."
7. Unfold the air mattress on top of the bottom sheet with the air hose at the head of the bed.
8. Apply a sheet over the air mattress. Tuck in loosely around the air hose.
9. Attach the air hose to the air pump and plug the pump into an electrical outlet.
10. Place the pump in a safe location near the head of the bed.
11. Adjust the air pump to the high setting.
12. Evaluate the firmness of the mattress in 20 minutes.
13. Adjust the air pump to a lower pressure if the air mattress is too firm.
14. Place a small pillow under the patient's head.
15. Assist the patient to a comfortable position.

PATIENT AND/OR FAMILY TEACHING
1. Explain the procedure and its purpose to the patient.
2. Instruct the patient to notify the nurse if any discomfort is experienced.
3. Provide instruction for the family regarding use of the air mattress if home use is anticipated.

DOCUMENTATION
1. Time the air mattress was applied.
2. The patient's reaction to the procedure.
3. Assessment of the patient's skin condition.
4. All patient teaching done and the patient's level of understanding.

Weighing the Ambulatory Patient

PURPOSE

1. Obtain an accurate weight as a parameter of patient assessment.
2. Assess the patient's response to treatment.

REQUISITES

1. Scale
2. Paper toweling

GUIDELINES

1. Weigh the patient at the same time each day, with the same scale and the same clothing.
2. The ambulatory patient should be weighed before breakfast and after voiding, if possible.
3. An accurate admission weight provides a baseline for subsequent daily weight measurements.
4. Daily weights are used in conjunction with, or instead of, intake and output to estimate the patient's fluid balance.
5. Any significant increase or decrease in the patient's weight should be reported.
6. The weight of the patient should be checked a second time if the result is inconsistent with previous weights or other assessment parameters.

NURSING ACTION/RATIONALE

1. Identify the patient.
2. Explain the procedure and instruct the patient to empty his/her bladder. If a Foley catheter is in place, empty the Foley drainage bag before weighing.
3. Balance the scale according to the directions from the manufacturer.
4. Place a clean piece of paper toweling on the scale platform.
5. Instruct the patient to remove his/her slippers and robe.
6. Assist the patient to step onto the weighing platform of the scale.
7. Follow any suggested manufacturer's directions for obtaining the proper weight reading.
8. Assist the patient off the scale.
9. Return the scale to the appropriate area.

PATIENT AND/OR FAMILY TEACHING

1. Instruct the patient on the proper techniques for obtaining an accurate weight, including the same time of day and the same clothing.
2. If the patient is to continue weighing at home, assess the type of scale that is available and teach the patient how to use it, if necessary.
3. Assist the patient to develop an accurate chart for recording weights at home.

DOCUMENTATION

1. Time of the procedure.
2. Patient's weight.
3. Any pertinent assessment parameters including edema, dyspnea, food and/or fluid intake, and urinary output.
4. All patient teaching done and the patient's level of understanding.

Weighing a Patient: Electronic Bedscale

PURPOSE
1. Obtain an accurate weight as a parameter of patient assessment.
2. Assess the patient's response to treatment.

REQUISITES
1. Bedscale (Figure 1-56)
2. Sheet
3. Disinfectant

GUIDELINES
1. Patients should be weighed on a bedscale when the patient is:
   a. Too ill to be out of bed.
   b. Non-weightbearing on one or both legs.
   c. Unable to stand independently.
   d. On bedrest per physician's order.
2. Other methods for weighing a patient with limitations are:
   a. Chairscale.
   b. Non-electric bedscale.
   c. Special bedframes with built-in scales.
3. A baseline assessment of the patient's weight should be obtained on admission to the health care facility.
4. To accurately detect weight changes, the patient should be weighed with the same clothing, on the same scale, and at the same time each day—preferably before breakfast and after voiding.
5. Significant weight loss or weight gain may indicate pathological problems and should be reported to the physician.
6. General principles apply to most electric hydraulic bedscales. Check the operator's manual for your scale.
   a. The weight of the stretcher should be determined initially and that weight subtracted from the scale weight before or after weighing the patient.

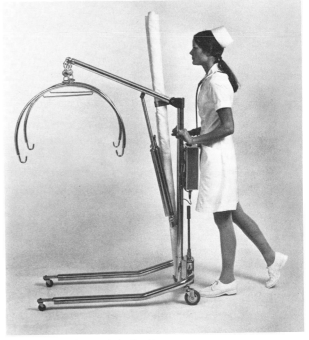

Figure 1-56. Electronic bedscale.

   b. The scales are usually plugged into an electrical outlet for recharging the battery when not in use, and unplugged to weigh a patient.
   c. The scale or stretcher must not be touching the bed, or weight will not be accurate.
   d. The legs of the bedscale should be spread whenever a patient is being weighed to maintain the stability of the apparatus.
   e. The bedscale should never be used to transport a patient from one area to another.
   f. At least two members of the nursing team should be available when a patient is being weighed, to alleviate patient fears and to ensure safety factors.

NURSING ACTION/RATIONALE

1. Assemble all equipment.
2. Identify the patient.
3. Explain the procedure to the patient.
4. Wash your hands.
5. Assist the patient as necessary to void or empty the urinary drainage bag, as appropriate.
6. Roll the bedscale to the patient's bedside and spread the base legs.
7. Obtain the weight of the stretcher by placing the empty stretcher on the scale and reading the weight. Make sure the digital readout is zero before attaching the stretcher.
8. Weigh any bed linen that will be covering the patient.
9. Remove the stretcher.
10. Set the digital readout for minus the weight of the stretcher and bed linen.
11. Fanfold all linen to the bottom of the bed.
12. Cover the patient with a sheet that has been preweighed.
13. Roll the patient to a side-lying position, with a nursing member on each side of the bed.
14. Place the stretcher on the bed, with one layer of preweighed linen between the stretcher and the patient.
15. Roll the patient back onto the stretcher. The patient should be centered on the stretcher.
16. Attach the stretcher to the bedscale frame.
17. Raise the stretcher off the bed at least 3 inches. No part of the patient or stretcher should be touching the bed.
18. Read the weight. Change the bottom sheets on the bed at this time, if necessary.
19. Lower the stretcher to rest on the mattress.
20. Remove the bedscale frame from over the bed.
21. Remove the stretcher by reversing the procedure.
22. Assist the patient to a comfortable position and replace the bed linen.
23. Clean the stretcher with a disinfectant.
24. Discard equipment or return it to the appropriate location.

PATIENT AND/OR FAMILY TEACHING

1. Explain the procedure to the patient. Answer any questions to alleviate patient fears.
2. Discuss the significance of weight gain or loss as it relates to the patient's disease process.

DOCUMENTATION

1. Time, procedure performed, and weight of patient.
2. Type of scale used.
3. The patient's tolerance of the procedure.
4. All patient teaching done and the patient's level of understanding.

Patient Education

PURPOSE

1. Assist patients to attain, maintain, or regain an optimal health status.
2. Assist the patient to adapt to the residual effects of illness by increasing cognitive, affective, and psychomotor skills.

REQUISITES

1. All applicable printed patient education material
2. Necessary equipment to demonstrate procedures or skills
3. Necessary audio/video equipment

GUIDELINES

1. The teaching/learning process is a dynamic process that is enhanced by the active participation of the teacher and learner.
2. Teaching/learning must be adapted to the individual learner through a thorough assessment of the learner's strengths, weaknesses, and needs.
3. Readiness to learn enhances the teaching/learning process.
4. The relevancy of the information as perceived by the patient affects the patient's motivation to learn.
5. The establishment of goals gives direction to the teaching/learning process.
6. Involvement of the patient in developing goals and choosing content to be learned facilitates learning.
7. Teaching should incorporate the use of a variety of teaching methods adapted to the patient's learning style and level of understanding.
8. When the information to be taught affects other individuals within a patient's life, those persons should be included in the teaching/learning process.
9. A learning environment free of distractions facilitates the teaching/learning process.
10. Evaluation and feedback provide both the teacher and learner with information concerning progress in achieving teaching/learning goals.

11. The teacher's role is to facilitate the teaching/learning process.
12. Teaching requires expertise in the subject to be taught and the ability to communicate that expertise effectively at the learner's level of understanding.

NURSING ACTION/RATIONALE

1. Identify the patient.
2. Assess the patient's present state of health. Learning needs are influenced by the comfort level and phase of illness.
3. Assess the patient's mental capacity. Level of consciousness, level of intelligence, and cognitive learning styles influence the patient's ability to learn.
4. Assess the patient's previous knowledge base. Learning is enhanced through utilization of previous experience and/or knowledge.
5. Assess the patient's motivation to learn. Motivation to learn enhances the teaching/learning process.
6. Assess the patient's level of stress. Mild anxiety is beneficial to learning, but moderate or severe anxiety will hinder learning.
7. Identify the patient's specific learning needs.
8. Establish mutually acceptable teaching/learning goals or expected outcomes. Goals or expected outcomes give direction to the teaching/learning process.
9. Select content and teaching strategies that are meaningful to the patient. Learning occurs more readily when the material is meaningful to the learner.
10. Establish an environment conducive to learning. Noise, interruptions, and distractions will hinder the active participation of the learner in the teaching/learning process.
11. Present material to the patient by proceeding from simple to complex and from the known to the unknown.

12. Evaluate the patient's progress in learning.
13. Provide feedback to the patient regarding his/her progress throughout the teaching/learning process.
14. Plan for reinforcement of material presented and/or future teaching based on an evaluation of the patient's progress.

DOCUMENTATION
1. Information or skill taught.
2. The patient's level of understanding or evidence of a change in behavior resulting from teaching.
3. Assessment of further learning needs.
4. Plans for reinforcement of teaching.
5. Plans for future teaching.

Medication Administration

Unit 2

Intramuscular Injection

PURPOSE

1. Provide a route for the administration of select medications.

REQUISITES

1. Sterile needle (19 to 22 gauge, 1½ to 3 inch)
2. Sterile syringe
3. Antiseptic wipes
4. Correct medication and dosage

GUIDELINES

1. Intramuscular injections are generally given when a more rapid absorption is desired or when the oral route is contraindicated.
2. As with all medications, observe the "five rights" of administration: the right patient, the right medication, the right dosage, the right route, and the right time.
3. Before administering any medication, the nurse should know the actions of the drug, the reason for giving the drug, the normal dosage and route of administration, incompatabilities, contraindications, and adverse reactions.
4. The amount of solution given via the intramuscular route varies with the medication. Usually no more than 5 cc is given in one site. Consideration should be given to dividing doses of 4 to 5 cc into two injection sites.
5. Rotation of injection sites is important for the patient's comfort to prevent unnecessary trauma to tissue and to aid in absorption.
6. A small air bubble of 0.2 cc for routine injections and 0.5 cc for the Z track method will force the last amount of medication into the muscle, ensuring the right dose was given and preventing leakage of medication into other tissue during needle withdrawal.
7. Preferred sites for injection include the dorsogluteal site, the ventrogluteal site, the vastus lateralis site, and the deltoid site (Figure 2-1 a through d).

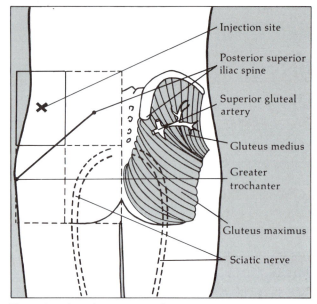

Figure 2-1. Sites for intramuscular injection.
(a) Dorsogluteal site.

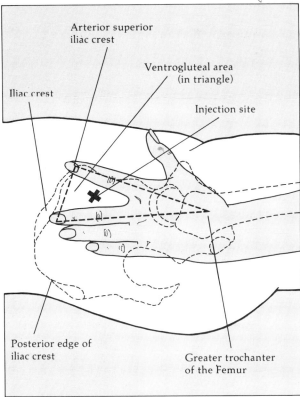

Figure 2-1(b). Ventrogluteal site.

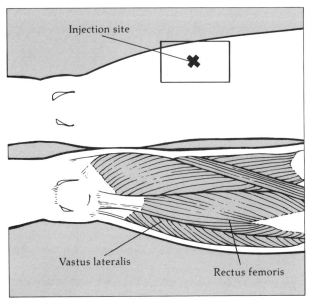

Figure 2-1(c). Vastus lateralis site.

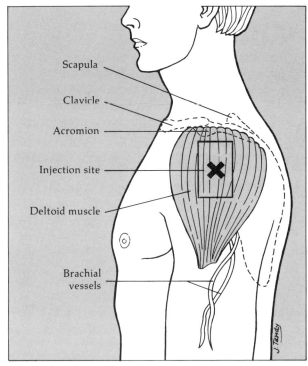

Figure 2-1(d). Deltoid site.

8. The position of the patient who is to receive an intramuscular injection should be safe, comfortable, and compatible with the patient's physical condition as well as offering an adequate exposure of the injection site.

9. A muscle that is painful or has hardened areas is not appropriate for an injection site.

10. A 22 gauge, 1½ inch needle is most commonly used for adult intramuscular injections. A 19 to 20 gauge, 2 to 3 inch needle is used for the Z track method.

11. The size of the needle and syringe vary depending on the amount of solution, the viscosity of the solution, the size of the patient, and the muscle selected for the injection. Select the smallest needle appropriate for the site and solution.

12. Medications that are injected slowly will absorb more effectively and cause less discomfort.

13. Before giving any new medication, assess for any patient allergies.

14. A Z track technique is used to inject certain medications that stain or cause superficial irritation to tissue. To prevent staining or irritation of superficial tissue from medication on the outside of the needle, the needle should be changed after the medication has been drawn up and before administration. Only the dorsogluteal site can be used for the Z track method.

NURSING ACTION/RATIONALE

1. Assemble all equipment.
2. Verify the medication order.
3. Wash your hands.
4. Prepare the medication, using aseptic technique.
5. Identify the patient.
6. Explain the procedure to the patient.
7. Provide privacy and position the patient as required.
8. Select an appropriate injection site, using anatomical landmarks.
9. Cleanse the injection site with an antiseptic wipe, using friction. Allow to dry.
10. Remove the needle cover, using aseptic technique.
11. Inform the patient that you are ready to give the injection.
12. Administer the injection.

Routine Method

a. Draw skin tissue taut, using the thumb and fingers of your non-dominant hand.
b. Thrust the needle quickly into the tissue to its full length at a 90 degree angle, using a dartlike motion.
c. Aspirate by pulling back on the plunger to ensure that a blood vessel has not been entered.
d. If blood has been aspirated, withdraw the needle and discard the medication. Prepare a new injection.
e. Inject the medication slowly by pushing on the plunger and holding the syringe steady.
f. Remove the needle quickly by following the line of insertion.
g. Apply pressure to the injection site with an antiseptic sponge.
h. Massage the site with a circular motion to enhance absorption.

Z Track Method

a. Displace the skin tissue laterally, using the side of your non-dominant hand (Figure 2-2).

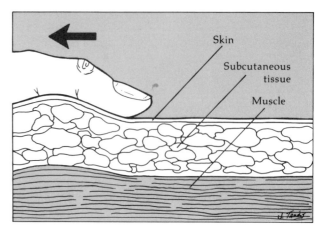
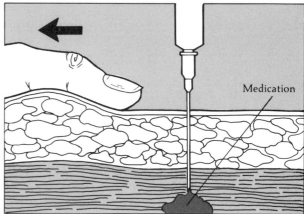
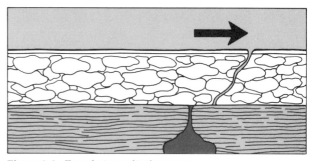

Figure 2-2. Z track tissue displacement.

b. Insert the needle, aspirate for placement, and inject the medication as described for a normal injection, maintaining tissue displacement.

c. Wait 10 seconds for the medication to disperse.

d. Remove the needle, allowing the displaced tissue to return to its normal position.

e. Apply pressure to the injection site with an antiseptic sponge. Do not massage the area.

13. Assess the injection site for bleeding. Apply additional pressure if necessary.

14. Assist the patient to a comfortable position, noting safety factors.

15. Discard equipment or return it to the appropriate area.

PATIENT AND/OR FAMILY TEACHING

1. Explain the reason for the injection and the type of medication, if appropriate.

2. Explain any untoward effects of the medication, if appropriate.

3. Instruct the patient to notify the nurse if unusual symptoms occur.

4. Explain the schedule for the administration of the medication, if appropriate.

5. Explain any activity restrictions.

6. Explain the need for the patient to notify the nurse if the medication is ordered P.R.N. (as necessary).

DOCUMENTATION

1. Medication, dosage, time, site, and route of administration.

2. Narcotics, using health care facility policies.

3. Any expected or unexpected effects of the medication, interventions, and results.

4. All patient teaching done and the patient's level of understanding.

⬛ Intradermal Injection

PURPOSE

1. Instill an allergen into the skin as a diagnostic measure to assess for an allergic reaction.
2. Test for histoplasmosis or tuberculosis.
3. Provide local anesthesia.

REQUISITES

1. Sterile needle (26 gauge, ⅝ inch needle)
2. Sterile syringe
3. Antiseptic wipes
4. Correct medication and dosage

GUIDELINES

1. As with all medications, observe the "five rights" of administration: the right patient, the right medication, the right dosage, the right route, and the right time.
2. Before administering any medication, the nurse should know the actions of the drug, the reason for giving the drug, the normal dosage and route of administration, incompatabilities, contraindications, and adverse reactions.
3. Preferred sites for diagnostic intradermal injections include the ventral forearms, the upper chest area, or the shoulder blades, since these areas are lightly pigmented, usually hairless, and thinly keratinized.
4. Results from diagnostic intradermal testing will not usually appear immediately, owing to the slow absorption rate of the dermis.
5. Before giving any new medications, assess for any patient allergies.
6. Giving the injection slowly will reduce the discomfort of the injection.
7. With any biological product, epinephrine should be immediately available in case of an anaphylactic reaction.
8. In highly sensitive individuals, strongly positive reactions including vesiculation, ulceration, or tissue necrosis may occur at the test site.
9. Never use an antiseptic skin preparation agent that will discolor the skin.

NURSING ACTION/RATIONALE

1. Assemble all equipment.
2. Verify the medication order.
3. Wash your hands.
4. Prepare the medication, using aseptic technique.
5. Identify the patient.
6. Explain the procedure to the patient.
7. Provide privacy, and position the patient as required.
8. Select an appropriate injection site, using anatomical landmarks.
9. Cleanse the site of injection with an antiseptic wipe, using friction. Allow to dry. For select diagnostic testing, 70% isopropyl alcohol is preferred.
10. Remove the needle cover, using aseptic technique.
11. Inform the patient that you are ready to give the injection.
12. Administer the injection:
    a. Pull the skin taut over the injection site, using the thumb of your non-dominant hand.
    b. Position the syringe so that the needle is almost parallel with the patient's skin (Figure 2-3).

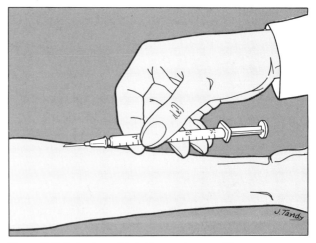

Figure 2-3. Intradermal injection syringe position.

c. Insert the needle, bevel up, into the most superficial layers of the skin. The point of the needle should be visible through the skin. Insert the needle approximately ⅛ inch below the skin surface between the epidermal and dermal layers.

d. Inject the medication slowly by pushing on the plunger and holding the syringe steady. Some resistance will be felt. If no resistance is felt, the needle is too deep and should be withdrawn slightly.

e. Leave the syringe in place for a moment and watch for a pale bleb or wheal to form about ¼ inch in diameter (Figure 2-4).

f. Withdraw the needle and apply light pressure to the site. Do not massage the area.

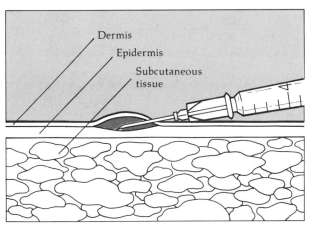

Figure 2-4. Formation of a small bleb after intradermal injection.

13. Assess the injection site for bleeding. Apply additional pressure if necessary.
14. Assist the patient to a comfortable position.
15. Discard equipment or return it to the appropriate area.
16. Assess the patient carefully for any symptoms of an allergic reaction if diagnostic testing has been done.

PATIENT AND/OR FAMILY TEACHING
1. Explain the reason for the injection and the type of medication, if appropriate.
2. Explain any untoward effects of the medication, if appropriate.
3. Instruct the patient to notify the nurse immediately if symptoms of an allergic reaction occur.

DOCUMENTATION
1. Medication, dosage, time, site, and route of administration.
2. Any expected or unexpected effects of the medication, interventions, and results.
3. Reaction, if administered for diagnostic purposes.
4. All patient teaching done and the patient's level of understanding.

Subcutaneous Injection

PURPOSE
1. Provide a route for the administration of select medications.

REQUISITES
1. Sterile needle (25 gauge, ⅝ inch)
2. Sterile syringe
3. Antiseptic wipes
4. Correct medication and dosage

GUIDELINES
1. Subcutaneous injections are generally given when a more rapid absorption is desired or when the oral route is contraindicated.
2. As with all medications, observe the "five rights" of administration: the right patient, the right medication, the right dosage, the right route, and the right time.
3. Before administering any medication, the nurse should know the actions of the drug, the reason for giving the drug, the normal dosage and route of administration, incompatabilities, contraindications, and adverse reactions.
4. Preferred areas of injection include (Figure 2-5):
   a. The dorsolateral aspect of the arm, 3 to 5 inches above the elbow.
   b. The abdomen, excluding the area 1 inch in diameter around the umbilicus and the belt line.
   c. The anterior and lateral thighs approximately 3 inches above the knee.
5. Injection sites must be rotated to avoid unnecessary trauma to tissues and to aid in medication absorption.
6. Tissue that is painful or has hardened areas is not appropriate for an injection site.
7. A 25 gauge, ⅝ inch needle is most commonly used for an adult subcutaneous injection.
8. Before giving any new medications, assess for any patient allergies.
9. When administering heparin or insulin, a diagram of common injection sites should be used to establish a precise record of sites used and sites remaining.

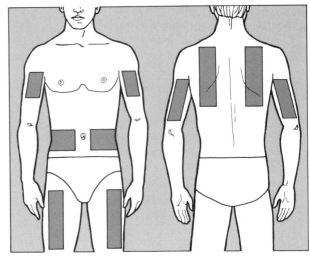

Figure 2-5. Sites for subcutaneous injection.

10. When administering heparin subcutaneously, follow the routine procedure with the following exceptions:
    a. Change the needle after drawing up the heparin, before administration.
    b. Do not aspirate the needle placement as this can cause tissue damage and hematoma formation.
    c. The abdomen is the preferred site for heparin administration.
    d. Never massage the site following a heparin injection, as this may cause hematoma formation.
    e. An ice cube may be applied to the injection site prior to injection to decrease the circulation to the area and thereby lessen the chance of hematoma formation.
    f. The injection should not be made within 2 inches of the umbilicus or a scar.
    g. Never inject heparin into an ecchymotic area.
11. A small air bubble of 0.2 cc may be used in the syringe if the subcutaneous injection is given at a 90 degree angle to force the last amount of medication into the tissue.

NURSING ACTION/RATIONALE

1. Assemble all equipment.
2. Verify the medication order.
3. Wash your hands.
4. Prepare the medication, using aseptic technique.
5. Identify the patient.
6. Explain the procedure to the patient.
7. Provide privacy, and position the patient as required.
8. Select an appropriate injection site, using anatomical landmarks.
9. Cleanse the injection site with an antiseptic wipe, using friction. Allow to dry.
10. Remove the needle cover, using aseptic technique.
11. Inform the patient that you are ready to give the injection.
12. Administer the injection:
    a. Gently accumulate a well-defined roll of skin with the thumb and index finger of your non-dominant hand.
    b. Insert the needle to its full length at a 45 to 90 degree angle depending on the amount of tissue available (Figure 2-6).

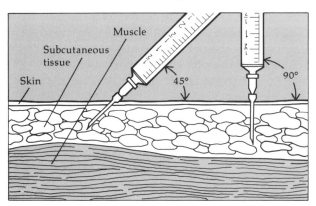

Figure 2-6. Angle for subcutaneous injection.

    c. Aspirate by pulling back on the plunger to ensure that a blood vessel has not been entered.
    d. If blood has been aspirated, withdraw the needle and discard the medication. Prepare a new injection.
    e. Inject the medication slowly by pushing on the plunger and holding the syringe steady.
    f. Remove the needle quickly by following the line of insertion.

    g. Apply pressure to the injection site with an antiseptic sponge.
    h. Massage the site with a circular motion to enhance absorption.
13. Assess the injection site for bleeding. Apply additional pressure if necessary.
14. Assist the patient to a comfortable position, noting safety factors.
15. Discard equipment or return it to the appropriate area.

PATIENT AND/OR FAMILY TEACHING

1. Explain the reason for the injection and the type of medication, if appropriate.
2. Explain any untoward effects of the medication, if appropriate.
3. Instruct the patient to notify the nurse if unusual symptoms occur.
4. Explain the schedule for the administration of the medication, if appropriate.
5. Explain any activity restrictions.
6. Explain the need for the patient to notify the nurse if the medication is ordered P.R.N. (as necessary).

DOCUMENTATION

1. Medication, dosage, time, site, and route of administration.
2. Narcotics, using health care facility policies.
3. Any expected or unexpected effects of the medication, interventions, and results.
4. All patient teaching done and the patient's level of understanding.

Subcutaneous Infusion (Hypodermoclysis)

PURPOSE

1. Infuse fluid into the subcutaneous tissue for absorption into the circulatory system.

REQUISITES

1. Hypodermoclysis administration set with two 2½ inch needles attached
2. Sterile injection solution (type and amount as ordered by the physician)
3. Prepared syringe of hyaluronidase (dosage as ordered by the physician) (optional)
4. Antiseptic wipes
5. 2 × 2 sterile gauze sponges
6. Tape
7. Clean sheet

GUIDELINES

1. Hypodermoclysis should be used only when intravenous therapy is contraindicated or unsuccessful.
2. Hypodermoclysis may be indicated for the obese patient, or for the very old or the very young whose veins are small and fragile.
3. Solutions used for hypodermoclysis should be isotonic or hypotonic. Hypertonic solution, such as 5% dextrose in water, draws electrolytes from the surrounding tissues and plasma. The decreased plasma volume can cause hypotension and shock.
4. Patients with hypovolemia and peripheral blood vessel collapse will not be able to absorb fluid from the subcutaneous tissue; consequently, hypodermoclysis is contraindicated in these patients.
5. Infusion sites that are most commonly used for hypodermoclysis include:
   a. Anterior and lateral aspects of the thigh.
   b. Upper back between the scapulae.
   c. Upper abdomen between the breasts and the iliac crests.
6. If the thighs are used, one needle is inserted into each thigh (Figure 2-7). In the other sites, the needles are inserted parallel to each other, one on each side of the trunk of the body.

7. The enzyme hyaluronidase may be ordered to be added to the solution or injected into the administration tubing. It promotes diffusion and consequently improves absorption of fluid in the tissues. The effects of hyaluronidase are maintained for 24 to 36 hours.
8. Aseptic technique must be used when performing hypodermoclysis. The subcutaneous tissue does not contain any antibodies against infection.
9. The fluid rate must be adjusted according to the patient's rate of absorption. Administering the solution too rapidly may cause edema at the site, with possible sloughing of the subcutaneous tissue.

NURSING ACTION/RATIONALE

1. Assemble all equipment.
2. Verify the physician's order.
3. Prepare the solution bottle, attach the administration set, and prime the tubing using the technique described in "Intravenous Therapy."
4. Identify the patient.
5. Explain the procedure to the patient.
6. Provide adequate lighting.
7. Provide privacy.
8. Position the patient appropriately with the site exposed. Drape the patient in two sections above and below the proposed infusion site using the extra sheet. Make the patient comfortable.
9. Wash your hands.
10. Cleanse the first infusion site with an antiseptic wipe, using friction.

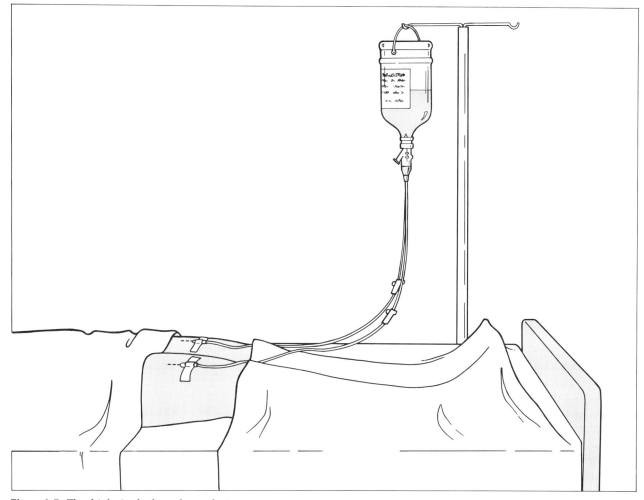

Figure 2-7. The thigh site for hypodermoclysis.

11. Insert one needle attached to the administration set:
   a. Gently accumulate a well-defined amount of tissue between your index finger and thumb.
   b. Tell the patient that you are ready to insert the needle.
   c. Insert the needle, bevel down, at a 30 degree angle into the tissue. The tip of the needle should be proximal to the insertion site.
   d. Assess for a backflash of blood into the administration tubing. If blood return is noted, withdraw the needle. Repeat the procedure, using a new needle and an adjacent site.

12. Unclamp the tubing attached to the needle inserted. Adjust the flow rate to one half of the prescribed rate.
13. Tape the needle in place.
14. Place a 2 × 2 gauze under the needle hub.
15. Apply antiseptic ointment and a 2 × 2 gauze dressing over the site. Tape the dressing securely.
16. Repeat the steps for insertion at the second site selected.
17. Unclamp the tubing attached to the second needle and adjust the flow rate to equal the prescribed rate.
18. Assess the sites for edema, which indicates too rapid an infusion rate in comparison to the absorption rate. Adjust the rate of the infusion accordingly.

19. Inject the hyaluronidase into each tubing, if ordered:
    a. Cleanse the rubber injection site with antiseptic.
    b. Insert the needle of the syringe into the rubber injection site.
    c. Pinch off the tubing to the solution.
    d. Aspirate for a blood return. If blood returns, *do not* inject the medication. Relocate the subcutaneous needles before continuing.
    e. Inject half of the prescribed dose.
    f. Unpinch the tubing.
    g. Repeat the procedure on the tubing attached to the other needle, using the other half of the prescribed hyaluronidase.
    h. Observe the injection sites for redness, which could be a sign of an allergic reaction to the hyaluronidase.
20. Assess the infusion every hour including the rate of flow, the site, and the surrounding tissue. Note the degree of absorption or engorgement. Assess for blanching, firmness, pain, and edema of the surrounding tissue. These signs may indicate poor absorption.
21. Clamp the tubing at intervals, if necessary, to allow excess fluid to be absorbed.
22. Change the patient's position regularly without disrupting the infusion.
23. At the conclusion of the treatment, clamp the tubing and remove the needles, following the path of insertion.
24. Apply an antiseptic ointment and a sterile 2 × 2 gauze sponge over the site, using aseptic technique.
25. Assist the patient to a comfortable position.
26. Discard equipment or return it to the appropriate location.

PATIENT AND/OR FAMILY TEACHING

1. Explain the procedure to the patient before starting.
2. Reinforce and clarify the physician's explanation of the disease process.
3. Explain any additional therapeutic orders.
4. Explain any activity restrictions during the infusion.
5. Instruct the patient to call the nurse if discomfort is experienced during the procedure.

DOCUMENTATION

1. Type of solution, rate of infusion, and amount of fluid infused.
2. Site used for the infusion.
3. All medication, dosage, route, and time of administration.
4. Assessment of infusion site, along with explanation of rate adjustments according to absorption rates.
5. The patient's reaction to the procedure during and after the infusion.
6. All patient teaching done and the patient's level of understanding.

Administration of Eye Drops/Eye Ointment

PURPOSE

1. Instill a medication into the eye for therapeutic effect.

REQUISITES

1. Eye drops or ointment as prescribed by the physician
2. Sterile saline
3. 2 × 2 sterile gauze sponges
4. Disposable tissue

GUIDELINES

1. Before administering any medication the nurse should know the actions of the drug, the reason for giving the drug, the normal dosage and route of administration, incompatibilities, contraindications, and adverse reactions.
2. The "five rights" of drug administration should be observed each time a medication is administered: the right medication, the right dosage, the right time, the right route, and the right patient.
3. The eye, especially the cornea, is a very sensitive area and is easily injured. Use extreme care when administering eye medication.
4. Sterile technique should be used whenever treating the eye. Use separate supplies for each eye.
5. Never instill eye drops or ointment directly onto the cornea.
6. Patient allergies should be assessed before administering any new medication.

NURSING ACTION/RATIONALE

1. Assemble all equipment.
2. Verify the physician's order.
3. Identify the patient.
4. Explain the procedure to the patient. Instruct the patient not to move during the procedure.
5. Provide adequate lighting.
6. Provide privacy.
7. Position the patient supine or sitting with the head tilted back.
8. Wash your hands.
9. Wipe the eyelid and lashes gently from the inner to the outer canthus, using a sterile 2 × 2 gauze sponge moistened with sterile saline for each stroke.
10. With one hand draw up the correct amount of solution in the medicine dropper or uncap the eye ointment.
11. Protecting your fingers with a sterile 2 × 2 gauze sponge, gently pull down the lower eyelid exposing the conjunctival sac.
12. Instruct the patient to look up toward the ceiling. This protects the cornea under the upper eyelid and prevents blinking at the approach of the medication dropper or ointment tube.
13. Rest the hand holding the medication on the patient's forehead above the eye. This avoids damaging the eye with the dropper or ointment tip if the patient should move. Hold the dropper or ointment tube 1 to 2 cm above the conjunctival sac (Figure 2-8).

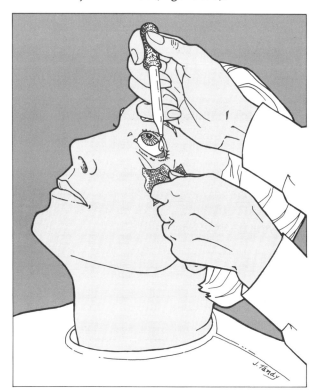

Figure 2-8. Administering eye drops.

14. Instill the prescribed number of drops or a 1 cm line of ointment onto the inner surface of the lower lid. Do not touch the dropper or tube to the patient's eye.
15. Release the lower lid. Instruct the patient to close the eye for a few seconds and move the eyeball to distribute the medication.
16. Absorb any excess medication around the eye with a tissue.
17. Wash your hands, and repeat the procedure on the other eye, if ordered.
18. Assist the patient to a comfortable position.
19. Discard equipment or return it to the appropriate area.

PATIENT AND/OR FAMILY TEACHING
1. Explain to the patient the nature and purpose of the procedure.
2. Instruct the patient to lie or sit still during the procedure and to close the eye and move the eyeball to distribute the medication after it has been instilled.

3. Reinforce and clarify the physician's explanation of the disease process.
4. Explain any additional therapeutic orders.
5. Teach the patient or a family member to administer the eye medication at home if needed.

DOCUMENTATION
1. Date, time, medication, dosage, and route of administration.
2. Assessment of the eye and any exudate.
3. The patient's reaction to the procedure.
4. All patient teaching done and the patient's level of understanding.

Administration of Ear Drops

PURPOSE
1. Instill a medication into the auditory canal for therapeutic effect.
2. Soften plugs of cerumen (ear wax).

REQUISITES
1. Medication as prescribed by the physician
2. Cotton balls
3. Normal saline (optional)

GUIDELINES
1. Before administering any medication the nurse should know the actions of the drug, the reason for giving the drug, the normal dosage and route of administration, incompatibilities, contraindications, and adverse reactions.
2. The "five rights" of drug administration should be followed each time a medication is administered: the right medication, the right dosage, the right time, the right route, and the right patient.

3. Ear drops should be administered at body temperature for patient comfort.
4. Instillation of eardrops is a clean procedure. If the tympanic membrane is ruptured, aseptic technique should be used.
5. The ear canal must be straightened to receive ear drops. The adult's ear canal is in a forward and downward direction, whereas an infant's ear canal is almost straight. This anatomical difference accounts for the different directions in which the adult's and infant's ears are pulled while administering ear drops.
6. Patient allergies should be assessed before administering any new medication.

NURSING ACTION/RATIONALE

1. Assemble all equipment.
2. Verify the physician's order.
3. Identify the patient.
4. Explain the procedure to the patient. Instruct the patient not to move during the procedure.
5. Provide adequate lighting.
6. Provide privacy.
7. Position the patient supine with the head to the side and the affected ear up.
8. Wash your hands.
9. Clean the external ear of exudate with cotton balls soaked in normal saline, if necessary.
10. Draw up the correct amount of the solution in the medicine dropper.
11. With one hand pull the auricle up and back _Adults_ (down and back for infants). Rest the other hand on the patient's head to avoid damaging the ear with the dropper if the patient should move (Figure 2-9).

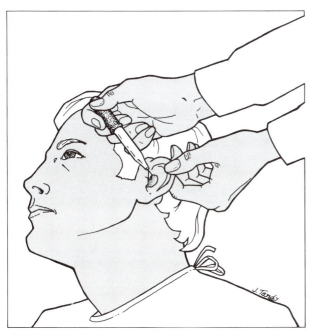

Figure 2-9. Administering ear drops.

12. Instill the prescribed amount of drops, one drop at a time, into the patient's ear, directing the flow toward the canal, rather than the eardrum. Do not allow the dropper to touch the ear.
13. Place a loose cotton ball in the outer ear to absorb any excess medication. Keep the patient's head turned to the side for 10 to 15 minutes.
14. Assist the patient to a comfortable position.
15. Discard or return all equipment to the appropriate area.
16. Wash your hands.

PATIENT AND/OR FAMILY TEACHING

1. Explain to the patient the nature and purpose of the procedure.
2. Instruct the patient to lie still during the procedure and for 10 to 15 minutes after the ear drops have been instilled.
3. Reinforce and clarify the physician's explanation of the disease process.
4. Explain any additional therapeutic orders.
5. Teach the patient or a family member to administer the ear drops at home if needed.

DOCUMENTATION

1. Date, time, medication, dosage, and route of administration.
2. An assessment of any exudate on the outer ear.
3. The patient's reaction to the procedure.
4. All patient teaching done and the patient's level of understanding.

Nasal Instillation

PURPOSE

1. Provide a route for administering medications used in treating nasal problems.

REQUISITES

1. Prescribed medication
2. Medication dropper
3. Disposable tissue

GUIDELINES

1. Nasal instillations of therapeutic agents may be administered to shrink edematous tissue, prevent or control bleeding, provide topical anesthesia, or treat infectious processes.
2. Although the nose is not a sterile cavity, its connection with the sinuses indicates a need for a medically aseptic technique.
3. The "five rights" of drug administration should be followed each time a medication is administered including the right medication, the right dosage, the right time, the right route, and the right patient.
4. Before administering any medication the nurse should know the actions of the drug, the reason for giving the drug, the normal dosage and route of administration, incompatibilities, contraindications, and adverse reactions.
5. The patient's head must be positioned over a pillow on the edge of the bed during nasal instillation. If the head is only tilted back, the medication will run into the throat and be swallowed, making the medication ineffective.
6. Touching the inner surface of the nose with the dropper should be avoided, since it may cause the patient to sneeze.
7. Nasal instillation preparations should be for single-patient use only.
8. Before giving any new medications, assess for any patient allergies.

NURSING ACTION/RATIONALE

1. Assemble all equipment.
2. Verify the physician's order.
3. Identify the patient.
4. Explain the procedure to the patient. Instruct the patient to avoid movement during the procedure to facilitate instillation.
5. Wash your hands.
6. Provide adequate lighting.
7. Place the patient in one of three positions to provide medication flow to the affected area.
   a. *Eustachian tube*—place the patient in a flat supine position with the head tilted slightly to the affected side.
   b. *Ethmoid and sphenoid sinuses*—place the patient in a flat supine position with the shoulders supported with a pillow to hyperextend the neck (Figure 2-10).

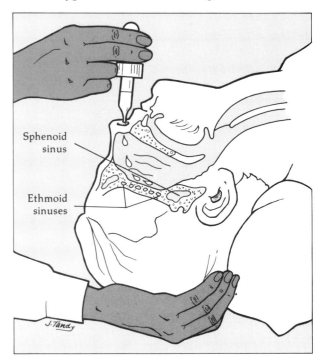

Figure 2-10. Proetz position for ethmoid or sphenoid sinus medications.

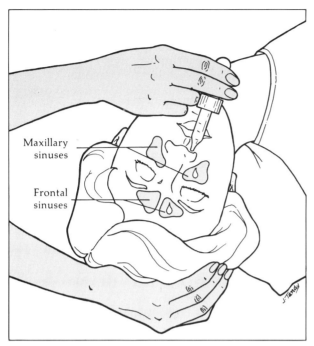

Figure 2-11. Parkinson position for maxillary and frontal sinus medications.

  c. *Frontal and maxillary sinuses*—place the patient in a flat supine position with the shoulders supported with a pillow and the head hyperextended and turned toward the affected side (Figure 2-11).
 8. Provide the patient with disposable tissue.
 9. Withdraw the appropriate amount of prescribed medication into the dropper.
10. Insert the tip of the dropper just inside the nares.
11. Instill the proper amount of medication by counting the drops.
12. Instruct the patient to maintain the position for 5 minutes to prevent the escape of medication.
13. Absorb the excess medication with disposable tissue but instruct the patient that nose blowing should be avoided.
14. Assist the patient to a comfortable position.
15. Return the medication and the dropper to the appropriate area.

PATIENT AND/OR FAMILY TEACHING

1. Explain the procedure and the required position for the nasal instillation.
2. Explain that for therapeutic effect, the patient must remain in the appropriate position for a minimum of 5 minutes.
3. Instruct the patient to notify the nurse if any unusual symptoms are experienced.
4. Demonstrate the nasal instillation procedure to the patient and/or family if the medication will be prescribed following discharge.
5. Caution the patient regarding the use of over-the-counter nasal preparations. Abuse of these medications can cause rebound congestion, decreasing the effectiveness of the drug.

DOCUMENTATION

1. Time of the procedure.
2. Type of medication, dosage, and route.
3. Any unusual reactions to the procedure or medication.
4. Any assessment parameters including the condition of the nasal mucosa and the nares as well as the ease of air passage through the nose.
5. Any patient teaching done and the patient's level of understanding.

Bladder Instillation

PURPOSE
1. Provide a route for the administration of medications into the bladder.

REQUISITES
1. Double or triple lumen Foley catheter in place in the patient
2. Antiseptic wipes
3. C clamp
4. Infusion method (with a triple lumen catheter)
   a. Solution bottle with medication (amount and dosage as ordered by the physician)
   b. Bladder irrigation tubing
   c. Sterile catheter plug
   d. Sterile gloves
   e. IV standard
5. Syringe method (double lumen Foley catheter)
   a. Prefilled syringe with medication (amount and dosage as ordered by the physician)
   b. Sterile 20 gauge needle

GUIDELINES
1. A physician's order is required to perform this procedure. The order should include the type and amount of medication to be administered, the frequency of instillation, and the length of time the medication should remain in the bladder.
2. Before administering any medication the nurse should know the actions of the drug, the reason for giving the drug, the normal dosage and route of administration, incompatibilities, contraindications, and adverse reactions.
3. The "five rights" of drug administration should be followed each time a medication is administered: the right medication, the right dosage, the right time, the right route, and the right patient.
4. Small amounts of medicated solution (50 to 100 cc) can be administered by the syringe method. Larger amounts of solution may require the infusion method with the triple lumen catheter.
5. Before administering any new medications, patient allergies should be assessed.
6. Aseptic technique must be maintained during this procedure.
7. To obtain maximum topical effect of the medication, the patient should remain supine during the time the medication is in the bladder. Turning the patient to the side, abdomen, and opposite side after one fourth, one half, and three fourths of the treatment time has passed, will also aid in ensuring contact of the medication with the entire bladder surface.

NURSING ACTION/RATIONALE
1. Assemble all equipment.
2. Verify the physician's order.
3. Identify the patient.
4. Explain the procedure to the patient.
5. Provide privacy.
6. Provide adequate lighting.
7. Position the patient supine and drape the patient to expose the connection of the catheter and drainage bag.
8. Wash your hands.

Infusion Method: Triple Lumen Catheter
1. Prepare the solution bottle and irrigation tubing and prime the tubing. Hang the bottle on the IV standard.
2. Put on the sterile gloves.
3. Cleanse the connection between the small lumen on the Foley and the catheter plug with an antiseptic wipe.
4. Remove the catheter plug and insert the irrigation tubing into the small lumen of the catheter.
5. Clamp the Foley drainage bag tubing.
6. Open the clamp on the irrigation tubing and allow the correct amount of solution to infuse into the bladder.
7. Close the clamp on the irrigation tubing.
8. Remove the sterile gloves.
9. Allow the solution to remain in the bladder the prescribed amount of time.
10. Open the clamp to the drainage bag and allow the bladder to drain completely. Assess the amount of drainage to ensure that all of the solution administered has returned.

11. When discontinuing the therapy, cleanse the connection between the irrigation tubing and the catheter.
12. Remove the tubing and insert a sterile catheter plug into the small lumen of the catheter, using aseptic technique.
13. Assist the patient to a comfortable position.
14. Discard equipment or return it to the appropriate location.

Syringe Method: Double Lumen Foley Catheter
1. Cleanse the injection port at the catheter-drainage tubing connection with alcohol wipes.
2. Clamp the Foley drainage tubing distal to the port.
3. Insert the needle of the prefilled syringe of medication into the injection port.
4. Inject the medication through the catheter.
5. Remove the needle when all medication has been administered.
6. Allow the solution to remain in the bladder the prescribed period of time.
7. Open the clamp on the drainage bag to allow the solution to drain. Assess that all solution has returned.
8. Reposition the patient comfortably.
9. Discard equipment or return it to the appropriate location.

PATIENT AND/OR FAMILY TEACHING
1. Explain the procedure to the patient.
2. Inform the patient of the medication to be administered and the purpose of the medication.
3. Instruct the patient to notify the nurse if experiencing any discomfort or urgency to void during the procedure.
4. Instruct the patient regarding the care of the catheter as described in "Care and Maintenance of an Indwelling Catheter."

DOCUMENTATION
1. Time, type of medication, dosage, and amount of medicated solution instilled into the bladder.
2. Length of time medication remained in bladder.
3. Amount, color, and clarity of return drainage.
4. Any discomfort the patient experienced during the procedure.
5. All patient teaching done and the patient's level of understanding.

Vaginal Instillation of Suppositories, Creams, and Medicated Tampons _____

PURPOSE

1. Provide a route for the administration of medications vaginally.

REQUISITES

1. Prescribed medication
2. Vaginal applicator, if appropriate
3. Sterile gloves
4. Exam gloves
5. Bed protector
6. Bath blanket
7. Disposable tissue
8. Washbasin
9. Towel and washcloth

GUIDELINES

1. Vaginal medications may be indicated to treat a vaginal infection, enhance the growth of normal bacteria in the vagina, or relieve discomfort and irritation.

2. Before administering any new medication, the nurse should know the actions of the drug, the reason for giving the drug, the normal dosage and route of administration, incompatibilities, contraindications, and adverse reactions.

3. The "five rights" of drug administration should be followed whenever a drug is administered: the right drug, the right dose, the right time, the right route, and the right patient.

4. Certain health care facility policies permit properly instructed patients to insert their own vaginal medications. Refer to your policy.

5. If both a vaginal irrigation and a vaginal medication have been ordered, the irrigation should be performed prior to inserting the medication unless otherwise ordered.

6. Although this is a clean procedure, sterile gloves should be worn.

7. Before administering any new medications, patient allergies should be assessed.

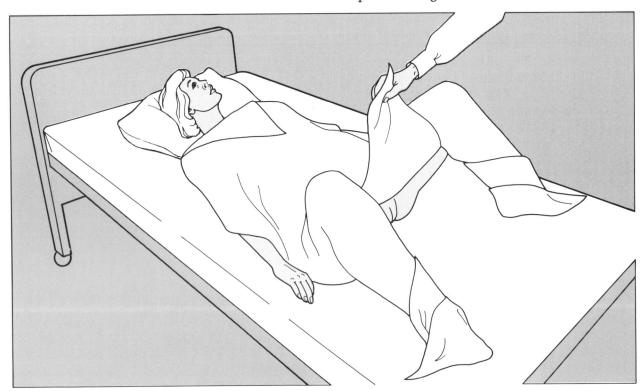

Figure 2-12. Dorsal recumbent position for vaginal instillation.

NURSING ACTION/RATIONALE

1. Assemble all equipment.
2. Verify the physician's order.
3. Identify the patient.
4. Explain the procedure and its purpose to the patient.
5. Provide privacy.
6. Instruct the patient to void in the toilet if ambulatory or in the bedpan if on bedrest.
7. Position the patient in the dorsal recumbent position. Drape the patient leaving only the perineum exposed. Place the bed protector under the patient's buttocks (Figure 2-12).
8. Provide adequate lighting.
9. Wash your hands.
10. Put on the exam gloves.
11. Examine the perineum assessing for drainage or irritation.
12. Cleanse the perineum with soap and water.
13. Remove the exam gloves.
14. Put on the sterile gloves.
15. Spread the patient's labia with one gloved hand. Gently insert the medication 2 inches into the vagina, using an applicator or gloved index finger (Figure 2-13).

16. Wipe the perineum with tissue, if necessary.
17. Instruct the patient to remain in bed for at least 30 minutes so the medication is not expelled and treatment can be facilitated.
18. Wash the applicator with warm soapy water if it is reusable, and store in a dry, clean area. Applicators are for single patient use only.
19. Remove the sterile gloves.
20. Assist the patient to a comfortable position.
21. Discard equipment or return it to the appropriate location.
22. Reassess the patient after 30 minutes to determine if the medication has been retained.

PATIENT AND/OR FAMILY TEACHING

1. Explain the procedure and the purpose of the medication.
2. Instruct the patient to remain in bed for 30 minutes following medication administration for maximum absorption of the medication.
3. Instruct the patient on perineal hygiene, including cleansing the perineal area from front to back.
4. Instruct the patient on self-administration of the medication, if appropriate.

DOCUMENTATION

1. Time, medication, dosage, and route of administration.
2. Assessment of the perineum including any drainage noted.
3. The patient's reaction to the procedure.
4. All patient teaching done and the patient's level of understanding.

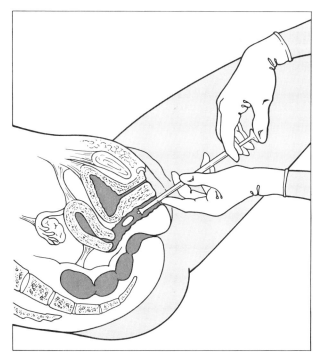

Figure 2-13. Correct insertion of vaginal medication.

Urethral Suppository

PURPOSE
1. Provide a route for the administration of medications into the urethra.

REQUISITES
1. Medication as prescribed
2. Sterile water-soluble lubricant
3. Sterile gloves
4. Cleansing towelette

GUIDELINES
1. Urethral suppositories are used in the treatment of urethritis to treat the infectious process and to control pain.
2. Patients are generally taught how to administer their own urethral suppositories since most treatment is in the outpatient setting.
3. Urethral suppositories are usually refrigerated until immediately before use to maintain firmness.
4. As with all medications, observe the "five rights" of administration: the right patient, the right medication, the right dosage, the right route, and the right time.
5. Before administering any medication, the nurse should know the actions of the drug, the reason for giving the drug, the normal dosage and route of administration, incompatibilities, contraindications, and adverse reactions.
6. Patient allergies should be assessed before administering any new medications.

NURSING ACTION/RATIONALE
1. Assemble all equipment.
2. Verify the medication order.
3. Identify the patient.
4. Explain the purpose and the nature of the procedure to the patient.
5. Provide privacy and adequate lighting.
6. Wash your hands.
7. Have the female patient lie supine with knees flexed and legs spread apart. Have the male patient lie supine with the legs flat.
8. Drape the patient.
9. Unwrap the urethral suppository partially and lubricate the tip, maintaining aseptic technique.
10. Put on sterile gloves.
11. Cleanse the meatus with the towelette. For females, separate the labia for cleansing and continue to hold the labia apart.
12. Insert the suppository gently through the meatus and into the urethral canal.
13. Position the patient in a comfortable position.
14. Discard equipment or return it to the appropriate area.

PATIENT AND/OR FAMILY TEACHING
1. Explain the purpose of the medication and why the urethral route is used.
2. Reinforce and clarify the physician's explanation of the disease process.
3. Teach perineal/genital hygiene.
4. Teach the patient self-administration of the suppository, if necessary, for discharge.

DOCUMENTATION
1. Medication, date, time, dosage, and route of administration.
2. Appearance of the perineum and urethral opening.
3. All patient teaching done and the patient's level of understanding.

Rectal Suppository

PURPOSE

1. Provide a route for the administration of medications to obtain local and systemic effects.

REQUISITES

1. Suppository as prescribed
2. Exam glove
3. Water-soluble lubricant
4. Toilet tissue
5. Waste receptacle

GUIDELINES

1. A history of any rectal pathology such as hemorrhoids, rectal bleeding, or rectal surgery should be assessed prior to initiating the procedure.
2. A rectal suppository is a medication in a firm base which is molded into a shape suitable for insertion into the rectum. It melts at body temperature.
3. Encouraging the patient to breathe through the mouth during suppository insertion helps relax the anal sphincter, thus facilitating the insertion of the suppository.
4. If a fecal impaction is suspected, a rectal assessment should be performed before administering the suppository. Inserting the suppository into fecal material may block the action and effect of the suppository.
5. As with all medications, observe the "five rights" of administration: the right patient, the right medication, the right dosage, the right route, and the right time.
6. Before administering any medication, the nurse should know the actions of the drug, the reason for giving the drug, the normal dosage and route of administration, incompatibilities, contraindications, and adverse reactions.
7. Patient allergies should be assessed before administering any new medications.

NURSING ACTION/RATIONALE

1. Assemble all equipment.
2. Verify the medication order.
3. Identify the patient.
4. Explain the procedure to the patient including the effect of the medication and whether the suppository should be retained or expelled.
5. Provide privacy.
6. Wash your hands.
7. Assist the patient into the left lateral position with the knees slightly bent, unless contraindicated (Figure 2-14).

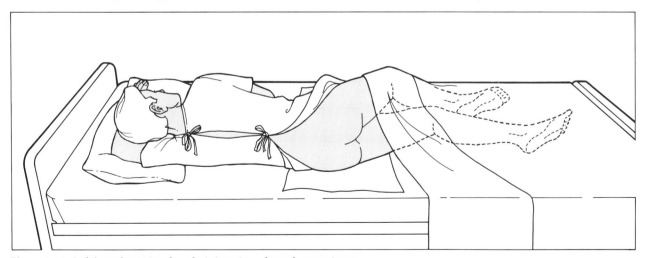

Figure 2-14. Left lateral position for administration of rectal suppository.

8. Put the exam glove on your dominant hand.
9. Remove the wrapper from the suppository and lubricate the suppository.
10. Separate the patient's buttocks with the ungloved hand to expose the anus.
11. Instruct the patient to take long deep breaths through the mouth.
12. Insert the suppository into the anus, tapered end first, with the gloved hand.
13. Advance the suppository beyond the sphincter muscle (approximately 2 inches).
14. Cleanse the anal area with toilet tissue.
15. Remove the exam glove.
16. Assist the patient to a comfortable position. Position the call signal within reach.
17. Instruct the patient to notify the nurse regarding the effect of the suppository. If given for a laxative effect, instruct the patient not to flush the toilet.
18. Discard equipment or return it to the appropriate location.
19. Wash your hands.

PATIENT AND/OR FAMILY TEACHING

1. Explain the procedure, the medication, and the effect of the medication to the patient.
2. Instruct the patient to defecate when the urge is felt if the suppository is being given to relieve constipation.
3. Instruct the patient to notify the nurse if the suppository results are to be assessed.
4. Instruct the patient to remain in bed in a supine position to aid in retaining a non-laxative suppository.
5. Teach the patient and/or family the procedure for administering the suppository if use will be continued following discharge.

DOCUMENTATION

1. Medication, date, time, dosage, and route of administration.
2. Effects of the suppository.
3. All patient and/or family teaching done and the level of understanding.

Intravenous Therapy

Unit 3

Intravenous Therapy

PURPOSE

1. Provide a route for the intravenous administration of medications, intravenous solutions, and blood and blood components.

REQUISITES

1. Intravenous administration tubing
2. Intravenous fluid, as ordered by the physician
3. Intravenous needle of choice
4. Sterile saline syringe, 5 cc
5. Tourniquet
6. Antiseptic wipes
7. Antiseptic ointment
8. Sterile 2 × 2 gauze—3
9. Tape
10. Bed protector
11. IV standard
12. Waste receptacle
13. Adequate lighting
14. Intravenous filter (optional)

GUIDELINES

1. Most health care facilities have policies governing the initiating of intravenous therapy. Refer to your facility's policy manual.
2. Aseptic technique must be maintained when performing this procedure.
3. Intravenous therapy is performed for a wide variety of reasons. The person initiating the intravenous therapy should have a clear understanding of the reason for the therapy.
4. Intravenous needles should not be introduced into the affected arm of a post-mastectomy patient, an arm with a functioning arteriovenous fistula, an affected arm of a paralyzed patient, or any arm that has circulatory or neurological impairment.
5. Lower extremity veins should not be used for intravenous therapy except when specifically ordered by the physician. Circulating blood in the lower extremities is more likely to pool and clot, resulting in an embolism.
6. Avoid using the patient's dominant arm for intravenous therapy, when possible, to help maintain the patient's independence.
7. Venipunctures should be initiated in the distal part of the upper extremities first (Figure 3-1). As the intravenous site is

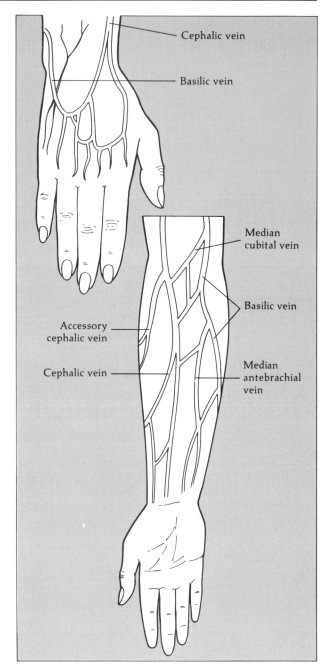

Figure 3-1. Dorsal and ventral view of the veins of the hand and forearm.

relocated for continuous therapy, the proximal veins can be used. Fluid flowing through a damaged or irritated vein can cause further damage.

8. Avoid locating intravenous needles over joints, since this will severely decrease the patient's mobility and can cause infiltration to occur more readily.

9. Intravenous needles should be relocated every 72 hours to help prevent the development of phlebitis.

10. Needles should be relocated promptly upon evidence of:
    a. Edema
    b. Redness or phlebitis
    c. Pain
    d. Subcutaneous infiltration

11. A functioning intravenous infusion in a critical patient should not be discontinued until another successful venipuncture has been performed.

12. A variety of intravenous needles are available. The type and size of needle used should be determined by the size of the patient's veins and the type of solution to be administered.

13. The use of intravenous filters varies in health care facilities. Intravenous filters remove particulate matter, which may cause irritation and phlebitis, from the solution.

14. Clear transparent occlusive dressings are available for use over the puncture site. The advantage of this type of dressing is that the dressing does not have to be changed as frequently because the site can be observed through the dressing.

15. Shaving the skin can promote bacterial growth if small cuts occur. Shaving should only be done when absolutely necessary to secure the intravenous needle in place.

16. All patients on intravenous therapy should have a regular assessment of their intake and output.

17. For further information on intravenous therapy, see the procedure "Care and Maintenance of the Intravenous Therapy System."

18. The following procedure demonstrates the proper set-up of an intravenous bottle. Set-up of an intravenous bag varies slightly in the method of inserting the spike of the tubing into the bag outlet.

19. The formula for determining the drip rate of an intravenous infusion is:

$$\text{drops/minute} = \frac{\text{Total cc to be infused} \times \text{drops/cc}}{\text{Total infusion time in minutes}}$$

The delivery rate in drops per cc is printed on all intravenous-tubing packaging.

NURSING ACTION/RATIONALE

1. Assemble all equipment.
2. Verify the intravenous infusion order.
3. Calculate the rate of infusion on the basis of the amount of solution and the length of infusion time.
4. Inspect the intravenous solution for:
   a. Color and clarity.
   b. Particulate matter.
   c. Defects in the bottle, cap, or hanging device.
   d. Expiration date.
5. Wash your hands.
6. Prepare the intravenous solution and tubing:
   a. Remove the overseal cap on the solution bottle.
   b. Cleanse the rubber stopper with an antiseptic wipe, using friction, and allow to dry.
   c. Close the clamp on the administration set and remove the protective cover over the spike.
   d. Place the solution bottle on a firm surface and insert the spike through the rubber stopper. Invert the bottle and hang it on the IV standard.
   e. Fill the drip chamber half full by squeezing and releasing it. Open the clamp and allow fluid to completely fill the tubing. Close the clamp.
7. Identify the patient.
8. Explain the procedure to the patient, including the reason for the therapy, sensations anticipated, length of therapy (if known), any activity restrictions, and the importance of remaining immobile during the venipuncture.
9. Position the patient in a semi-Fowler's or supine position. Remove the sleeve of the patient's garment and any watch or other constriction.

10. Provide adequate lighting and privacy.
11. Place a bed protector under the selected arm.
12. Wash your hands.
13. Lower the selected arm and apply the tourniquet about 6 inches above the planned venipuncture site. Assess if a radial pulse is palpable. If not, remove the tourniquet and reapply with less tension. Return the arm to a resting position.
14. Select the vein by sight and palpation. If the veins are not distended, have the patient open and close the hand to increase the blood supply. If unable to locate a vein, remove the tourniquet and wrap the extremity in a warm moist towel for 10 minutes. Reapply the tourniquet and select the vein.
15. Cleanse the skin around the venipuncture site with antiseptic wipes. Start at the planned venipuncture site and rub in a circular motion outward for 2 inches in diameter (Figure 3-2). Allow the area to dry for 1 minute.

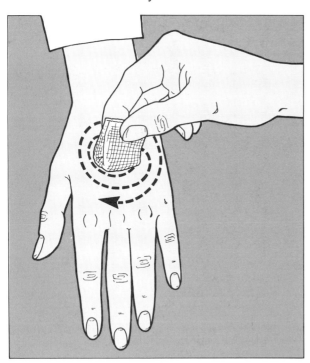

Figure 3-2. Use friction and prep the skin in a circular motion, moving away from the insertion site.

16. Remove the needle from the protector and inspect it for flaws. If using a scalp vein needle, attach a syringe of sterile saline to the end of the short tubing and flush the needle with saline. Leave the syringe attached.

17. Perform the venipuncture:
    a. Retract the skin and stabilize the vein distal to the puncture site with the thumb of your free hand.
    b. Hold the needle bevel up at a 30 to 45 degree angle to the skin directly over the vein (Figure 3-3). Insert the needle in one smooth motion through the skin and the vein wall. A flashback of blood in the flashback chamber of a plastic catheter needle indicates the vein has been entered. If using a scalp vein needle, aspirate the sterile saline syringe to observe for a blood return. If the vein has not been entered, reassess the location of the vein and the tip of the needle. Do not remove the needle, but advance the needle into the vein.

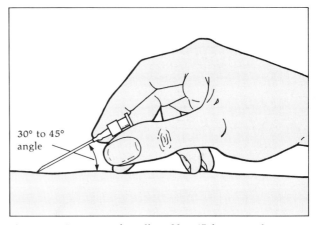

Figure 3-3. Insertion of needle at 30 to 45 degree angle.

    c. Remove the tourniquet.
    d. Lower the angle of the needle and advance it along the vein wall. For a plastic catheter, advance the plastic sheath while holding the metal stylet stable. When the plastic catheter has been completely advanced, remove the stylet.
    e. Attach the IV tubing to the hub of the needle, using aseptic technique.

f. Open the clamp on the tubing and allow the fluid to flow slowly. Watch the insertion site for signs of any infiltration. If an infiltration is noted, clamp the tubing, remove the intravenous needle, and repeat the venipuncture at a different site with new sterile equipment.

g. Anchor the intravenous needle with tape, securely (Figure 3-4). Do not tape over the insertion site or the junction of the needle and tubing.

h. Apply antiseptic ointment to the insertion site and cover with a 2 × 2 gauze sponge. Tape securely. Apply an additional 2 × 2 gauze sponge under the hub of the plastic cannula. Tape the intravenous tubing and gauze sponges to the patient's arm. Label the intravenous site dressing with the date, time, type of needle, size of needle, and your initials (Figure 3-5).

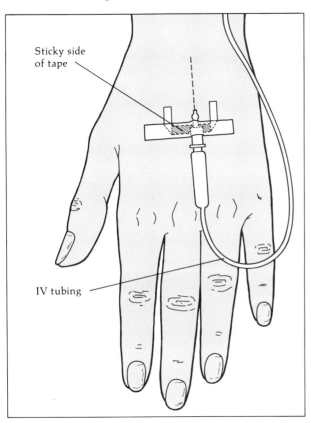

Figure 3-4. Tape the plastic catheter securely.

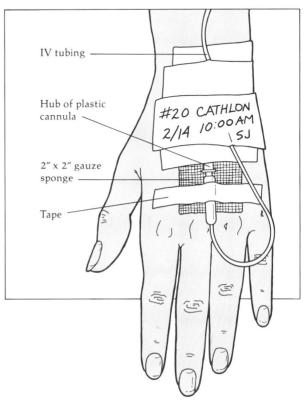

Figure 3-5. IV site dressing.

18. Regulate the drip rate of the infusion with the roller clamp as ordered.
19. Mark the solution bottle at appropriate time intervals and label with the patient's name, room number, date, and bottle number (Figure 3-6).

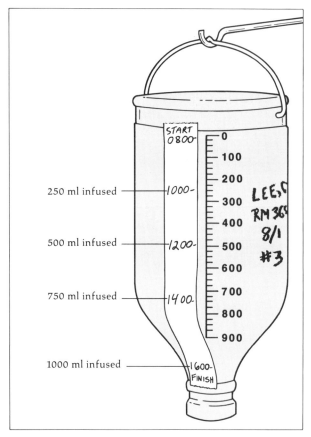

250 ml infused
500 ml infused
750 ml infused
1000 ml infused

START
0800
1000
1200
1400
1600
FINISH

0
100
200
300
400
500
600
700
800
900

LEE, C
RM 369
8/1
#3

Figure 3-6. Marked solution bottle.

20. Discard or return all equipment to the appropriate area.
21. Reassess the infusion site, drip rate, and patient condition frequently during the infusion.

PATIENT AND/OR FAMILY TEACHING
1. Explain the procedure to the patient as described in the "Nursing Action/Rationale" section.
2. Instruct the patient not to adjust the flow rate or bend or pinch the tubing.
3. Instruct the patient to call the nurse if any sensations of swelling, heat, burning, pain, or drainage are noted at the puncture site or if blood is backing up into the tubing.
4. Instruct the patient not to manipulate the dressings or the needle.
5. Demonstrate precautions for ambulating with an intravenous infusion if ambulation is allowed.
6. Explain related therapeutic orders as appropriate.
7. Warn the patient that an increase in urination is likely to occur, and is normal.

DOCUMENTATION
1. Date, time, and site of venipuncture.
2. Type and size of needle used.
3. Type, amount, lot number, and rate of flow of intravenous solution.
4. Any problems encountered with the procedure.
5. All patient teaching done and the patient's level of understanding.

Care and Maintenance of the Intravenous Therapy System _____

PURPOSE
1. Decrease the possibility of complications related to the intravenous therapy system.

REQUISITES
1. Sterile 2 × 2 gauze sponge—2
2. Antiseptic wipes
3. Antiseptic ointment
4. Tape
5. Waste receptacle
6. Other equipment as appropriate to the specific procedure. (Refer to related intravenous procedures.)

GUIDELINES
1. Aseptic technique must be maintained whenever procedures involving the intravenous therapy system are performed.
2. Whenever a break in technique occurs while working with the intravenous therapy system resulting in contamination of part or all of the system, the part involved or the entire system should be changed.
3. Intravenous administration tubing should be changed every 24 to 48 hours, depending on how often the closed system is entered. The more frequently the system is entered, the greater the possibility of contamination and the more frequently the tubing should be changed. (Refer to the procedure "Intravenous Therapy" for correct set-up of the system.)
4. Intravenous needles should be routinely relocated every 72 hours to decrease the possibility of irritation to the vein and the development of a phlebitis. (Refer to the procedure "Intravenous Therapy" for the correct method of venipuncture.)
5. Intravenous solutions infusing at a very slow rate should be changed at least every 24 hours to decrease the possibility of bacterial growth in the solution. (Refer to the procedure "Continuous Intravenous Medication Infusion Drip" for the correct method of changing a solution bottle.)

6. Intravenous dressings should be changed once every 24 hours and the site cleansed and assessed for signs of inflammation, including:
   a. Redness
   b. Edema
   c. Tenderness or pain
   d. Drainage
7. The venipuncture site should be assessed for signs of subcutaneous infiltration at least every 2 hours, or more often if the intravenous solution is infusing at a rapid rate.
8. The intravenous needle should be relocated immediately upon any signs of inflammation or infiltration.
9. Any patient complaint of discomfort at the venipuncture site should be investigated thoroughly.
10. The dressing change, tubing change, and solution bottle change should be done at the same time whenever possible.

NURSING ACTION/RATIONALE
Dressing Change
1. Assemble all equipment.
2. Identify the patient.
3. Explain the procedure to the patient, assuring the patient that there will be minimal discomfort.
4. Provide adequate lighting.
5. Position the patient comfortably with the venipuncture extremity in a resting position.
6. Wash your hands.
7. Remove the dressing tape carefully, holding the skin taut to decrease discomfort.
8. Lift the dressing off, touching only the outer surface of the dressing.
9. Assess the venipuncture site.
10. Remove the tape securing the needle if it is loose or soiled, or if it is covering the venipuncture site or the tubing and needle hub junction. Apply new tape.

11. Change the administration tubing at this time if a tubing change is indicated:
    a. Cleanse the junction of the tubing and needle with an antiseptic wipe.
    b. Close the clamp on the tubing.
    c. Grasp the needle hub and loosen the old tubing from the needle by twisting it.
    d. Remove the protector cap from the new primed tubing, maintaining aseptic technique.
    e. Remove the old tubing from the needle hub and insert the new tubing quickly, maintaining aseptic technique.
    f. Open the clamp and adjust the flow rate.
12. Cleanse the insertion site with antiseptic wipes, using one wipe for each stroke and discarding in the waste receptacle. Remove all old antiseptic ointment remaining.
13. Apply antiseptic ointment to the venipuncture site.
14. Place a sterile 2 × 2 gauze over the puncture site, and another 2 × 2 gauze under the hub of the needle.
15. Tape the dressings in place securely.
16. Loop the tubing distal to the puncture site, allowing some slack. Tape the tubing to the arm.
17. Label the dressing with a piece of tape, indicating type and size of needle, date, and your initials.
18. Assist the patient to a comfortable position.
19. Discard equipment or return it to the appropriate location.

Troubleshooting

1. Blood backed up in the tubing:
    a. Check the tubing for any kinks or bends. Check the clamp to make sure it is open.
    b. Raise the height of the bottle.
    c. Open the clamp to increase the flow rate temporarily.
    d. Place the tubing between your thumb and a hard surface such as a pencil, and strip the tubing in the direction of the needle in one smooth movement.
    e. Relocate the intravenous needle if unable to regain a solution flow. Never irrigate an occluded intravenous needle.

2. A sluggish flow rate, or no flow rate:
    a. Assess the site for subcutaneous infiltration.
    b. Try steps a, b, c, and d listed in item 1 under "Troubleshooting."
    c. Reposition the patient's extremity.
    d. Apply a warm compress over the venipuncture site if the solution infusing is cool. Cool solution can cause constriction of the blood vessel around the needle.
    e. Perform a tubing change if the system has a filter. The filter may be occluded.
    f. Relocate the intravenous needle if unable to regain an adequate solution flow. Never irrigate an occluded intravenous needle.

3. Tubing disconnected:
    a. Cleanse the ends of the tubing with an antiseptic wipe, using friction.
    b. Reconnect the tubing.
    c. Prepare new tubing and perform a tubing change immediately.

4. Solution bottle broken:
    a. Clamp off the tubing immediately.
    b. Perform a solution bottle and tubing change immediately.
    c. Relocate the intravenous needle if it has occluded. Never irrigate an occluded intravenous needle.

PATIENT AND/OR FAMILY TEACHING

1. Explain all procedures to the patient before starting. Warn the patient if discomfort is anticipated.
2. Explain any activity restrictions.
3. Instruct the patient to keep the affected extremity lower than the solution bottle.
4. Instruct the patient to avoid getting the venipuncture site wet.
5. Instruct the patient not to manipulate the tubing, dressing, or flow clamp.
6. Reinforce any previous instructions to notify the nurse if:
    a. Discomfort is experienced at the site.
    b. Blood is backed up in the tubing.
    c. The tubing has become disconnected.
    d. The venipuncture site dressing becomes wet.

DOCUMENTATION

1. Any procedure performed with the intravenous therapy system. (See related intravenous procedures.)
2. Assessment of the venipuncture site and functioning of the system.
3. Any complications, interventions, and results.
4. Any patient teaching done and the patient's level of understanding.

 # Removal of the Intravenous Device

PURPOSE

1. Remove the intravenous device.

REQUISITES

1. Sterile 2 × 2 gauze sponges—2
2. Antiseptic ointment
3. Tape
4. Waste receptacle

GUIDELINES

1. Intravenous devices are removed for a number of reasons including:
   a. A physician's order to discontinue intravenous therapy.
   b. Relocating the intravenous site every 72 hours for continuous intravenous therapy.
   c. An intravenous site having signs of redness, edema, pain, or subcutaneous infiltration.
2. The nurse discontinuing the intravenous device should be aware of the type of needle being used before attempting to terminate it.

3. Adhesive strips should not be used to cover the intravenous puncture site after termination, because they do not apply sufficient pressure to prevent bleeding or hematoma formation.
4. Never remove a functioning intravenous device from a critical patient until another successful venipuncture has been performed.

NURSING ACTION/RATIONALE

1. Assemble all equipment.
2. Verify the intravenous termination order, if appropriate.
3. Identify the patient.
4. Provide adequate lighting.
5. Explain the procedure to the patient and warn the patient that a slight burning sensation may be felt.
6. Wash your hands.
7. Stop the flow of the infusion by closing the roller clamp, if a solution is infusing.
8. Remove all tape and lift off the existing dressing. Discard into the waste receptacle. Note the condition of the puncture site and surrounding tissue.
9. Loosen or remove the tape securing the needle.

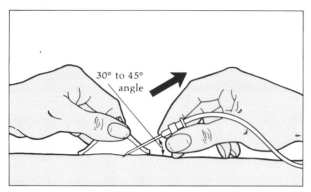

Figure 3-7. Removal of needle at 30 to 45 degree angle.

10. Place a sterile 2 × 2 gauze sponge over the puncture site, applying slight pressure. Remove the intravenous needle, following the path of insertion (Figure 3-7). Immediately apply more pressure to the 2 × 2 gauze over the puncture site and elevate the extremity.
11. Assess that the intravenous device is intact.
12. Remove the 2 × 2 gauze sponge when the bleeding has stopped, and discard in the waste receptacle. Return the extremity to a resting position.
13. Apply antiseptic ointment to the puncture site.
14. Apply a sterile 2 × 2 gauze sponge, using aseptic technique, and tape securely.
15. Discard equipment or return it to the appropriate area.
16. Assess the puncture site in 15 minutes to ensure that no bleeding has occurred.

PATIENT AND/OR FAMILY TEACHING

1. Explain the procedure to the patient and warn the patient that a burning sensation may be experienced.
2. Instruct the patient to avoid vigorous activity with the extremity for at least 15 minutes following removal of the device.
3. Instruct the patient to call the nurse if bleeding from the site occurs.
4. Explain any other changes in the treatment plan.
5. Encourage the patient to increase fluid intake, if appropriate.

DOCUMENTATION

1. Time, site, and type of needle terminated and reason for termination.
2. Condition of catheter or needle.
3. Assessment of the venipuncture site.
4. Amount of solution infused, if appropriate.
5. All patient teaching done and the patient's level of understanding.

Administration of Intravenous Piggyback Medications

PURPOSE

1. Administer a diluted medication intravenously through an existing intravenous line at prescribed intervals over a prescribed period of time.

REQUISITES

1. Existing intravenous line with Primary Piggyback tubing (Abbott Laboratories)
2. Premixed bottle of medication in dilutant
3. Secondary Piggyback tubing with a needle and extension hanger (Abbott Laboratories)
4. Antiseptic wipes
5. Tape
6. IV administration set with a needle attached (for heparin lock)
7. Prefilled sterile saline syringes— 2 (for heparin lock)
8. Prefilled syringe of heparin (100 U/cc) (for heparin lock)
9. IV standard

GUIDELINES

1. Before administering any medication the nurse should know the actions of the drug, the reason for giving the drug, the normal dosage and route of administration, incompatibilities, contraindications, and adverse reactions.
2. The "five rights" of drug administration should be followed each time a medication is administered: the right medication, the right dosage, the right time, the right route, and the right patient.
3. A drug that is incompatible with the primary intravenous solution cannot be administered via intravenous piggyback through that line unless the line is flushed with a compatible solution.
4. There are a variety of products on the market for administering piggyback medications. Follow the manufacturer's recommendations for the product being used. The procedure described here is based on the use of Abbott Laboratories equipment.
5. It is best to have intravenous admixtures prepared in the pharmacy under sterile conditions to prevent bacterial contamination of the solution.

6. Since the onset of action of a medication given intravenously is more rapid than with other routes of administration, the patient should be assessed closely for the therapeutic effect of the drug and any adverse reactions.
7. Patient allergies should be determined prior to initiating administration of any medication.

NURSING ACTION/RATIONALE

1. Assemble all equipment.
2. Verify the medication order.
3. Wash your hands.
4. Check the expiration date on the prepared piggyback solution.
5. Prepare the piggyback bottle and tubing:
    a. Remove the covering from the bottle.
    b. Cleanse the stopper with an antiseptic wipe, using friction.
    c. Close the clamp on the Secondary Piggyback tubing.
    d. Insert the spike of the tubing into the bottle.
    e. Invert the bottle and fill the drip chamber halfway by squeezing the drip chamber.
    f. Attach the needle to the tubing and remove the protective cover.
    g. Unclamp the tubing, flush carefully to prevent loss of solution, and reclamp.
    h. Cover the needle with the protector.
6. Identify the patient.
7. Explain the procedure, medication, and purpose to the patient.
8. Assess the intravenous site for patency.
9. Lower the primary intravenous bottle on the IV standard with the extension hanger.
10. Hang the secondary bottle with tubing on the IV standard. The secondary bottle will be higher than the primary bottle.
11. Rewash your hands.
12. Cleanse the port closest to the primary bottle with an antiseptic wipe. Allow it to dry.

13. Insert the needle on the piggyback tubing into the primary tubing port up to the hub. Tape the needle securely (Figure 3-8).

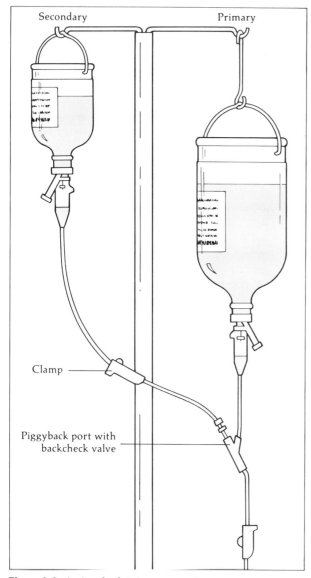

Secondary   Primary

Clamp

Piggyback port with backcheck valve

Figure 3-8. A piggyback intravenous set-up.

14. Open the clamp on the piggyback tubing completely. The rate of the infusion will be controlled by the clamp on the primary solution tubing.
15. Adjust the flow to the prescribed rate.
16. Assess the patient, the intravenous infusion, and the infusion site frequently during the administration of the intravenous medication.

17. Discontinue the piggyback infusion by clamping the Secondary Piggyback tubing, removing the needle, and covering with the protector, after all medication is infused. The primary bottle will automatically start infusing when the fluid in the secondary line is lower than the fluid level of the primary bottle.
18. Return the primary bottle to the original position and adjust the flow rate as prescribed.
19. Perform the following steps for administration of an intravenous piggyback medication through a heparin lock device. (See also, "Insertion and Management of a Heparin Lock").
    a. Follow nursing action steps 1, 2, and 3.
    b. Set up the piggyback solution and tubing as described in "Intravenous Therapy," adding the needle to the tubing before flushing.
    c. Identify the patient.
    d. Explain the procedure to the patient.
    e. Assess the intravenous site for patency.
    f. Wash your hands.
    g. Cleanse the diaphragm of the heparin lock device with an antiseptic wipe, and allow it to dry.
    h. Insert the needle of the sterile saline syringe through the diaphragm. Aspirate to check the patency of the heparin lock device. Inject the saline to flush the heparin out of the heparin lock device. Remove the syringe and needle.
    i. Insert the needle on the end of the solution tubing into the diaphragm of the heparin lock device.
    j. Regulate the flow of the medication solution as prescribed. Tape the needle to the heparin lock to secure it.
    k. Close the clamp on the tubing when the solution has infused, and remove the needle from the diaphragm.
    l. Cleanse the diaphragm with an antiseptic wipe and flush the heparin lock device with the second syringe of sterile saline if the medication is incompatible with heparin.
    m. Inject the heparin into the diaphragm of the heparin lock.
20. Discard equipment or return it to the appropriate location.

PATIENT AND/OR FAMILY TEACHING

1. Explain the procedure to the patient, and explain that no discomfort will be felt.
2. Inform the patient of the medication to be given and its purpose.
3. Explain to the patient that when the small bottle empties, the large bottle will begin to drip.
4. Explain any anticipated therapeutic effects of the drug, such as an increase in urination.
5. Instruct the patient to call the nurse for any unusual symptoms.

DOCUMENTATION

1. Medication, dosage, time, route, and rate of administration.
2. Total amount of intravenous administered on the patient's intake record.
3. Therapeutic effect of the drug, if any.
4. Any adverse reactions, interventions, and results.
5. All patient teaching done and the patient's level of understanding.

Continuous Intravenous Medication Infusion Drip

PURPOSE

1. Administer a medication on a continuous basis intravenously.

REQUISITES

1. Premixed intravenous solution with medication
2. Antiseptic wipes
3. An existing intravenous infusion, or equipment for initiating intravenous therapy (see "Intravenous Therapy")

GUIDELINES

1. Before administering any drug the nurse should know the actions of the drug, the reason for giving the drug, the normal dosage and route of administration, incompatibilities, contraindications, and adverse reactions.
2. The "five rights" of drug administration should be followed each time a medication is administered: the right medication, the right dosage, the right time, the right route, and the right patient.
3. Since the onset of action of a medication given intravenously is more rapid than with other routes of administration, the patient should be assessed closely for the therapeutic effect of the drug and any adverse reactions.
4. Intravenous solutions with medications are generally administered through a filter unless contraindicated by the drug manufacturer. Refer to your institution's policy manual or pharmacist.
5. Medications reconstituted and mixed in an intravenous solution should be discarded after 24 hours.
6. It is desirable to have intravenous admixtures prepared in the pharmacy under sterile conditions to prevent bacterial contamination of the solution.
7. Medications that require precise infusion rates, such as heparin, lidocaine, and aminophylline, should be placed in an intravenous pump or controller to ensure an accurate infusion.
8. To determine the compatibility of medications, refer to the *Physician's Desk Reference (PDR)*, *The American Hospital Formulary Service*, or your hospital pharmacist.
9. For further information regarding the initiation and care of an intravenous infusion, refer to the procedures "Intravenous Therapy" and "Care and Maintenance of the Intravenous Therapy System."
10. Patient allergies should be determined prior to initiating administration of any medication.

NURSING ACTION/RATIONALE

1. Assemble all equipment.
2. Verify the premixed intravenous solution with the physician's order for correct medication, dosage, time, and route.
3. Follow the procedure "Intravenous Therapy" if there is no existing intravenous infusion. A venipuncture will need to be done and the intravenous lines prepared.
4. Identify the patient.
5. Explain the procedure to the patient, including the medication to be administered, its purpose, and any anticipated effects.
6. Wash your hands.
7. Assess the infusion site for irritation or infiltration.
8. Remove the protective cover from the prepared intravenous solution.
9. Cleanse the seal with an antiseptic wipe, using friction, and allow it to dry.
10. Clamp the tubing on the existing intravenous line.
11. Remove the bottle from the intravenous standard and carefully remove the tubing spike from the existing bottle. Do not touch or contaminate the spike.
12. Insert the spike into the new bottle, using aseptic technique.
13. Hang the new bottle on the IV standard.
14. Open the clamp and adjust the flow rate.
15. Mark the bottle with times, indicating where the level of fluid should be at a specific time.
16. Discard equipment or return it to the appropriate location.
17. Assess the patient frequently for signs and symptoms of phlebitis or infiltration at the infusion site and response to the infusion.
18. Continue to assess the flow rate of the infusion.

PATIENT AND/OR FAMILY TEACHING

1. Explain the procedure to the patient, including the medication, its purpose, and anticipated effects.
2. Instruct the patient to call the nurse for any unusual symptoms.
3. See "Intravenous Therapy" and "Care and Maintenance of the Intravenous Therapy System" for further teaching areas.

DOCUMENTATION

1. Medication, dosage, time, route, and rate of administration.
2. Total amount of intravenous solution administered (on the patient's intake record).
3. Therapeutic effect of the drug, if any.
4. Any adverse reactions, interventions, and results.
5. All patient teaching done and the patient's level of understanding.

Administration of Intravenous Push Medications

PURPOSE
1. Administer a medication intravenously for immediate effect.
2. Administer a medication that cannot be given by another route.

REQUISITES
1. Sterile syringe, with correct medication and dosage and a 22 gauge, 1 inch needle attached
2. Antiseptic wipes
3. Watch with a second indicator
4. Sterile syringe and needle filled with 3 to 5 cc of sterile saline—2 (if medication is incompatible with heparin or the intravenous solution infusing)
5. Sterile syringe and needle with 1 cc of heparin 100 U/cc (for heparin lock only)

GUIDELINES
1. Before administering any medication, the nurse should know the actions of the drug, the reason for giving the drug, the normal dosage and route of administration, incompatibilities, contraindications, and adverse reactions.
2. The "five rights" of drug administration should be followed each time a medication is administered: the right medication, the right dosage, the right time, the right route, and the right patient.
3. Since the onset of action of a medication given via intravenous push is more rapid than with other routes of administration, the patient should be assessed closely for the therapeutic effect of the drug and any adverse rections.
4. Certain drugs have recommended rates of administration for the intravenous push route. Consult with the *Physician's Desk Reference (PDR), The American Hospital Formulary Service,* or the hospital pharmacist for specific information. If no specific rate is recommended, the rate of one (1) cc per minute is generally considered standard.

5. See the related intravenous procedures for insertion and management of the various intravenous devices.
6. Patient allergies should be determined prior to initiating administration of any medication.

NURSING ACTION/RATIONALE
1. Assemble all equipment.
2. Verify the medication order.
3. Calculate the rate of injection. See Guideline 4.
4. Determine any incompatibilities with heparin or with the intravenous solution presently infusing.
5. Identify the patient.
6. Explain the procedure, medication, and purpose to the patient, if appropriate.
7. Wash your hands.
8. Perform the following steps if the medication is to be given through an existing continuous intravenous infusion:
   a. Inspect the venipuncture site to determine that the infusion is patent, with no infiltration or phlebitis. If either condition is found, the intravenous needle must be relocated before continuing.
   b. Cleanse the port of the tubing closest to the needle with an antiseptic wipe, using friction. Allow to dry.
   c. If the medication to be administered is incompatible with the intravenous solution, insert the needle of the prefilled saline syringe into the injection port. Clamp the tubing close to the medication port, aspirate for blood to check for patency, and flush the tubing with the sterile saline. Remove the needle and syringe.

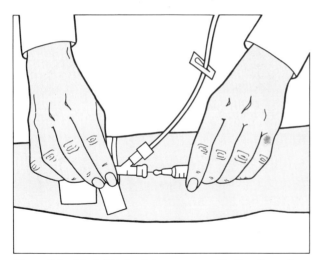

Figure 3-9. Administering intravenous medication through an intravenous line.

d. Insert the needle of the syringe with the medication into the port (Figure 3-9).
e. Clamp the tubing, if not already clamped.
f. Aspirate for a blood return to determine patency of the intravenous needle.
g. Inject the medication at the correct rate.
h. Remove the needle and syringe when the administration is complete.
i. For an incompatible drug, flush the intravenous tubing again with the second syringe of sterile saline, using the same method.
j. Unclamp the tubing and establish the previous infusion flow rate.
k. Discard or return all equipment to the proper location.

9. Perform the following steps if the medication is to be given through a heparin lock:
a. Assess the infusion site for phlebitis or inflammation and relocate the heparin lock as necessary.
b. Cleanse the injection site with an antiseptic swab. Allow to dry.
c. If the medication is incompatible with heparin, insert the needle with the syringe of sterile saline into the port.
d. Aspirate to determine patency.
e. Flush the intravenous needle with saline and remove.

f. Insert the needle with the syringe of medication into the port and inject the medication at the correct rate (Figure 3-10). Remove the syringe and needle.

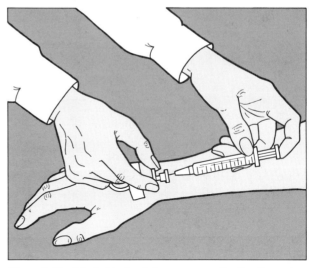

Figure 3-10. Administering intravenous medication through a heparin lock.

g. For an incompatible medication, insert the needle of the second saline syringe into the port and flush the intravenous needle. Remove the syringe and needle.
h. Insert the needle and syringe with the prefilled heparin, aspirate for patency, and instill the heparin into the heparin lock device. Remove the needle and syringe.
i. Discard equipment or return it to the appropriate location.

10. Assess the patient closely following intravenous push administration to determine the effectiveness of the drug or any adverse reactions.

PATIENT AND/OR FAMILY TEACHING

1. Explain the reason for the injection and the type of medication, if appropriate.
2. Explain any untoward effects of the medication, if appropriate.
3. Instruct the patient to report any pain or burning at the infusion site during or after the procedure.
4. Instruct the patient to notify the nurse if unusual symptoms occur.
5. Explain the schedule for administration of the medication, if appropriate.

DOCUMENTATION

1. Medication, dosage, time, route, and rate of administration.
2. Therapeutic effect of the drug, if any.
3. Any adverse reactions, interventions, and results.
4. All patient teaching done and the patient's level of understanding.

 # Insertion and Management of a Heparin Lock Device

PURPOSE

1. Provide an established venous access route.
2. Decrease the possibility of complications that may occur with the heparin lock device.

REQUISITES

Insertion

1. Intermittent infusion needle, or an intravenous needle and an adapter plug
2. Prefilled syringe of sterile saline for injection, with a needle attached.
3. Prefilled syringe of heparin (100 U/cc) with a needle attached
4. Tourniquet
5. Antiseptic wipes
6. Antiseptic ointment
7. 2 × 2 sterile gauze sponges—2
8. Tape

Converting

1. A functioning intravenous therapy system
2. Adapter plug
3. Prefilled syringe of sterile saline for injection, with a needle attached
4. Prefilled syringe of heparin (100 U/cc), with a needle attached
5. Antiseptic wipes

Anticoagulating

1. Prefilled syringe of heparin (100 U/cc), with a needle attached
2. Antiseptic wipes

GUIDELINES

1. A heparin lock is established as a precautionary measure for patients whose conditions could change rapidly, requiring an immediate access to the venous system for emergency use, or for patients who require intermittent infusion therapy. The heparin lock eliminates the need for multiple venipunctures.
2. The advantages of the heparin lock over continuous intravenous therapy are:
   a. It allows the patient to be more mobile while maintaining the venous access route.
   b. It allows for a readily available venous access route without increasing the patient's fluid intake when that is contraindicated.
3. A continuous intravenous therapy needle can be converted to a heparin lock device, or a new venipuncture with an intermittent infusion needle can be performed for the purpose of establishing a heparin lock.

4. Special heparin lock devices are available; these are butterfly needles with short tubing and a rubber diaphragm over the end of the tubing (Figure 3-11a). Also available is a hard plastic plug with a rubber diaphragm over one end, used to convert a regular intravenous needle to a heparin lock (Figure 3-11b).

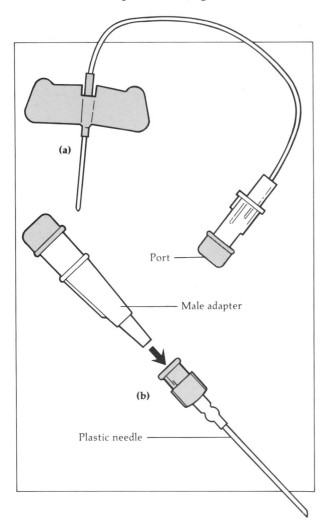

(a)

Port

Male adapter

(b)

Plastic needle

Figure 3-11. Types of heparin locks. (a) Butterfly heparin lock. (b) Male adapter plug.

5. A venipuncture for inserting a heparin lock needle is performed in the same manner as described in "Intravenous Therapy."
6. Care of the venipuncture site for a heparin lock is the same as described in "Care and Maintenance of the Intravenous Therapy System."

7. Administration of medications through the heparin lock device is described in the procedures, "Administration of Intravenous Push Medications" and "Administration of Intravenous Piggyback Medications."
8. The procedure for removal of the heparin lock device is the same as for all intravenous needles. Refer to the procedure "Removal of the Intravenous Device."
9. A heparin lock device that is not being entered for medication or intravenous fluid administration at regular intervals should be anticoagulated regularly to maintain the patency of the system. The frequency for anticoagulating the device depends upon the concentration of heparin being used, the health care facility's policy, and/or the physician's order.

NURSING ACTION/RATIONALE
Insertion
1. Assemble all equipment.
2. Verify the physician's order.
3. Identify the patient.
4. Explain the procedure to the patient. Explain the specific purpose of the heparin lock for the individual patient.
5. Position the patient comfortably.
6. Wash your hands.
7. Follow the steps in the procedure "Intravenous Therapy" for performing a venipuncture with a butterfly needle or a plastic needle.
8. Perform the following steps after a successful venipuncture:
   a. Butterfly intermittent infusion needle (a saline syringe with a needle should be in place in the rubber diaphragm when performing the venipuncture):
      (1) Aspirate the saline syringe plunger to check for a blood return.
      (2) Inject the saline slowly into the vein. Remove the syringe and needle.
      (3) Tape the needle in place.
      (4) Cleanse the rubber diaphragm with an antiseptic wipe and allow it to dry.
      (5) Insert the heparin syringe with needle into the rubber diaphragm.
      (6) Inject the heparin. Remove the syringe and needle.

(7) Apply a dressing to the site. (See "Intravenous Therapy.")

(8) Discard equipment or return it to the appropriate location.

b. Regular plastic catheter intravenous needle:

(1) Using aseptic technique, remove the metal stylet after advancing the plastic catheter into the vein. Insert the male end of the adapter plug into the hub of the needle.

(2) Tape the needle in place.

(3) Cleanse the rubber diaphragm of the plug with an antiseptic wipe and allow it to dry.

(4) Insert the sterile saline syringe needle into the diaphragm.

(5) Aspirate to remove all air from the plug and to check the needle for patency.

(6) Remove the syringe and needle.

(7) Expel all air from the saline syringe.

(8) Reinsert the syringe needle into the diaphragm and inject the sterile saline. Remove the syringe and needle.

(9) Insert the needle of the heparin syringe into the diaphragm. Inject the heparin slowly. Remove the syringe and needle.

(10) Dress the venipuncture site. (See "Intravenous Therapy.")

(11) Discard or return all equipment to the appropriate location.

Conversion (changing a continuous intravenous infusion to a heparin lock device)

1. Assemble all equipment.
2. Verify the physician's order.
3. Explain the procedure and its purpose to the patient.
4. Position the patient comfortably.
5. Wash your hands.
6. Cleanse the junction of tubing and needle with an antiseptic wipe.
7. Close the roller clamp on the intravenous tubing.

8. Loosen the tubing from the hub of the needle.
9. Remove the tubing from the needle and quickly insert the adapter plug into the hub, using aseptic technique.
10. Cleanse the adapter plug with an antiseptic wipe and allow it to dry.
11. Follow the steps for anticoagulating the needle as listed for insertion of a regular plastic catheter intravenous needle.

Anticoagulation (performed when the heparin lock device is not being used at regular intervals for medication or intravenous solution administration)

1. Assemble all equipment.
2. Verify the physician's order.
3. Identify the patient.
4. Explain the procedure to the patient.
5. Position the patient comfortably.
6. Wash your hands.
7. Cleanse the rubber diaphragm with an antiseptic wipe. Allow it to dry.
8. Insert the needle of the heparin syringe through the diaphragm.
9. Aspirate to assess for patency.
10. Inject the heparin slowly and remove the needle and syringe.
11. Discard equipment or return it to the appropriate location.

PATIENT AND/OR FAMILY TEACHING

1. Explain the procedure for inserting or converting a heparin lock, as appropriate.
2. Explain the purpose of the heparin lock.
3. Explain the care that will be given to the heparin lock and lock site, including anticoagulating it.
4. Explain any other therapeutic orders as appropriate, such as medications or intravenous solutions ordered to be administered through the heparin lock.
5. Instruct the patient to call the nurse if any redness, swelling, or pain is noted at the venipuncture site.

DOCUMENTATION

1. Type and size of needle inserted and location of venipuncture site, as appropriate.
2. Time intravenous system was converted to a heparin lock, as appropriate.
3. Medication, time, dosage, and route of all medications administered, including the heparin.
4. Assessment of the venipuncture site.
5. The patient's reaction to the procedure.
6. All patient teaching done and the patient's level of understanding.

 # Blood Transfusion Therapy

PURPOSE

1. Provide a route for the administration of blood or blood components.

REQUISITES

1. Unit of whole blood or blood component, as prescribed
2. Intravenous normal saline solution 0.9%
3. Y type blood administration tubing
4. Extension tubing, 20 inch
5. Antiseptic wipes
6. Blood pressure cuff, stethoscope, thermometer
7. Equipment for initiating a venipuncture, if necessary. Refer to the procedure "Intravenous Therapy."
8. IV standard

GUIDELINES

1. This procedure is appropriate for transfusion of whole blood, packed red blood cells, fresh frozen plasma, and leukocyte-free or poor red blood cells.
2. Accurate identification of the patient and donor blood to avoid error in administration is imperative. Each hospital has its own policy regarding blood donation, the type and crossmatch, and identification of the patient and the blood. Refer to your hospital's policy manual.
3. When a hematalogic deficit is related to a specific component in the blood, a transfusion of that specific component is advised rather than a transfusion of whole blood.
4. The venipuncture for blood transfusion therapy should be performed in a vein large enough to accommodate an 18 or 19 gauge needle. Intravenous needles vary in the size of the lumen of the needle. With some products, large amounts of blood can be infused well through a 20 gauge needle.
5. Blood tranfusions require a sterile filter of 170 microns to screen out any particulates and fibrin clots. This helps to prevent red cell hemolysis and infection.
6. Intravenous normal saline 0.9% should always be administered with a blood transfusion. Intravenous fluids containing glucose may cause hemolysis of red cells and are contraindicated.
7. Due to the possibility of bacterial growth in the recipient set and filter, most health care facilities have policies governing the frequency for changing the blood tubing.
8. The blood should remain in the blood bank refrigerator until immediately before the transfusion is begun. Blood should not remain at room temperature for more than 30 minutes before the infusion is started. Prewarming is not necessary unless large amounts of blood are to be given rapidly.

9. The rate of the blood transfusion is dependent upon the patient's condition and the product being transfused. If the patient is at risk of circulatory overload because of age or heart disease, the transfusion should be administered more slowly. One unit of whole blood should be transfused within 2 to 4 hours. Fresh frozen plasma should be transfused within 2 hours of thawing. One unit of packed red blood cells should be transfused within 2 to 3 hours.

10. Before and during the transfusion of whole blood the blood should be mixed gently by inverting it several times to evenly distribute the cells and plasma.

11. No medications should be given into an intravenous line through which blood is running.

12. The nurse must be aware of the clinical manifestations of transfusion reactions or complications so that there is no delay in diagnosis and intervention. Types of transfusion reactions and complications are described below.

    a. *Hemolytic reaction.* This reaction occurs when incompatible red cells are injected into the patient's circulating blood. This is the most life-threatening reaction and can cause renal failure and death. Signs and symptoms occur almost immediately and include flank pain, a feeling of fullness in the head, chest pressure, chills, neck vein distention, hypotension, tachypnea, and tachycardia.

    b. *Pyrogenic reaction.* This reaction is due to the presence of bacterial contamination in the blood, and symptoms usually occur near the end of the transfusion or after completion. Symptoms include sudden chilling, fever, headache, nausea, and vomiting. The mortality rate is high with this complication.

    c. *Allergic reaction.* This reaction occurs when antibodies in the patient's blood react to allergens in the donor's blood. The reaction may occur anytime during the transfusion. Symptoms include pruritis, urticaria, chills, fever, nausea, vomiting, asthmatic wheezing, and in severe cases, anaphylaxis.

    d. *Circulatory overload.* This complication is due to excessive volumes of blood being administered at a rate faster than the heart can accept. Symptoms include a rise in venous pressure, distended neck veins, dyspnea, cough, and râles heard in the base of the lungs.

    e. *Hyperkalemia.* This complication results when stored blood develops an abnormally high potassium level due to red blood cell lysis. Symptoms include muscle cramping and weakness, cardiac arrhythmias, nausea, vomiting, and diarrhea. As serum potassium levels rise, cardiac arrest may occur.

    f. *Hypocalcemia.* This complication is a reaction to toxic proportions of sodium citrate, which is used as a preservative in blood. The citrate ion binds with the calcium, and when the citrate is excreted the calcium is also excreted from the body. Symptoms include tingling sensations in fingers and toes, muscle cramps, convulsions, hypotension, and tetany. As serum calcium levels fall, cardiac arrest may occur.

    g. *Air embolism.* This complication may occur when a transfusion is given under pressure and air is introduced into the system. Symptoms include hypotension, tachycardia, and tachypnea.

13. Whenever a blood transfusion reaction or complication is suspected, the following measures should be implemented:

    a. Immediately stop the transfusion by closing the roller clamp; prime new intravenous tubing with the normal saline; disconnect the blood tubing at the extension and connect the normal saline tubing; open the clamp and infuse the normal saline to maintain the patency of the line.

    b. Monitor the patient closely and provide emergency treatment as necessary.

    c. Notify the physician immediately.

    d. Save the blood and the tubing and notify the blood bank personnel of the possible reaction.

    e. Send the first voided urine specimen of the patient following the reaction to the laboratory for analysis. Following a hemolytic reaction, red blood cells are found in the urine.

14. Before beginning the transfusion inspect the blood for gas bubbles and changes in color. Check the expiration date on the label. Never administer blood beyond its expiration date.
15. When administering blood to a comatose patient, extra precautions should be taken in observing for transfusion reactions or complications.
16. When administering blood transfusion therapy, assess the patient's vital signs, including temperature, frequently. Under normal circumstances, the vital signs should be assessed before the transfusion is started, 15 minutes after the transfusion is started, every hour during the transfusion, 1 hour following the transfusion, and every 4 hours for the next 24 hours. Vital signs should be assessed more frequently when the patient's condition is unstable.

NURSING ACTION/RATIONALE

1. Assemble all equipment.
2. Verify the physician's order.
3. Notify the blood bank of the order for whole blood or the blood component.
4. Identify the patient.
5. Explain the nature and purpose of the impending procedure to the patient.
6. Wash your hands.
7. Prepare the normal saline and tubing:
   a. Close all three roller clamps on the blood administration tubing. Attach the extension tube to the distal end.
   b. Cleanse the top of the normal saline with an antiseptic wipe and allow it to dry.
   c. Remove the protective cover from the intravenous solution tubing spike.
   d. Insert the spike into the bottle of normal saline.
   e. Invert the normal saline and hang it on the IV standard.
   f. Open the clamp on the Y tubing to the bottle.
   g. Fill the drip chamber with normal saline to just above the filter by squeezing and releasing the drip chamber.
   h. Open the clamp on the primary line and fill the tubing with normal saline.
   i. Close the clamp

8. Provide privacy.
9. Provide adequate lighting.
10. Position the patient for a venipuncture, if necessary.
11. Perform a venipuncture, if necessary. Refer to the procedure "Intravenous Therapy."
12. If an intravenous is infusing, cleanse the needle and tubing connection, close the clamp on the present tubing, disconnect the tubing from the needle, and attach the blood administration tubing to the needle. Open the roller clamp and adjust the flow of normal saline.
13. Follow your hospital's policy for verifying the patient identification and the blood component with laboratory personnel when the blood arrives.
14. Assess the patient's baseline vital signs, including temperature.
15. Wash your hands.
16. Prepare the unit of whole blood or blood component for infusion (Figure 3-12):
    a. Separate the tabs over the port on the blood unit.
    b. Remove the cover from the spike on the second Y tubing.
    c. Insert the spike into the port using a twisting motion, invert the blood unit, and hang it on the IV standard.
    d. Close the clamp on the Y tubing to the normal saline.
    e. Open the clamp on the Y tubing to the unit of blood.
    f. Squeeze the drip chamber to begin the flow of blood.

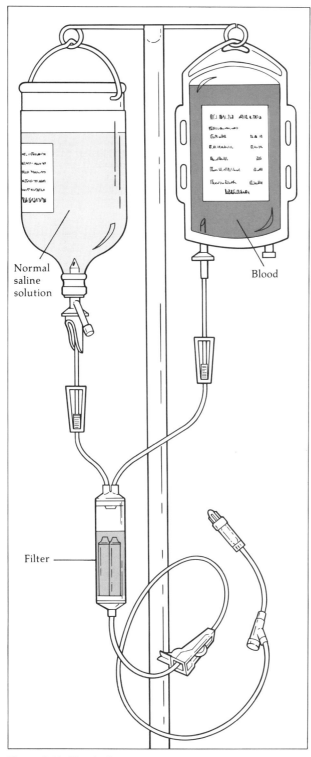

Normal saline solution

Blood

Filter

Figure 3-12. Blood administration set-up.

17. Adjust the flow rate as prescribed.
18. Stay with the patient for the first 15 minutes. Assess the patient for any untoward reactions.
19. Assess vital signs after 15 minutes.
20. Instruct the patient to notify the nurse of any unusual symptoms.
21. Reassess the patient frequently. Reassess the patient's vital signs as described in the guidelines or more frequently if necessary.
22. If a life-threatening complication occurs, stop the transfusion, attach a new intravenous line with normal saline and infuse the normal saline. Provide emergency treatment as necessary and notify the physician immediately.
23. After the infusion is completed, clear the tubing with normal saline and either discontinue the intravenous device or hang the prescribed solution with new tubing.
24. Discard equipment or return it to the appropriate location.

PATIENT AND/OR FAMILY TEACHING

1. Explain the nature and purpose of the transfusion.
2. Explain the possible reactions to the transfusion that can occur and the monitoring that will be done during the procedure.
3. Instruct the patient to notify the nurse if any of the following complications occur:
   a. Chills.
   b. Urticaria.
   c. Feeling of warmth.
   d. Breathing difficulty.
   e. Lightheadedness.
   f. Pain in the venipuncture site.
   g. Flank pain.
4. Explain additional therapeutic orders as appropriate.

DOCUMENTATION

1. Date, time the transfusion was started and discontinued, blood component administered, donor numbers, and approximate volume.
2. Normal saline hung and amount infused.
3. Any medications administered.
4. All parameters of assessment.
5. Any reactions, interventions, and results.
6. All patient teaching done and the patient's level of understanding.

Administration of White Blood Cells

PURPOSE

1. Provide a route for the administration of leukocytes and granulocytes.

REQUISITES

1. Unit of white blood cells
2. Intravenous normal saline 0.9%
3. Y type blood administration tubing
4. Extension tubing—20 inch
5. Antiseptic wipes
6. Blood pressure cuff, stethoscope, and thermometer
7. Equipment for initiating a venipuncture, if necessary. Refer to the procedure "Intravenous Therapy."
8. IV standard

GUIDELINES

1. Administration of white blood cells is indicated as supportive therapy for patients with neutropenia who have infections and are not responsive to antibiotic therapy. A great number of patients receiving white blood cells are oncology patients with severe bone marrow depression and progressive infections.

2. White blood cells obtained from a unit of whole blood contain numerous red blood cells. It is necessary for the patient to be ABO and Rh compatible to the donor because of the red blood cells.
3. The volume of one unit of white blood cells varies, depending on the method used in preparation. The volume is printed on the unit label.
4. Immediate transfusion following collection is recommended. In any case, the white cells must be transfused within 48 hours of collection.
5. White blood cell therapy usually includes 1 unit of white cells administered daily for 4 to 5 days. The effectiveness of the therapy is determined by the clinical improvement of the patient.
6. White blood cells should be administered slowly, and the patient should be assessed closely for any untoward reactions. The unit should be infused over a period of 2 to 4 hours.
7. The patient's vital signs should be taken before the transfusion, 15 minutes after the transfusion is started, every hour during the transfusion, and 1 hour following the transfusion.

8. The usual reactions related to blood transfusions can also be seen in white blood cell administration.

9. Some non-life-threatening problems with white blood cells call for close assessment and treatment, but not necessarily a discontinuation of treatment:

   a. *Chills and fever.* Shaking chills and temperature elevation are not serious. These reactions are usually treated symptomatically.

   b. *Urticaria.* Urticaria (hives) is an allergic reaction and is usually treated with an antihistamine. When urticaria appear on the face or neck, be alert for laryngeal edema. Patients are usually premedicated with an antihistamine to decrease the reaction.

   c. *Persistent cough.* The patient should be assessed closely since a persistent cough may indicate an impending respiratory reaction.

10. Other complications related to the administration of white blood cells are life-threatening and include:

    a. *Moderate hypotension.* The transfusion rate should be slowed, and the patient's vital signs should be monitored every 10 minutes until the blood pressure returns to normal.

    b. *Severe hypotension.* A significant fall in blood pressure accompanied by an increased pulse rate and lightheadedness is a reaction that requires immediate response. Stop the transfusion, maintain the intravenous line with normal saline, and notify the physician.

    c. *Severe pulmonary reaction.* This reaction is seen most frequently in patients with pulmonary infections. Symptoms may include cough, dyspnea, and hyperpnea. Stop the transfusion, maintain the intravenous line with normal saline, and notify the physician. Provide emergency treatment as indicated.

    d. *Anaphylactic reaction.* This is a medical emergency. Stop the transfusion, provide emergency treatment as indicated, and notify the physician.

NURSING ACTION/RATIONALE

1. Assemble all equipment.
2. Verify the physician's order.
3. Notify the blood bank of the order for white blood cells.
4. Identify the patient.
5. Explain the nature and purpose of the impending procedure to the patient. Explain the purpose of any prophylactic medication to the patient.
6. Wash your hands.
7. Prepare the normal saline and tubing:

   a. Close all three roller clamps on the blood administration tubing. Attach the extension tube to the distal end.

   b. Cleanse the top of the normal saline with an antiseptic wipe and allow it to dry.

   c. Remove the protective cover from the intravenous solution tubing spike.

   d. Insert the spike into the bottle of normal saline.

   e. Invert the normal saline and hang it on the IV standard.

   f. Open the clamp on the Y tubing to the bottle.

   g. Fill the drip chamber with normal saline to just above the filter by squeezing and releasing the drip chamber.

   h. Open the clamp on the primary line and fill the tubing with normal saline.

   i. Close the clamp.

8. Provide privacy.
9. Provide adequate lighting.
10. Position the patient for a venipuncture, if necessary.
11. Perform a venipuncture, if necessary. Refer to the procedure "Intravenous Therapy."
12. If an intravenous is infusing, cleanse the needle and tubing connection, close the clamp on the present tubing, disconnect the tubing from the needle, and attach the blood administration tubing to the needle. Open the roller clamp and adjust the flow of normal saline.
13. Follow your hospital's policy for verifying the patient's identification and the blood component with laboratory personnel when the blood arrives.

14. Assess the patient's baseline vital signs, including temperature.
15. Wash your hands.
16. Prepare the unit of white blood cells for infusion:
    a. Separate the tabs over the port on the blood unit.
    b. Remove the cover from the spike on the second Y tubing.
    c. Insert the spike into the port using a twisting motion, invert the white blood cell unit, and hang it on the IV standard.
    d. Close the clamp on the Y tubing to the normal saline.
    e. Open the clamp on the Y tubing to the unit of white blood cells.
    f. Squeeze the drip chamber to begin the flow of white cells.
17. Adjust the flow rate as prescribed.
18. Stay with the patient for the first 15 minutes. Assess the patient for any untoward reactions.
19. Assess vital signs after 15 minutes.
20. Instruct the patient to notify the nurse of any unusual symptoms.
21. Reassess the patient frequently. Reassess the patient's vital signs as described in the guidelines or more frequently if necessary.
22. If a life-threatening complication occurs, stop the transfusion, attach a new intravenous line with normal saline, and infuse the normal saline. Provide emergency treatment as necessary and notify the physician immediately.
23. After the infusion is completed, clear the tubing with normal saline and either discontinue the intravenous device or hang the prescribed solution with new tubing.
24. Discard equipment or return it to the appropriate location.

PATIENT AND/OR FAMILY TEACHING
1. Explain the nature and purpose of the transfusion.
2. Explain the possible reactions to the transfusion that can occur and the monitoring that will be done during the procedure.
3. Instruct the patient to notify the nurse if any of the following complications occur:
    a. Chills.
    b. Urticaria.
    c. Feeling of warmth.
    d. Breathing difficulty.
    e. Lightheadedness.
    f. Pain at the venipuncture site.
    g. Flank pain.
4. Explain additional therapeutic orders as appropriate.

DOCUMENTATION
1. Date, time the transfusion was started and discontinued, blood component administered, donor numbers, and approximate volume.
2. Normal saline hung and amount infused.
3. Any medications administered.
4. All parameters of assessment.
5. Any reactions, interventions, and results.
6. All patient teaching done and the patient's level of understanding.

Administration of Normal Serum Albumin

PURPOSE

1. Provide a route for the administration of normal serum albumin.

REQUISITES

1. Albumin (amount and concentration as ordered by the physician)
2. Albumin administration set with needle
3. Antiseptic wipes
4. Equipment for initiating intravenous therapy, if necessary
5. Tape
6. Blood pressure cuff, stethoscope, and thermometer
7. IV standard

GUIDELINES

1. Normal serum albumin expands the blood volume by drawing fluid from the surrounding tissue. Its administration is indicated in the emergency treatment of shock, severe burns, hypoproteinemia with or without edema, cerebral edema, and hepatic cirrhosis.
2. Human serum albumin 25% is a sterile solution composed of human albumin in an aqueous diluent buffered with sodium carbonate. It is pasteurized at 60°C for 10 hours and is free of viral hepatitis contamination.
3. Human serum albumin does not require typing and crossmatching. Because albumin is stable, soluble, and free of cellular components, there is no danger of sensitization with repeated transfusions.
4. Human serum albumin is supplied in 5% and 25% concentrations. The 5% solution is isotonic. The 25% solution is salt-poor and is osmotically equal to five times its volume of whole blood.
5. Administration of serum albumin results in a rapid interstitial fluid shift into the circulatory system; 20 cc of 25% albumin will draw approximately 70 cc of additional fluid into the circulation within 15 minutes. It should be used cautiously in patients susceptible to fluid overload.

6. The intravascular pressure rise occurring during albumin infusion may produce pulmonary edema, congestive heart failure, or excessive bleeding in the trauma patient.
7. The patient's vital signs should be assessed every 15 minutes during the transfusion and at least every hour for 4 hours following the transfusion.
8. The rate of infusion should be prescribed by the physician. In general, the rate for a patient with a normal blood volume should not exceed 1 cc per minute. Patients with low blood volumes can receive albumin at a much faster rate.
9. Laboratory studies including hemoglobin, hematocrit, electrolytes, and serum protein should be used to monitor the patient during the course of albumin therapy.
10. Serum albumin is compatible with most intravenous solutions and may be administered by piggyback into an already established intravenous line. Compatibility of intravenous solutions should always be determined prior to administration.
11. Normal serum albumin contains no preservatives and should be used immediately after the bottle is opened. It should not be used if the solution appears turbid or if sediment is present.
12. Normal serum albumin is packaged with its own administration tubing.

NURSING ACTION/RATIONALE

1. Assemble all equipment.
2. Verify the physician's order.
3. Notify the blood bank of the order for normal serum albumin.
4. Identify the patient.
5. Explain the nature and purpose of the procedure to the patient.
6. Provide privacy.
7. Provide adequate lighting.
8. Position the patient comfortably.
9. Wash your hands.
10. Establish an intravenous therapy system and perform a venipuncture if the patient does not have an established intravenous. Refer to the procedure "Intravenous Therapy."

11. Obtain baseline vital signs.
12. Follow the procedure in your facility for correctly identifying the patient and the normal serum albumin.
13. Rewash your hands.
14. Attach the needle to the administration set, spike the normal serum albumin vial, and prime the tubing according to the directions on the normal serum albumin package. Use aseptic technique.
15. Cleanse the port on the primary intravenous tubing and allow it to dry.
16. Insert the needle of the albumin tubing into the port and tape it securely.
17. Close the roll clamp on the primary tubing.
18. Open the roll clamp on the albumin tubing and adjust the flow rate as prescribed.
19. Assess the patient's vital signs every 15 minutes during the infusion. Assess the patient for signs of circulatory overload and pulmonary edema. Monitor urinary output every hour, or more frequently. Stop the infusion and notify the physician immediately if complications occur.
20. Discontinue the infusion when complete:
    a. Close the roll clamp on the albumin tubing.
    b. Remove the needle from the port.
    c. Open the roll clamp on the primary tubing and reestablish the prescribed rate.
21. Discard equipment or return it to the appropriate location.

PATIENT AND/OR FAMILY TEACHING

1. Explain the nature and purpose of the procedure to the patient.
2. Explain to the patient the frequent monitoring that will be done during the therapy.
3. Instruct the patient to notify the nurse regarding any untoward symptoms such as:
    a. Nausea
    b. Vomiting
    c. Shortness of breath
    d. Pruritus
    e. Chills
    f. Pain at the venipuncture site

DOCUMENTATION

1. Date, time, type, rate, and amount of solution administered.
2. All assessment parameters including vital signs.
3. The patient's response to therapy.
4. Any complications, interventions, and results.
5. All patient teaching done and the patient's level of understanding.

Administration of Platelets

PURPOSE

1. Provide a route for the administration of normally functioning platelets.

REQUISITES

1. Platelet donor pack (concentration as ordered by the physician)
2. Component infusion kit containing:
   a. Infusion set with filter
   b. 60 cc syringe
   c. Needle
3. Intravenous normal saline 0.9%
4. Equipment for initiating a venipuncture, if necessary. Refer to the procedure "Intravenous Therapy."
5. Watch with second indicator
6. Blood pressure cuff, stethoscope, and thermometer
7. Antiseptic wipes
8. IV standard

GUIDELINES

1. Platelets are a concentrate of megakaryocyte cytoplasmic fragments separated from one unit of whole blood and suspended in a small amount of plasma.
2. Platelet transfusions may be indicated in the treatment of bleeding due to thrombocytopenia or functionally abnormal platelets. They may also be useful in patients with low platelet counts secondary to cancer chemotherapy.
3. Side effects and possible complications of platelet transfusions are chills, fever, and allergic reactions. Viral hepatitis can be transmitted through platelets.
4. ABO compatible platelets should be administered whenever possible. Rh antigens are not found on platelets; therefore Rh compatibility is not necessary unless the platelet preparation is contaminated with numerous red blood cells.
5. Platelets contain HLA antigens. Patients who receive numerous platelet transfusions may develop antibodies to the HLA or platelet antigens. For these select patients, platelets from a compatible HLA donor may be necessary.

6. Platelet counts should be done before the transfusion, 1 hour after the transfusion, and 24 hours after the transfusion to assess the patient's response to the platelet therapy.
7. Platelets should be administered through a clot filter. Microaggregate filters remove platelets and should not be used for platelet transfusions.
8. One unit of platelets can be transfused over a period of 10 minutes, or the rate as prescribed by the physician.
9. Platelets must be administered within 4 hours of the time of pooling.
10. Platelets can be administered through a Y type blood administration set. See the procedure "Blood Transfusion Therapy." The small volume of platelets makes it imperative that all platelets be infused into the patient. To facilitate this, follow the platelet transfusion with 100 cc of normal saline to flush the platelets from the tubing.

NURSING ACTION/RATIONALE

1. Assemble all equipment.
2. Verify the physician's order.
3. Notify the blood bank of the order for platelets.
4. Identify the patient.
5. Explain the nature and purpose of the procedure to the patient.
6. Provide adequate lighting.
7. Provide privacy.
8. Position the patient comfortably for a venipuncture, if a venipuncture will be necessary.
9. Wash your hands.
10. Prepare the normal saline solution for infusion and either perform a venipuncture if necessary, or replace the present intravenous infusion solution with normal saline. Refer to the procedure "Intravenous Therapy."
11. Obtain baseline vital signs, including temperature.
12. Follow your hospital's procedure for correctly identifying the patient and the blood component with blood bank personnel.
13. Rewash your hands.

14. Assemble the component infusion set using aseptic technique (Figure 3-13):
    a. Use the wrapper of the kit as a sterile field.
    b. Close the clamps on the set.
    c. Pull the tabs apart to expose the port of the platelet pack.
    d. Remove the cover of the spike on the infusion set.
    e. Insert the spike into the port, using a twisting motion.
    f. Remove the protector from the syringe adapter on the set.
    g. Attach the 60 cc syringe to the set.
    h. Open the slide clamp and aspirate the contents of the platelet pack into the syringe. Close the slide clamp.
    i. Attach the needle to the distal end of the infusion set.
    j. Remove the cover over the needle and open the roll clamp.
    k. Depress the syringe plunger and fill the set with platelets, expelling all the air.
    l. Replace the protective cover over the needle.

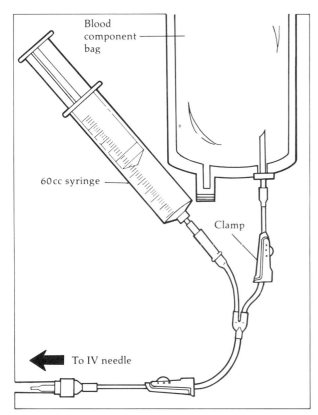

Figure 3-13. Blood component infusion set.

15. Cleanse the distal port on the patient's existing intravenous tubing with an antiseptic wipe. Allow it to dry.
16. Remove the needle cover from the infusion set, and insert the needle into the intravenous tubing port.
17. Clamp off the primary line of normal saline.
18. Infuse the platelets at the correct rate by depressing the syringe plunger.
19. After the platelets have been infused, close the clamp on the infusion set and open the clamp to the normal saline solution.
20. Remove the infusion set from the normal saline tubing and replace the protective cover over the needle.
21. Change the intravenous solution to the prescribed solution, or discontinue the intravenous needle, whichever is appropriate.
22. Reassess the patient's vital signs, then reassess every hour for the next 4 hours, then every 4 hours for 24 hours.
23. Instruct the patient to notify the nurse of any unusual symptoms.
24. Reposition the patient comfortably.
25. Discard equipment or return it to the appropriate location.

PATIENT AND/OR FAMILY TEACHING
1. Explain the nature and purpose of the procedure to the patient.
2. Instruct the patient on the possible side effects of the platelet transfusion.
3. Instruct the patient to notify the nurse of any unusual symptoms.
4. Explain other therapeutic orders as appropriate.

DOCUMENTATION
1. Date, time the transfusion was started, and time completed, number of units transfused, donor numbers, and volume of fluid infused.
2. Method used for transfusion.

3. Amount of normal saline solution hung and infused.
4. Venipuncture site and needle type and size, if appropriate.
5. Baseline and succeeding vital signs.
6. Any reactions to the blood component.
7. All patient teaching done and the patient's level of understanding.

Administration of Cryoprecipitate

PURPOSE
1. Provide a route for the administration of Factors VIII, XIII, and fibrinogen.

REQUISITES
1. Cryoprecipitate pack (number of units as ordered by the physician)
2. Sterile component infusion kit containing:
   a. Infusion set with filter
   b. 60 cc syringe
   c. Needle
3. Intravenous normal saline 0.9%
4. Equipment for initiating intravenous therapy, if necessary. Refer to "Intravenous Therapy."
5. Watch with second indicator
6. Blood pressure cuff, stethoscope, thermometer
7. Antiseptic wipes
8. IV standard

GUIDELINES
1. Cryoprecipitate is prepared from fresh-frozen plasma and is used in the treatment of hemophilia A and von Willebrand's disease. It is used for the control of bleeding in Factor VIII deficiency and for the replacement of Factor XIII and fibrinogen.
2. Side effects of the administration of cryoprecipitate include febrile and allergic reactions and the transmission of hepatitis. Hyperfibrinogenemia is possible in patients transfused with large amounts of this component.
3. Compatibility testing is not essential for this component; however, ABO compatibility is preferred. The Rh factor compatibility need not be considered. Type AB is the universal donor.

4. Cryoprecipitate is stored frozen and is thawed for 15 minutes in a waterbath. Thawed cryoprecipitate may be kept at room temperature for 6 hours if the bag has not been entered. If the bag is entered after thawing, the component should be administered within 4 hours of thawing.
5. The amount of solution in a pack of cryoprecipitate will depend on the concentration and amount of the component ordered by the physician and the number of units per pack. Generally the rate of infusion is 1 unit over a period of 5 minutes, but the rate may vary according to the physician's preference.
6. All cryoprecipitate should be administered through a filter.

NURSING ACTION/RATIONALE
1. Assemble all equipment.
2. Verify the physician's order.
3. Notify the blood bank of the order for cryoprecipitate.
4. Identify the patient.
5. Explain the nature and purpose of the procedure to the patient.
6. Provide adequate lighting.
7. Provide privacy.
8. Position the patient comfortably for a venipuncture, if a venipuncture will be necessary.
9. Wash your hands.

10. Prepare the normal saline solution for infusion and either perform a venipuncture if necessary, or replace the present intravenous infusion solution with normal saline. Refer to the procedure "Intravenous Therapy."
11. Obtain baseline vital signs, including temperature.
12. Follow your hospital's procedure for correctly identifying the patient and the blood component with blood bank personnel.
13. Rewash your hands.
14. Assemble the component infusion set using aseptic technique (see Figure 3-13):
    a. Use the wrapper of the kit as a sterile field.
    b. Close the clamps on the set.
    c. Pull the tabs apart to expose the port of the cryoprecipitate pack.
    d. Remove the cover of the spike on the infusion set.
    e. Insert the spike into the port, using a twisting motion.
    f. Remove the protector from the syringe adapter on the set.
    g. Attach the 60 cc syringe to the set.
    h. Open the slide clamp and aspirate the contents of the cryoprecipitate pack into the syringe. Close the slide clamp.
    i. Attach the needle to the distal end of the infusion set.
    j. Remove the cover over the needle and open the roll clamp.
    k. Depress the syringe plunger and fill the set with cryoprecipitate, expelling all the air.
    l. Replace the protective cover over the needle.
15. Cleanse the distal port on the patient's existing intravenous tubing with an antiseptic wipe. Allow it to dry.
16. Remove the needle cover from the infusion set, and insert the needle into the intravenous tubing port.
17. Clamp off the primary line of normal saline.
18. Infuse the cryoprecipitate at the correct rate by depressing the syringe plunger.
19. After the cryoprecipitate has been infused, close the clamp on the infusion set and open the clamp to the normal saline solution.

20. Remove the infusion set from the normal saline tubing and replace the protective cover over the needle.
21. Change the intravenous solution to the prescribed solution, or discontinue the intravenous needle, whichever is appropriate.
22. Reassess the patient's vital signs, then reassess every hour for the next 4 hours, then every 4 hours for 24 hours.
23. Instruct the patient to notify the nurse of any unusual symptoms.
24. Reposition the patient comfortably.
25. Discard equipment or return it to the appropriate area.

PATIENT AND/OR FAMILY TEACHING

1. Instruct the patient about the purpose of cryoprecipitate, the method of administration, and possible side effects.
2. Instruct the patient to notify the nurse of any unusual symptoms.
3. Explain other therapeutic orders as appropriate.

DOCUMENTATION

1. Date, time started and completed, unit numbers of the cryoprecipitate, rate of infusion, and approximate volume infused.
2. Amount of normal saline hung and infused.
3. Venipuncture site and size and type of needle inserted, if appropriate.
4. Baseline and succeeding vital signs.
5. Any reactions to the blood component.
6. All patient teaching done and the patient's level of understanding.

Assisting the Physician with Insertion of a Cutdown Catheter

PURPOSE
1. Assist the physician to insert a catheter into a vein surgically for therapeutic or diagnostic purposes.

REQUISITES
1. Sterile cutdown tray
2. Intravenous catheter (type and size as ordered by the physician)
3. Intravenous fluid (type and amount as ordered by the physician)
4. Administration tubing
5. Sterile gloves
6. Antiseptic solution
7. 2 × 2 sterile gauze sponges
8. Antiseptic ointment
9. Tape
10. Gauze roll (optional)
11. Armboard
12. Bed protector
13. IV standard
14. Waste receptacle

GUIDELINES
1. A cutdown is used when peripheral veins are not accessible. This may be when the veins are constricted from shock, collapsed from multiple venipunctures, or too small or fragile as in elderly or newborn patients.
2. A cutdown may also be used when prolonged intravenous therapy is planned for the purpose of antibiotic therapy or hyperalimentation.
3. The preferred veins for an elective cutdown are the cephalic and basilic veins of the antecubital fossa.
4. The complications to be considered with a cutdown are phlebitis, pulmonary embolus, and infection, especially when the saphenous vein is used.
5. The requirement for a signed consent for an invasive procedure varies among hospitals. Refer to your hospital's policy.
6. Health care facilities vary as to the qualifications of persons allowed to discontinue a cutdown catheter. Refer to your hospital's policy.

7. Guidelines and nursing care described in "Intravenous Therapy" apply to intravenous therapy with a cutdown catheter site. If the catheter will be used for hyperalimentation, refer to the procedures related to hyperalimentation therapy.

NURSING ACTION/RATIONALE
1. Assemble all equipment.
2. Verify the physician's order.
3. Wash your hands.
4. Prepare the intravenous solution and tubing. Refer to the procedure "Intravenous Therapy."
5. Identify the patient.
6. Explain the procedure to the patient. Reinforce and clarify the physician's explanation of the procedure.
7. Obtain an informed consent if required.
8. Provide adequate lighting.
9. Provide privacy.
10. Assist the patient to a supine position exposing the site of the cutdown. Tape the extremity to an armboard to limit mobility if desired. Place a bed protector under the extremity.
11. Rewash your hands.
12. Open the sterile supplies using aseptic technique.
13. Assist the physician as required.
14. Reassure the patient frequently during the procedure.
15. Attach the intravenous tubing to the catheter when indicated.
16. Adjust the intravenous flow rate as prescribed.
17. Dress the insertion site:
    a. Apply antimicrobial ointment.
    b. Secure the catheter to the skin with tape.
    c. Apply a 2 × 2 sterile gauze over the insertion site, using aseptic technique. Do not obstruct the point where the tubing is attached to the catheter.
    d. Secure the dressing and the tubing with tape.
    e. Wrap the extremity with gauze to further protect it, if desired.
18. Assist the patient to a comfortable position.
19. Discard equipment or return it to the appropriate area.

PATIENT AND/OR FAMILY TEACHING

1. Explain the procedure to the patient.
2. Remind the patient to notify the nurse of any discomfort at the cutdown site.
3. Reinforce and clarify the physician's explanation of the disease process.
4. Explain any activity restrictions necessary to protect the cutdown site.

DOCUMENTATION

1. Date, time, vein used, insertion site, and catheter size.
2. Type and amount of solution hung and rate of infusion.

3. The patient's reaction to the procedure.
4. Assessment of the cutdown site as the dressing is changed each day.
5. All teaching done and the patient's level of understanding.

Assisting the Physician with Insertion of a Central Venous Catheter

PURPOSE

1. Assist the physician with insertion of the central venous catheter.
2. Minimize the possibility of complications.

REQUISITES

1. Sterile subclavian insertion tray with a subclavian catheter
2. Intravenous solution (type as ordered by the physician)
3. Primary administration tubing
4. Intravenous filter
5. 30 inch extension tubing
6. Antiseptic scrub sponge
7. Sterile gloves
8. Sterile hemostat with covered teeth
9. Pour bottle sterile water
10. Antiseptic ointment
11. Sterile drape
12. Sterile gloves
13. Masks
14. Alcohol wipes
15. Sterile basin
16. Sterile 4 × 4 gauze sponges
17. Washbasin with soap and water
18. Towel and washcloth
19. Prep razor
20. Intravenous infusion pump or IV standard
21. 70% alcohol
22. Scissors

GUIDELINES

1. Subclavian catheters are inserted for a variety of reasons and patient conditions. The procedure for inserting the catheter is the same regardless of the purpose for the line. Any equipment needed, such as central venous pressure tubing for central venous pressure readings, should be obtained before the procedure is begun.
2. Administration of hyperalimentation solutions requires a vein that has optimal blood flow to rapidly dilute the highly concentrated solution.
3. The sites of choice for the insertion of a line for hyperalimentation are the left or right subclavian veins. Other sites that can be used include the left or right internal or external jugular veins or the brachial approach to the superior vena cava.
4. The Trendelenburg position is used for insertion of the subclavian catheter because it increases venous pressure, dilates blood vessels, and makes the subclavian vein easier to locate.

5. The Valsalva maneuver is used to increase central venous pressure and prevent air emboli as the stylet is removed from the catheter and the catheter is connected to the intravenous tubing.

6. To do the Valsalva maneuver, the patient takes a deep breath and bears down as if to have a bowel movement. For the unconscious or uncooperative patient, the nurse may need to compress the patient's abdomen to raise the diaphragm, which also increases central venous pressure.

7. A chest x-ray is done immediately following the insertion of a subclavian catheter to ensure that the tip of the subclavian catheter is in the superior vena cava.

8. Signs and symptoms of catheter misplacement include dyspnea, decreased breath sounds, chest pain, edema of the surrounding tissue, and hematoma formation at the insertion site.

9. An isotonic glucose solution or normal saline is usually administered by slow gravity drip or slow pump infusion until the placement of the catheter is confirmed by x-ray.

10. Strict aseptic technique must be maintained during the insertion of the subclavian catheter.

11. The nurse, physician, and patient should mask during this procedure to prevent infection from airborne contaminants from nasopharyngeal secretions.

12. The requirement for a signed consent form for invasive procedures varies among health care facilities. Refer to your hospital's policy.

NURSING ACTION/RATIONALE
Prepare the Patient:
1. Assemble all equipment.
2. Wash your hands.
3. Prepare the intravenous solution and prime the tubing, including the filter and extension tubing. Refer to the procedure "Intravenous Therapy." Attach the intravenous tubing to the infusion pump, following manufacturer's recommendations. Set the controls on the infusion pump.
4. Identify the patient.

5. Reinforce the physician's explanation of the procedure including:
   a. The anticipated cool sensation of the local anesthetic.
   b. The Valsalva maneuver.
   c. The necessary positioning for the procedure.
   d. The necessity for masking all persons in the area including the patient.
6. Obtain an informed consent, if required.
7. Provide adequate lighting.
8. Provide privacy.
9. Assist the patient to a supine position.
10. Wash your hands.
11. Clip hair at the site for insertion if indicated and wash and dry thoroughly.
12. Instruct the patient to turn his/her head away from the insertion site.
13. Open sterile prep supplies, using aseptic technique.
14. Pour sterile water over the gauze in the sterile basin.
15. Apply a mask to your face.
16. Apply sterile gloves.
17. Scrub the subclavian insertion site and 6 inches around the site with an antiseptic scrub sponge for 5 minutes.
18. Rinse the site with a sterile 4 × 4 gauze soaked in sterile water.
19. Dry the area with sterile 4 × 4 sponges.
20. Cover the site with sterile drapes.
21. Remove the sterile gloves.

Assist the Physician:
1. Place the patient in a Trendelenburg position and place a rolled towel under the patient's back.
2. Place a mask on the patient, or instruct the patient to keep his/her head turned away from the insertion site.
3. Wash your hands.
4. Cleanse the bedside table with 70% alcohol.
5. Open the sterile supplies, using aseptic technique.
6. Assist the physician as necessary.
7. Reassure the patient frequently.
8. Assist the patient with the Valsalva maneuver when necessary.
9. Turn on the infusion pump when the catheter is placed and the tubing is connected.

10. Assist the physician as necessary to apply antiseptic ointment and an occlusive dressing to the site.
11. Tape all intravenous tubing connections.
12. Assess the patient for signs and symptoms of catheter misplacement.
13. Reposition the patient comfortably.
14. Obtain an x-ray to verify location.
15. Discard equipment or return it to the appropriate location.

PATIENT AND/OR FAMILY TEACHING

1. Reinforce and clarify the physician's explanation of the central venous catheter insertion including:
   a. The cool sensation of the anesthetic.
   b. The position required for the procedure.
   c. The Valsalva maneuver.
   d. Masking.
2. Explain activity restrictions.
3. Instruct the patient to avoid touching the subclavian dressing and to notify the nurse if the dressing becomes soiled, wet, or loose.
4. Explain the use of the intravenous pump, if appropriate, and demonstrate the alarm sound.
5. Explain the hyperalimentation therapy and its purpose to the patient. Refer to the procedure "Initiation of Hyperalimentation."
6. Instruct the patient to notify the nurse of any discomfort or shortness of breath.
7. Explain all additional therapeutic orders as appropriate.

DOCUMENTATION

1. Date, time, size of the catheter, site, and name of physician who inserted the catheter.
2. Type of solution hung and rate of infusion.
3. The patient's reaction to the procedure, any untoward reactions, and action taken.
4. Chest x-ray confirming location of catheter.
5. All patient teaching done and the patient's level of understanding.

Initiation of Hyperalimentation

PURPOSE

1. Provide necessary protein, calories, and nutrients.
2. Minimize complications with hyperalimentation.

REQUISITES

1. Central venous line in place in the patient with an intravenous infusing on an infusion pump
2. Hyperalimentation solution (type and amount as ordered by the physician)
3. Alcohol wipes
4. Blood pressure cuff and stethoscope
5. Thermometer
6. Glucose and acetone test kit
7. Scale

GUIDELINES

1. Hyperalimentation, or total parenteral nutrition, is the administration of sufficient nutrients, calories, protein, and fatty acids by the intravascular route to support life and maintain growth and development.
2. Hyperalimentation is used in the treatment of patients who cannot, because of their disease, ingest or absorb sufficient nutrients to maintain growth and development.
3. Hyperalimentation solutions are prescribed by the physician on the basis of the patient's needs. Generally, the solution contains 20 to 50% glucose, electrolytes, water, amino acids, carbohydrates, vitamins, minerals, and in some instances insulin.
4. The body's response to the high glucose concentration of solution is to secrete more insulin to utilize the glucose. Hyperglycemia and hypoglycemia are common complications related to the therapy as the pancreas adjusts to the change in serum glucose.
5. Symptoms of hyperglycemia are nausea, headache, lassitude, and diuresis. This can occur if the rate of infusion of the hyperalimentation solution is increased suddenly.
6. Symptoms of hypoglycemia are confusion, restlessness, tremors, diaphoresis, weakness, and hunger. This can occur if the rate of infusion of the hyperalimentation solution is suddenly decreased.
7. Infusing the hyperalimentation solution at a constant rate, as prescribed, can help to prevent these metabolic complications. An intravenous infusion pump should be used to help ensure a constant rate of infusion.
8. The high concentration of glucose infusing into a central vein, together with the weakened condition of the patient, makes the patient very susceptible to infection. Infection control precautions should be taken with these patients, including:
   a. Using aseptic technique when handling any part of the system.
   b. Performing good handwashing before and after contact with the patient.
   c. Maintaining a dry occlusive dressing over the insertion site at all times.
   d. Segregating the patient from any infected patients.
   e. Preparing the solution in the pharmacy under sterile conditions.
   f. Refrigerating the solution until ready to use.
   g. Using solutions within 24 hours after preparation.
   h. Using an intravenous filter to prevent bacteria and particulate contamination.
   i. Changing hyperalimentation dressings and inspecting the insertion site every 48 hours.
   j. Changing intravenous tubing every 24 hours.
   k. Maintaining the line exclusively for hyperalimentation. Blood should not be drawn from the line, and the line should not be used for administering blood transfusions or piggyback medications.
9. Vital signs should be assessed every 4 hours, and any elevation in temperature should be reported to the physician.
10. Urine tests for glucose and acetone should be performed every 6 hours to evaluate the patient's metabolic response to the hyperalimentation.

11. Accurate intake and output measurements should be maintained to evaluate the patient's fluid balance.
12. Daily weights should be obtained to evaluate the patient's response to the increased calories. A steady, constant weight gain is indicative of a positive response to therapy. Any substantial weight gain or loss should be reported to the physician.
13. Daily laboratory serum studies indicate the patient's response to therapy and guide the physician in determining the formula for further solution preparations.
14. Most patients on hyperalimentation have had extensive hospitalizations, prolonged food restrictions, and an altered body image. These patients have special psychological and emotional needs.
15. Since most hyperalimentation patients receive nothing by mouth, good oral hygiene every 4 hours is essential.
16. Since the hyperalimentation solution flows into a central line, the connections on the tubing should be taped to maintain a closed system. The patient should wear a special intravenous hospital gown to avoid excessive manipulation of the system.
17. Patients may be discharged on hyperalimentation therapy with a subclavian catheter or a Hickman catheter in place. The patients and their families require extensive teaching to maintain the therapy without complications.
18. Hyperalimentation flow sheets can be used for documenting all assessment parameters related to hyperalimentation therapy (Figure 3-14).
19. Hyperalimentation therapy can be initiated immediately after insertion, providing x-ray films demonstrate correct location of the central line.

NURSING ACTION/RATIONALE

1. Assemble all equipment.
2. Verify the physician's order.
3. Allow the hyperalimentation solution to warm to room temperature.
4. Identify the patient.
5. Explain the hyperalimentation therapy and its purpose to the patient.

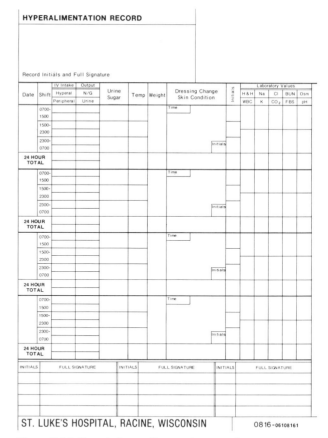

Figure 3-14. Sample hyperalimentation record.

6. Provide privacy.
7. Provide adequate lighting.
8. Obtain baseline vital signs.
9. Wash your hands.
10. Open the seal on the hyperalimentation solution bottle.
11. Cleanse the rubber stopper with an alcohol wipe and allow it to dry.
12. Turn the infusion pump off.
13. Remove the spike of the administration tubing from the previous solution bottle.
14. Insert the spike into the hyperalimentation bottle, using aseptic technique.
15. Hang the bottle on the IV standard.
16. Set the infusion pump to the prescribed rate, following manufacturer's recommendations.
17. Turn the pump on.
18. Assess the function of the pump.
19. Mark the bottle for the infusion times.
20. Assess the dressing site.
21. Continue to monitor and assess all parameters of assessment as described in the guidelines.

22. Assess the infusion rate and entire system every hour for correct functioning.
23. Discard equipment or return it to the appropriate location.

PATIENT AND/OR FAMILY TEACHING

1. Explain the procedure for hyperalimentation to the patient including:
   a. The purpose.
   b. The anticipated results.
   c. The type and frequency of assessments that will be done.
   d. The dressing changes and care of the insertion site.
2. Explain any activity restrictions.
3. Explain the purpose of the intravenous pump and demonstrate the alarm system.
4. Instruct the patient to notify the nurse of any new symptoms or discomfort.
5. Instruct the patient to avoid touching the dressing and to notify the nurse if the dressing becomes loose, soiled, or wet.

6. Explain any other therapeutic orders, as appropriate.
7. Instruct the patient regarding all the details involved in home care, if the patient will be discharged on hyperalimentation therapy.

DOCUMENTATION

1. Date, time, type, amount, and rate of solution hung.
2. Use of the intravenous pump.
3. Baseline vital signs.
4. All other parameters of assessment, including condition of dressing.
5. All patient teaching done and the patient's level of understanding.

 # Hyperalimentation Central Venous Catheter Dressing Change

PURPOSE

1. Promote stability of the catheter.
2. Minimize the potential for mechanical and septic complications.
3. Assess the catheter insertion site.
4. Preserve skin integrity at the catheter insertion site.

REQUISITES

1. Sterile central venous pressure catheter dressing change kit containing:
   a. Plastic bag with tie
   b. Gloves
   c. Large non-woven drape
   d. Acetone/alcohol swabs
   e. Swab sticks
   f. Povidone-iodine solution
   g. Disposable scissors
   h. 2 × 2 inch gauze sponges—2
   i. 3 × 3 inch gauze sponge
   j. Adhesive non-porous patch—5 × 6 inches
2. Antiseptic ointment

3. Masks—2
4. Adhesive tape—1 inch
5. Sterile gloves
6. Exam gloves

GUIDELINES

1. Hyperalimentation dressing changes should be done with strict aseptic technique. The nutrients and high concentration of glucose in the solution increase the susceptibility of the patient to bacterial infection.
2. Certain health care facilities may require certification of personnel performing hyperalimentation procedures, including dressing changes. Refer to your hospital's policy manual.
3. If possible, the first dressing change should be performed by the two staff members who will be responsible for the dressing changes while the patient is receiving treatment. This provides continuity in the observation of the site.

4. Hyperalimentation dressings should be changed at least every 48 hours or as ordered by the physician.
5. The dressing should always be kept clean, dry, and air occlusive.
6. Dressings that become wet or loose should be considered contaminated and changed immediately.
7. Care should be taken to prevent contamination of the subclavian insertion site with drainage from other proximal wounds.
8. During the dressing change, assess the insertion site for suture integrity and any redness, edema, skin ulceration, or drainage.
9. During the dressing change, the nurse and the patient should each wear a mask to prevent cross infection due to airborne contaminants from nasopharyngeal secretions. If the patient is unable to tolerate a mask, instruct the patient to turn his/her head away from the insertion site during the dressing change.
10. New air-occlusive bandages made of non-porous materials are being used in some hospitals, necessitating less frequent dressing changes. These dressings make it possible to observe the site without removing them.
11. Some physicians have specific orders for dressing changes. When necessary, alter the procedure to follow the specific order while maintaining aseptic technique.

NURSING ACTION/RATIONALE
1. Assemble all equipment.
2. Identify the patient.
3. Explain the procedure to the patient.
4. Provide adequate lighting.
5. Provide privacy.
6. Place unopened supplies on a clean bedside table adjusted to waist level.
7. Place the patient in a supine position. Remove the gown on the side where the catheter is located.
8. Apply a mask to the patient and yourself.
9. Wash your hands.
10. Open sterile supplies, using aseptic technique.
11. Unfold the sterile drape, touching only the underside. Place it close to the catheter insertion site.
12. Remove the plastic bag from the kit. Place the open bag close to the patient.
13. Put on the exam gloves.
14. Remove the existing dressing, taking care not to dislodge the catheter. Leave the piece of tape on the extension tubing just outside the dressing site to maintain the security of the catheter.
15. Discard the dressings in the plastic bag.
16. Remove the exam gloves and discard.
17. Apply the sterile gloves.
18. Cleanse the catheter insertion site with acetone/alcohol swabs in a circular motion, starting from the catheter insertion site and moving to the periphery.
19. Continue cleansing until all the exudate, adhesive, debris, and old ointment are removed. Use a new swab each time you return to the insertion site.
20. Assess the site for redness, inflammation, edema, catheter placement, and suture integrity.
21. Open the povidone-iodine packet and pour the solution over the swab sticks.
22. Prep the insertion area with the povidone-iodine soaked swabs, using a circular cleansing motion and moving from the insertion site to the periphery. Cleanse the catheter hub and connection site of the catheter and tubing with the last swab.
23. Allow the povidone-iodine solution to dry naturally. After 3 to 5 minutes, any excess may be lightly blotted off with sterile gauze.
24. Apply antiseptic ointment to the catheter insertion site.
25. Fold the 2 × 2 inch gauze sponges and place one on each side of the catheter at the insertion site. This creates a barrier between the skin and the catheter without having to cut the 2 × 2 gauze sponges.
26. Place the 3 × 3 gauze sponge over the 2 × 2 gauze dressing.
27. Remove the sterile gloves.
28. Apply the adhesive patch over the proximal end of the extension tubing and the dressings, making sure all sides are secured to the skin.
29. Change the one piece of tape that was not changed earlier. This piece of tape is secured outside the dressing.

30. Loop the tubing over the adhesive patch and secure it to the dressing with a piece of tape.
31. Label the new dressing with the date, the time of the dressing change, and your name (Figure 3-15).

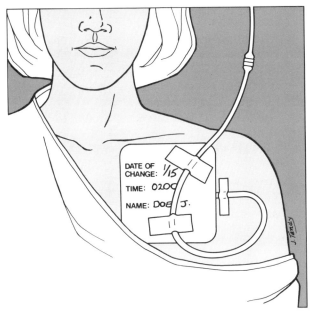

DATE OF CHANGE: 1/15
TIME: 0200
NAME: DOE J.

Figure 3-15. Hyperalimentation dressing.

32. Remove the masks.
33. Ensure that all connection sites are secure and taped.
34. Assist the patient to a comfortable position.
35. Discard all equipment in the appropriate location.

PATIENT AND/OR FAMILY TEACHING

1. Explain the procedure and the aseptic technique that will be used.
2. Explain to the patient the frequency of the dressing changes.
3. Instruct the patient to avoid touching the dressing or getting it wet.
4. Instruct the patient to inform the nurse if the dressing becomes wet.
5. Instruct a family member regarding the dressing change technique if the patient will go home on hyperalimentation therapy. A satisfactory return demonstration is evidence that the family member has learned.

DOCUMENTATION

1. Date and time of dressing change.
2. Assessment of the site.
3. The patient's reaction to the procedure.
4. All teaching done and the patient's level of understanding.

Hyperalimentation Central Venous Tubing and Bottle Change

PURPOSE
1. Maintain patency of the line.
2. Decrease the possibility of complications.

REQUISITES
1. Hyperalimentation solution as ordered
2. Sterile administration tubing for the intravenous pump, including a sterile filter
3. Hemostat with protective tubing over the teeth, or a smooth clamp
4. Adhesive tape, 1 inch
5. Antiseptic wipes

GUIDELINES
1. Hyperalimentation tubing should be changed at least every 24 hours to maintain the sterility of the line. The solution bottle should be changed at least every 12 hours. Since the solution is high in sugar, it is an excellent media for bacterial growth.
2. If any of the tubing becomes contaminated, the whole intravenous set-up should be changed.
3. Before hanging a new intravenous solution bottle, inspect it carefully for clarity of the solution and integrity of the bottle and note the expiration date.
4. To prevent the complication of air embolism when disconnecting and reconnecting the tubing, the patient should be placed in the Trendelenburg position and instructed to perform the Valsalva maneuver. Refer to the procedure, "Assisting the Physician with Insertion of a Central Venous Catheter." If the patient is unable to perform the Valsalva maneuver, a protected hemostat can be applied to the extension tubing during the tubing change.
5. If an extension tubing is applied to the catheter hub, it need not be changed unless it becomes contaminated. If an extension tubing is not used, the tubing and bottle change procedure must be done at the same time as the dressing change.
6. Daily tubing changes should coordinate with a solution bottle change to decrease the frequency that the closed system is entered.

7. An intravenous filter should be used in the administration of hyperalimentation solutions to remove any particulate matter from the solution.
8. If a filter obstructs the flow of solution, this is either because it is defective or because it has filtered a large amount of particulate matter. In either case, a new tubing change, including the filter, should be performed.
9. Some intravenous filters are unable to withstand the pressure of the "purging" mechanism on certain intravenous pumps. Refer to the manufacturer's recommendations for priming the intravenous filter.
10. To prevent puncturing the intravenous tubing during a tubing change, the ribbed edges of the hemostat should be covered with plastic, or a smooth clamp should be used on the extension tubing.
11. All connections on the intravenous tubing should be taped to eliminate the possibility of disconnection, which could cause contaminants or air to enter the system.
12. Hyperalimentation solution should be prepared in the pharmacy, shortly before the bottle is to be hung. If prepared ahead of time, it should be refrigerated. If the hyperalimentation solution has not been prepared and solution must be hung, a solution of 10% dextrose can be hung for a short time to maintain the patency of the system until the hyperalimentation solution is ready.

NURSING ACTION/RATIONALE
1. Assemble all equipment.
2. Verify the list of additives in the solution bottle with the physician's order. Check the solution expiration date.
3. Provide adequate lighting.
4. Wash your hands.
5. Prepare the solution bottle and prime the tubing. Refer to the "Intravenous Therapy" procedure.
6. Identify the patient.
7. Explain the procedure to the patient, if appropriate.

8. Remove the existing tubing from the infusion pump and adjust the rate of infusion for gravity flow.
9. Attach the prepared intravenous tubing to the infusion pump or controller according to manufacturer's instruction.
10. Check the new intravenous tubing for air bubbles. Tap the tubing and filter as necessary to remove any air.
11. Assist the patient to a supine position close to the edge of the bed, and remove the pillow.
12. Remove the tape from the junction of the extension and administration tubing.
13. Wash your hands.
14. Cleanse the connection between the extension tubing and the administration tubing with an antiseptic wipe.
15. Loosen the tubing at the connection site but do not disconnect.
16. Apply a protected hemostat or a smooth clamp to the distal end of the extension tubing, if the patient is unable to perform the Valsalva maneuver.
17. Close the clamp on the existing hyperalimentation tubing.
18. Remove the protective cover from the new tubing.
19. Instruct the patient to perform the Valsalva maneuver.
20. Disconnect the existing tubing from the extension.
21. Hold the end of the extension tubing straight up.
22. Turn the infusion pump on.
23. Drip 2 or 3 drops of solution from the new tubing into the extension tubing and connect the tubings, using aseptic technique.
24. Instruct the patient to relax.
25. Remove the protected hemostat from the extension tubing, if appropriate.
26. Assess the settings on the infusion pump and adjust as necessary.
27. Cleanse the connection site with an antiseptic wipe. Allow to dry.
28. Tape the connection sites.
29. Loop the tubing over the dressing. Secure the tubing to the dressing with tape.
30. Label the intravenous tubing with the date and time of the change and your initials. Label the solution bottle with the date and the infusion times.
31. Assist the patient to a comfortable position.
32. Discard equipment or return it to the appropriate location.

PATIENT AND/OR FAMILY TEACHING
1. Explain the procedure to the patient and the patient participation required.
2. Reinstruct your patient as often as necessary on how to perform the Valsalva maneuver.
3. Instruct the patient to notify the nurse if experiencing any unusual symptoms.
4. Explain additional therapeutic orders as appropriate.

DOCUMENTATION
1. Date, time, type, amount, and rate of infusion.
2. All assessment parameters.
3. Amount of solution absorbed.
4. The patient's reaction to the procedure.
5. All patient teaching done and the patient's level of understanding.

Hickman Catheter Dressing Change

PURPOSE
1. Maintain the patency and integrity of the catheter.
2. Minimize the potential for mechanical and septic complications.

REQUISITES
1. Sterile precut 4 × 4 gauze sponge
2. Sterile 4 × 4 gauze sponges—2
3. Antiseptic swabs
4. Antiseptic ointment
5. Sterile gloves
6. Tape
7. Luer Lock cap
8. Smooth cannula clamp (on the catheter)
9. Masks
10. Hydrogen peroxide (optional)
11. Sterile applicators
12. Alcohol wipes
13. Exam gloves
14. Waste receptacle

GUIDELINES
1. The Hickman catheter is a right atrial indwelling catheter that is inserted into the cephalic vein. The tip of the catheter is at the entrance to the right atrium. The Hickman catheter is different than other central lines, since it is inserted through a long tunnel in the subcutaneous tissue. The distal end of the catheter exits between the nipple and the sternum. The catheter has a Dacron cuff that lies within the tunnel. The subcutaneous tissue eventually fibroses around the cuff. The tunnel and the cuff serve as barriers to infection (Figure 3-16).
2. Once the entrance site over the cephalic vein heals, the only opening left on the skin is the exit site of the catheter.
3. The Hickman catheter can be used for any type of intravenous therapy. It provides ready access to the circulation for blood samples and for monitoring central venous pressure.
4. Patients may be discharged with the Hickman catheter in place. They are taught to administer their own parenteral nutrition and to care for the catheter.

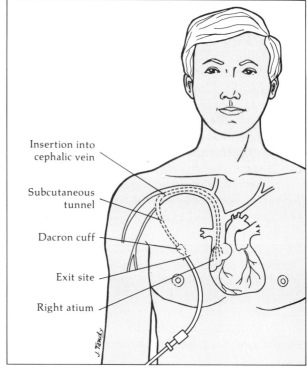

Figure 3-16. Placement of the Hickman catheter.

Labels: Insertion into cephalic vein; Subcutaneous tunnel; Dacron cuff; Exit site; Right atium

5. The catheter can be used for continuous or intermittent therapy. When therapy is intermittent, a heparin lock can be established to maintain the patency of the line. Refer to the procedure "Hickman Catheter Flush."
6. Dressings over the sites should be changed every 48 hours, using aseptic technique. Dressings should be maintained so that they are aseptic, dry, and air-occlusive.
7. The first dressing change should be done by the two nurses who will be responsible for the dressing changes while the patient is receiving therapy. This will provide continuity in the assessment of the site.
8. A smooth cannula clamp should be in place on the catheter at all times except when injecting into the catheter. Only smooth clamps should be used, and the clamp should be placed over a piece of flagged tape to prevent puncturing or severing the line.
9. Clotting and severing of the catheter are the two most common problems. The catheter

should be thoroughly inspected during each dressing change.

10. If the catheter breaks, the emergency procedure is to immediately clamp the line proximal to the break and to notify the physician. A repair kit is available, and the catheter can be repaired by the physician if enough catheter tubing remains.

11. Refer to the procedure "Drawing Blood from the Hickman Catheter," for the specific steps for obtaining a serum specimen for laboratory analysis.

NURSING ACTION/RATIONALE

1. Assemble all equipment.
2. Verify the physician's order.
3. Identify the patient.
4. Explain the procedure to the patient.
5. Provide privacy.
6. Provide adequate lighting.
7. Place the patient in a supine position and expose the dressing site. Drape the patient as necessary.
8. Mask all persons in the area, including the patient. If the patient cannot tolerate a mask, instruct the patient to turn his/her head away from the site during the dressing change.
9. Wash your hands.
10. Open sterile supplies on a clean table.
11. Put on exam gloves.
12. Remove the old dressings and discard. Leave one piece of tape to secure the catheter.
13. Remove exam gloves and discard.
14. Put on sterile gloves.
15. Cleanse the suture line at the entrance site with one antiseptic swab. (The entrance site is cleansed and dressed until completely healed.)
16. Cleanse around the catheter at the exit site with an antiseptic swab in a circular motion, moving away from the catheter. Use a new swab each time you return to the exit site. Remove any encrusted drainage with a sterile applicator soaked in hydrogen peroxide.
17. Allow the area to dry. Assess the site and the catheter.
18. Apply antiseptic ointment to the entrance and exit sites using a separate applicator for each site.
19. Apply a sterile 4 × 4 gauze sponge over the entrance site.

20. Apply the precut 4 × 4 gauze sponge over the exit site and cover with another 4 × 4 gauze sponge, ensuring that the cannula clamp and catheter end are exposed.
21. If the catheter is capped, change the Luer Lock cap at this time:
    a. Assess that the clamp is closed.
    b. Cleanse the cap with an alcohol wipe.
    c. Remove the cap.
    d. Insert a sterile cap.
22. Remove the sterile gloves.
23. Loop any excess catheter tubing over the dressing and tape the dressing occlusively. Tape the entrance site dressing securely.
24. Label the dressing with the date, the time, and your initials.
25. Reposition the patient comfortably.
26. Discard equipment or return it to the appropriate location.

PATIENT AND/OR FAMILY TEACHING

1. Explain the procedure to the patient, including the need for the mask.
2. Instruct the patient to avoid touching the dressing or pulling on the catheter.
3. Instruct the patient to notify the nurse if:
    a. Any discomfort is experienced at the site.
    b. The cannula clamp is lost.
    c. The Luer Lock cap (if any) is lost.
    d. Any leakage from the catheter occurs.
    e. The dressing becomes loose, wet, or soiled.
4. Instruct the patient regarding the dressing change procedure if the patient will be discharged with the catheter in place. (Home care dressing changes are usually clean procedures.)

DOCUMENTATION

1. Date, time, and dressing change procedure.
2. Assessment of the sites.
3. Assessment of the condition of the catheter.
4. All patient teaching done and the patient's level of understanding.

Hickman Catheter Flush

PURPOSE

1. Maintain patency of the catheter.
2. Prevent the formation of precipitate between incompatible infusions.

REQUISITES

1. Prefilled syringe of heparinized saline (amount and concentration as ordered by the physician)
2. Needle—25 gauge, ⅝ inch
3. Antiseptic wipes
4. Prefilled saline syringes—2 (if medications are incompatible)
5. Bed protector

GUIDELINES

1. When the Hickman catheter is used for intermittent infusions, it must be heparinized (flushed) to maintain patency.
2. The Hickman catheter must be flushed with 6 cc of normal saline, or the amount ordered by the physician, between incompatible injections. If the injectate is incompatible with heparin, normal saline must be used before and after the administration of the medication.
3. A heparin flush should be performed on a Hickman catheter not being used for continuous infusion in the following circumstances:
   a. Immediately after the catheter is inserted.
   b. After medication administration.
   c. After an intravenous infusion.
   d. After drawing blood samples.
   e. Every 8 hours or as ordered by the physician for a catheter not being used.
4. A ⅝ inch needle is used whenever injections are made through the Luer Lock cap. The length of this needle minimizes the possibility of puncturing the catheter.
5. Any flush or direct push medication should be done with a needle and syringe. Any infusion drip should be done by attaching the tubing to the catheter, with the cap removed.

NURSING ACTION/RATIONALE

1. Assemble all equipment.
2. Verify the physician's order.
3. Identify the patient.
4. Explain the procedure to the patient.
5. Provide privacy.
6. Provide adequate lighting.
7. Position the patient comfortably and expose the catheter.
8. Place the bed protector under the distal end of the catheter.
9. Wash your hands.
10. Cleanse the Luer Lock cap with an antiseptic wipe, using friction. Allow it to dry.
11. Insert the needle attached to the syringe through the bull's-eye of the Luer Lock cap:
    a. Use the saline syringe if flushing because of medication incompatibility.
    b. Use the heparinized saline syringe if incompatibility is not a problem.
12. Open the clamp on the catheter.
13. Ensure the patency of the line by aspirating for a blood return.
14. Inject the medication into the catheter.
15. Close the clamp as the last 0.5 cc of injectate is instilled. This will ensure forward pressure and prevent backflow of blood and clotting at the tip of the catheter.
16. Remove the needle and syringe.
17. Repeat the procedure using the heparin concentration if a saline flush was done first.
18. Position the patient comfortably.
19. Discard equipment or return it to the appropriate location.

PATIENT AND/OR FAMILY TEACHING

1. Explain the nature and purpose of the procedure to the patient.
2. Instruct the patient on the actions and side effects of the medications.
3. Instruct the patient to notify the nurse if:
   a. Any discomfort is experienced at the site.
   b. The cannula clamp opens.
   c. The Luer Lock cap is lost.
   d. Any leakage from the catheter occurs.
   e. The dressings become loose, wet, or soiled.
4. Instruct the patient thoroughly on the procedure if the patient will be discharged with the catheter in place.

DOCUMENTATION

1. Date, time, and medication instilled, including amount and concentration.
2. Any problems with the procedure.
3. Assessment of the catheter.
4. All patient teaching done and the patient's level of understanding.

 # Drawing Blood from a Hickman Catheter

PURPOSE

1. Obtain serum for laboratory analysis without performing a venipuncture.

REQUISITES

1. 10 cc sterile glass syringes—3
2. Appropriate laboratory tubes
3. Blood transfer needles
4. Exam gloves (optional)
5. Antiseptic wipes
6. Bed protector

Continuous Infusion with a Multiport Adapter

1. Prefilled syringe of normal saline, 10 cc—2

Heparin Lock Hickman Catheter

1. Prefilled syringe of heparinized saline with a 25 gauge, ⅝ inch needle (amount and concentration as ordered by the physician)

GUIDELINES

1. Drawing blood from the Hickman catheter allows for withdrawal of serum samples for analysis without performing repeated venipunctures.
2. Blood should be drawn from a Hickman catheter only under specific order of the physician.
3. Blood can be drawn from a heparin lock Hickman catheter or from a Hickman catheter with a continuous infusion. An accessory adapter can be used on a catheter with a continuous flow infusion. The adapter has two or three ports. This facilitates drawing blood from one port without disconnecting the infusion tubing on another port (Figure 3-17).
4. Occasionally it is difficult to obtain a sufficient blood return from the catheter for samples. The following measures may enhance blood withdrawal:
   a. Assist the patient to change position by moving from side to side or sitting up.
   b. Instruct the patient to perform the Valsalva maneuver.
   c. Instruct the patient to lift one or both arms.
5. A smooth cannula clamp should be in place on the catheter at all times, except when injecting medication or withdrawing blood.

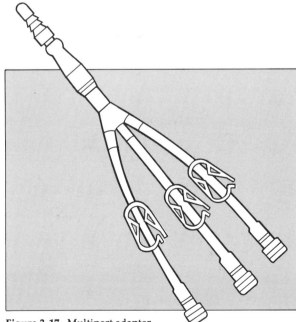

Figure 3-17. Multiport adapter.

6. Laboratory personnel should be present and should assist with the blood specimen collection by procuring the correct collection tubes, transferring the blood into the tubes, labeling the tubes, and delivering the tubes to the laboratory.
7. If an attempt at obtaining the blood samples is unsuccessful, the physician should be notified.
8. Good handwashing should be done before and after this procedure. Necessary precautions should be taken if the patient has an infectious blood disease.

NURSING ACTION/RATIONALE
1. Assemble all equipment.
2. Verify the physician's order.
3. Identify the patient.
4. Explain the procedure to the patient.
5. Provide privacy.
6. Provide adequate lighting.
7. Position the patient and expose the catheter.
8. Place the bed protector under the catheter.
9. Wash your hands.

Continuous Infusion with a Multiport Adapter
1. Cleanse the cap and tubing of the port to be used, using an antiseptic wipe and friction.
2. Clamp the port to be used, if not already clamped.
3. Clamp the port of the continuous infusion.
4. Remove the cap from the blood-drawing port, maintaining the sterility of the inside of the cap.
5. Attach the prefilled 10 cc syringe of sterile saline, unclamp the port, and flush the catheter. Reclamp the port.
6. Remove the saline syringe.
7. Attach one empty, sterile glass 10 cc syringe to the catheter, unclamp the port, and withdraw 10 cc of blood. Reclamp the port.
8. Remove the syringe. This amount of blood will be discarded.
9. Attach a second empty, sterile glass 10 cc syringe, unclamp the port, and withdraw 10 cc of blood or the amount needed. Reclamp the port.
10. Remove the syringe and hand it to the laboratory technician so the blood can be transferred to the blood collection tube.

11. Repeat the procedure with another empty, sterile 10 cc syringe if more blood is needed.
12. Attach the second prefilled saline syringe, unclamp the port, and flush the catheter with saline. Reclamp the port.
13. Remove the syringe.
14. Reattach the port cap, maintaining the sterility of the inside.
15. Open the clamp on the port to the infusion and reestablish the correct infusion rate.
16. Reposition the patient comfortably.
17. Discard equipment or return it to the appropriate location.
18. Wash your hands.

Heparin Lock Hickman Catheter
1. Cleanse the connection of the Luer Lock cap and catheter with an antiseptic wipe, using friction.
2. Close the cannula clamp if not already closed.
3. Remove the Luer Lock cap, maintaining the sterility of the inside of the cap.
4. Attach an empty, sterile glass 10 cc syringe to the catheter.
5. Open the clamp.
6. Withdraw 10 cc of blood and clamp the catheter.
7. Remove the syringe. This blood will be discarded, since it contains heparin.
8. Attach a second empty, sterile glass 10 cc syringe to the catheter and open the clamp.
9. Withdraw 10 cc of blood or the amount necessary for the specimen. Close the cannula clamp.
10. Remove the syringe of blood and hand it to the laboratory technician so the blood can be transferred to the collection tube.
11. Repeat the procedure using a new syringe, if more blood needs to be drawn.
12. Replace the Luer Lock cap, maintaining the sterility of the inside.
13. Cleanse the cap with an antiseptic wipe, using friction.
14. Insert the needle of the syringe of heparinized saline through the cap. Open the clamp.

15. Instill the heparin into the catheter. Close the clamp as the last 0.5 cc of injectate is instilled. This will ensure forward pressure and prevent backflow of blood and clotting at the tip of the catheter.
16. Remove the syringe.
17. Reposition the patient comfortably.
18. Discard equipment or return it to the appropriate location.

PATIENT AND/OR FAMILY TEACHING

1. Explain the nature and purpose of the procedure to the patient.
2. Instruct the patient on the measures for facilitating blood withdrawal, as necessary. See the guidelines.
3. Instruct the patient to notify the nurse if:
   a. Any discomfort is felt at the site.
   b. The cannula clamp opens.
   c. The Luer Lock cap is lost.
   d. The dressings become loosened, wet, or soiled.

DOCUMENTATION

1. Time, procedure, blood volume aspirated, tests ordered, and disposition of specimens.
2. Any problems with the procedure, interventions, and results.
3. The patient's tolerance of the procedure.
4. All medications administered, including dosages.
5. All patient teaching done and the patient's level of understanding.

Administration of Intravenous Chemotherapy

PURPOSE

1. Provide a route for the administration of intravenous chemotherapy.
2. Administer intravenous chemotherapeutic agents safely.

REQUISITES

Administration through an Existing Intravenous Infusion

1. Intravenous solution, if existing solution incompatible
2. Medication as prescribed in prefilled syringe with a 22 gauge, 1½ inch needle
3. Antiseptic wipes
4. 2 × 2 sterile gauze sponges—2
5. Tape

Administration by Direct Intravenous Push

1. Medication as prescribed in prefilled syringe
2. Prefilled syringes with normal saline—2
3. Scalp vein needle—22, 25, or 27 gauge, individualized for patient
4. Tourniquet
5. Antiseptic wipes
6. 2 × 2 sterile gauze sponges—2
7. Tape
8. Bed protector

GUIDELINES

1. A physician's order is required for the administration of intravenous chemotherapy. Policy may vary regarding nursing personnel permitted to administer chemotherapy. Refer to your health care facility's policy.
2. Patients receiving chemotherapy who are involved in a research study may need to sign an informed consent. It is the physician's responsibility to fully explain the regimen to the patient prior to obtaining the consent. Refer to your health care facility's policy for other requirements.
3. The "five rights" of drug administration should be followed each time a medication is administered: the right medication, the right dosage, the right time, the right route, and the right patient.
4. No medication should be given until the order is checked by two registered nurses. The nurse administering the medication should be familiar with the medication, acceptable dosage, potential side effects, and toxic effects.
5. Chemotherapy administration routes include oral, intravenous, intrathecal, intracavity, and intraarterial infusion and perfusion.
6. Intravenous chemotherapy administration is accomplished through an intravenous infusion line or by direct intravenous push. The intravenous infusion line method is the preferred method because this allows interruption of treatment without loss of the vein, and it allows intravenous access in cases of anaphylaxis. Flushing of the tubing and vein is more easily accomplished, and it is less confining for the patient.
7. Chemotherapeutic agents for intravenous administration are preferably prepared in the pharmacy department where air circulation routes and safety measures can be maintained. In some clinics and hospitals the registered nurse mixes these agents. Skin irritation and inhalation dangers should be minimized by the use of gloves, masks, and strict handwashing.
8. Disposal of equipment used in chemotherapy is best accomplished by isolation of such equipment and incineration.
9. Each chemotherapeutic agent has specific guidelines. The nurse must refer to these before chemotherapy administration.
10. When chemotherapy is to be administered, current laboratory serum studies should be available for the physician since the decision to administer certain chemotherapeutic agents is dependent on these studies.
11. Extravasation and anaphylaxis orders (either standing orders or individual orders) should be signed and on the patient's chart prior to the administration of chemotherapeutic agents.

12. Extravasation and anaphylaxis medications should be available and in the patient's room during chemotherapy administration. Resuscitation equipment and an oxygen source should be readily available.
13. When vesicant (irritating) medications are administered, the patient must remain immobile and the arm vein must be stabilized. Aspiration for placement must be performed frequently to assess needle placement and prevent tissue infiltration.
14. When a combination of chemotherapeutic agents is given, the most vesicant (irritating) medications are generally given first.
15. Choice of intravenous sites is preferably on the dorsum of the hand or the lower forearm. Since these drugs are toxic, it is important to choose locations that will not compromise venous circulation.
16. When chemotherapeutic agents are administered through an existing intravenous line, it is preferable that it be a recently or newly started infusion in a vein site recommended for chemotherapy.
17. The chemotherapy injection should be discontinued immediately if signs of extravasation or anaphylaxis occur. Refer to the procedure "Treatment for Chemotherapy Drug Extravasation" or your anaphylaxis protocol for treatment.
18. When administering more than one type of medication, the tubing and needle must be flushed between injections.

NURSING ACTION/RATIONALE
Preparation
1. Verify the physician's order. Verify the drug order with another registered nurse.
2. Assemble all equipment.
3. Identify the patient.
4. Explain the procedure and any activity restrictions to the patient.
5. Provide privacy.
6. Assist the patient to a comfortable position.
7. Provide adequate lighting.
8. Wash your hands.

Administration through an Existing Intravenous Line
1. Change the intravenous solution and tubing if the existing solution is incompatible with the medication. Refer to the procedure "Intravenous Therapy."
2. Remove the intravenous site dressing in order to observe the needle insertion site during medication administration.
3. Cleanse the injection port on the intravenous tubing with an antiseptic wipe. Allow to dry.
4. Remove the needle protector from the medication syringe.
5. Insert the medication syringe into the injection port.
6. Clamp off the intravenous tubing above the injection port.
7. Aspirate to ensure a blood return.
8. Instill the medication, using the time factor recommended by the drug manufacturer. Aspirate after each 1 cc to ensure a blood return.
9. Stop the injection immediately if any signs of extravasation or anaphylaxis occur. Provide emergency treatment according to procedure and protocol.
10. Remove the syringe from the injection port when administration has been completed.
11. Open the clamp on the intravenous tubing and flush the tubing and the vein.
12. Repeat steps 4 through 11 if administering more than one medication.
13. Reestablish the intravenous rate as prescribed.
14. Reapply the needle site dressing, using aseptic technique.
15. Reposition the patient comfortably.
16. Discard equipment or return it to the appropriate location.

Administration by Direct Intravenous Push
1. Perform a venipuncture, using a small scalp vein needle. Refer to the procedure "Intravenous Therapy."
2. Detach the normal saline syringe and connect the medication syringe, using aseptic technique.
3. Instill the medication, using the time factor recommended by the drug manufacturer. Aspirate after each 1 cc to ensure a blood return.

4. Stop the injection immediately if any signs of extravasation or anaphylaxis occur. Provide emergency treatment according to procedure and protocol.
5. Detach the medication syringe when administration has been completed, and attach the second saline filled syringe.
6. Flush the scalp vein needle and vein with the saline solution.
7. Repeat steps 2 through 6 if administering more than one medication.
8. Remove the scalp vein needle, apply pressure to the site, and apply a small dressing. Refer to "Removal of the Intravenous Device" for the procedure describing the method for discontinuing an intravenous infusion.
9. Reposition the patient comfortably.
10. Discard equipment or return it to the appropriate location.

Patient Assessment
1. Instruct the patient to report immediately any sensations of burning or pain at the needle site that may indicate extravasation.
2. Assess the needle site for edema or redness during the administration of the medication.
3. Instruct the patient to report any symptoms such as vertigo, nausea, flushing, itching, or shortness of breath that may indicate anaphylaxis.
4. Report any signs or symptoms to the physician immediately.
5. Observe the patient every 15 to 30 minutes following medication administration for signs of untoward reactions to the drug.

PATIENT AND/OR FAMILY TEACHING
1. Explain the procedure to the patient and family.
2. Reinforce and clarify the physician's explanation of the chemotherapy, including the frequency of treatments, administration techniques, side effects, and long-term treatment plan.

3. Instruct the patient to report immediately any sensations of burning or pain at the needle site.
4. Instruct the patient to report immediately any symptoms such as vertigo, nausea, itching, or shortness of breath.
5. Reinforce nutritional counseling to minimize anorexia during chemotherapy.

DOCUMENTATION
1. Medication, dosage, time, and route of administration.
2. Type of administration method, including the intravenous flow rate, if appropriate.
3. Needle size and site.
4. Any assessment parameters including vital signs.
5. Any complications such as extravasation or anaphylaxis, your interventions, and the results.
6. The patient's reaction to the procedure, including any side effects.
7. All patient teaching done and the patient's level of understanding.

Treatment for Chemotherapy Drug Extravasation _____

PURPOSE
1. Prevent tissue damage and necrosis following drug extravasation.

REQUISITES
1. 5 cc syringe with a 22 gauge needle
2. 2 cc syringe with a 27 gauge needle
3. Antiseptic wipes
4. Solu-Cortef, 100 mg/cc Mix-O-Vial for IV use only
5. Hydrocortisone cream, 1% topical
6. Sterile 3 × 3 gauze sponges
7. Tape
8. Exam glove
9. Ice
10. Bath towel

GUIDELINES
1. Equipment for the drug extravasation procedure should be kept on the chemotherapy unit in a box labeled "Emergency Extravasation Box." The box should be taken into the patient's room when administering chemotherapy.
2. Recognize and suspect extravasation of specific vesicant drugs such as doxorubicin sulfate, daunorubicin, vincristine, vinblastine sulfate, actinomycin-D, and mitomycin-C when:
   a. The patient complains of pain and/or burning at the injection site.
   b. A venous blood return is not obtained during aspiration of the intravenous tubing.
   c. Erythema or swelling occurs at the intravenous site.
3. Treatment of extravasation, which is an emergency procedure, is best provided for with standing orders from a physician or with a hospital policy. The following nursing action describes a method of handling extravasation; however, it should not be implemented without a physician's specific order.
4. Chemotherapy may be given through an existing intravenous line or directly into the vein.
5. Cold applications are generally applied to the site for 24 hours after extravasation.

NURSING ACTION/RATIONALE
1. Aspirate the chemotherapy syringe to remove as much of the drug from the venipuncture site as possible. Leave the needle in place.
2. Initiate treatment of the site, using standing extravasation orders, while another team member notifies the physician.
3. Open the "Emergency Extravasation Box."
4. Explain the procedure to the patient.
5. Remove the chemotherapy syringe from the needle and attach a syringe containing 100 to 150 mg of Solu-Cortef. Inject the Solu-Cortef through the IV needle.
6. Remove the IV needle.
7. Administer 50 to 200 mg of Solu-Cortef intradermally and subcutaneously from the periphery of the bleb inward toward the area of erythema. The dosage will vary according to the size of the bleb.
8. Apply a film of hydrocortisone 1% topical cream to the area.
9. Cover the area with a sterile 3 × 3 gauze dressing and secure with tape.
10. Apply an ice glove to the area and secure it in place. The ice glove should be applied for 24 hours.
11. Follow the physician's orders for further treatment.
12. Continue assessing the extravasation site for tissue damage with each dressing change.
13. Discard equipment or return it to the appropriate area.

PATIENT AND/OR FAMILY TEACHING

1. Instruct the patient to notify the nurse if the pain becomes intense or is not relieved by the ice glove and steroid cream.
2. Instruct the patient to exercise the affected area to prevent restricted joint mobility.
3. Instruct the patient and/or family regarding the care of the extravasation site if dressing changes and treatment will be necessary after discharge.
4. Instruct the patient regarding the importance of follow-up care with the physician following discharge.

DOCUMENTATION

1. Time of the procedure, type of procedure, and person performing the procedure.
2. Any medications given during the procedure.
3. The patient's reaction to the treatment, including specific assessment parameters such as pain.
4. Appearance of extravasation site.
5. Name of physician notified.
6. All patient teaching done and the patient's level of understanding.

Infusion Pumps and Controllers

PURPOSE

1. Accurately infuse a prescribed amount of fluid or medication in a given time through the intravenous route.
2. Provide nursing management of intravenous infusion pumps and controllers.

REQUISITES

1. Infusion pump or controller
2. Tubing appropriate for the infusion pump or controller
3. Intravenous solution or medication as prescribed
4. Antiseptic wipes
5. Equipment for initiating intravenous therapy, if necessary
6. Tape

GUIDELINES

1. Infusion pumps or controllers can be divided into three main types: the syringe pump, the nonvolumetric pump, and the volumetric pump.
2. Syringe pumps are generally used for the administration of small volumes of intravenous fluids or medications such as chemotherapy, critical care drugs, or insulin. The plunger of the syringe is automatically depressed at a constant set rate.
3. The nonvolumetric pump measures the drop rate and is used for the administration of larger volumes of solutions. A conversion chart accompanies the machine to calculate the number of cc per hour.
4. The volumetric pump measures the volume of solution infused. It operates by drawing the solution into a metered chamber and exerting pressure to infuse the solution into the vein at a prescribed rate.
5. Most intravenous infusion pumps and controllers can be used with either glass bottles or plastic bags. Refer to the manufacturer's recommendations for the appropriate tubing and solution container.

6. Intravenous infusion pumps work by gravitational force. The solution container must be suspended above the venipuncture site, as with a straight gravity infusion. A drop sensor attached to the drip chamber activates the alarm when the flow rate is not as prescribed.

7. Intravenous infusion pumps work by exerting positive pressure on the intravenous fluid or intravenous line, preventing back flow of blood into the intravenous tubing.

8. All infusion pumps and most controllers have an alarm system to alert the nurse of any infusion problems.

9. Most intravenous infusion pumps and controllers can be attached to an IV standard to enhance their portability. Some syringe pumps require a stationary position on a table.

10. Most infusion pumps have a rechargeable battery, which will usually operate the pump away from an electrical source for a period of time. The battery should not be used except temporarily; that is, when an electrical outlet is not accessible.

11. Many infusion pumps need to be plugged into an electrical outlet when in storage. Refer to the manufacturer's instructions.

12. All infusion pumps and controllers need to be inspected and serviced regularly.

13. Many infusion filters cannot withstand the pressure exerted by a pump. Filter limitations and pump pressures should always be assessed.

14. Infusion pumps or controllers do not take the place of good nursing care. The pump will accurately infuse the solution only if it is assembled properly and is in good working order. The nurse must carefully assess the patient during any fluid or medication infusion.

NURSING ACTION/RATIONALE

1. Assemble all equipment.
2. Verify the physician's order for the appropriate solution or medication.
3. Wash your hands.

4. Attach the solution or medication to the infusion tubing according to the manufacturer's directions.
5. Prime the pump attachments and tubing according to the manufacturer's directions.
6. Identify the patient.
7. Explain the purpose of the infusion pump to the patient. Demonstrate the alarm and explain the purpose of the alarm.
8. Connect the unit to an electrical outlet, if appropriate.
9. Perform a venipuncture if the patient does not have an established infusion. Refer to the procedure "Intravenous Therapy."
10. Attach the infusion pump tubing to the intravenous device, using aseptic technique.
11. Turn on the infusion pump.
12. Set the prescribed rate.
13. Check for proper functioning of the infusion pump and ensure that all alarms are on.
14. Tape all connections.
15. Assess the intravenous insertion site.
16. Discard equipment or return it to the appropriate location.

PATIENT AND/OR FAMILY TEACHING

1. Explain the purpose and function of the infusion pump.
2. Demonstrate the alarm on the infusion pump and explain the purpose of the alarm.
3. Explain any activity restrictions as appropriate.
4. Instruct the patient not to change the settings on the machine.
5. Explain all other therapeutic orders as appropriate.
6. Refer to the "Intravenous Therapy" procedure for patient teaching related to intravenous therapy.

DOCUMENTATION

1. Date, time, type, amount, and rate of solution to be infused.
2. Type of infusion pump being used.
3. The patient's reaction to the intravenous therapy and the infusion pump.
4. All patient teaching done and the patient's level of understanding.

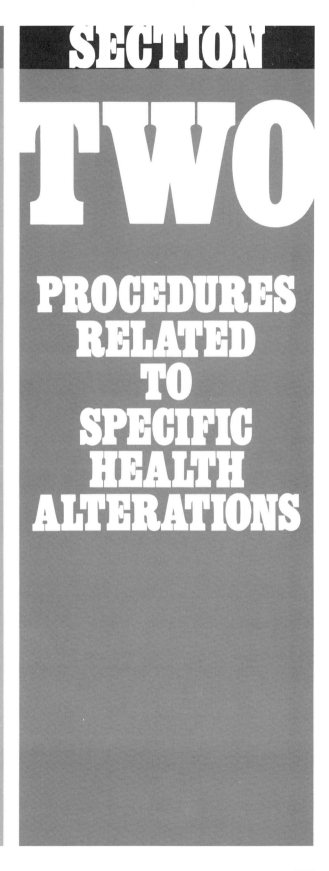

SECTION

TWO

PROCEDURES RELATED TO SPECIFIC HEALTH ALTERATIONS

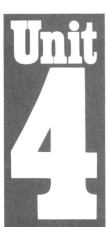

Unit 4

Cardiopulmonary Procedures

PROCEDURES

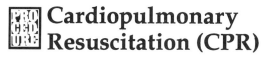

Cardiopulmonary Resuscitation (CPR)

PURPOSE

1. Diagnose cardiopulmonary arrest.
2. Maintain cardiac and respiratory function until definitive treatment can be given.

REQUISITES

None

GUIDELINES

1. Many causes of sudden death require cardiopulmonary resuscitation including suffocation, choking, electrocution, drowning, drug overdose, anaphylaxis, and heart failure. The most common cause is myocardial infarction followed by ventricular arrhythmias or asystole.
2. The procedure for resuscitation is the same regardless of the cause. A determination must be made whether the victim is unconscious, whether the victim is breathing, and whether the victim has a pulse.
3. Clinical death occurs when a victim is not breathing and has no heart beat. Biological death occurs when brain tissue dies after lack of oxygen for 4 to 6 minutes.
4. By utilizing the correct procedure for cardiopulmonary resuscitation, a victim's respirations and circulation can be adequately supported until:
   a. A physician stops the procedure.
   b. Someone as qualified or better qualified relieves you.
   c. You are physically exhausted and cannot continue.
   d. The victim regains adequate circulation and respirations.
5. An unconscious patient can develop an obstructed airway very easily, since the tongue falls back into the pharynx and obstructs the upper airway. The airway must be opened to establish a state of breathlessness.
6. The carotid pulse should be palpated on the side nearest the rescuer to prevent compressing both carotids simultaneously.
7. Correct hand placement during chest compression is essential to avoid injury to the ribs and surrounding organs.

8. The rhythm and rate of chest compressions should be even to produce an adequate blood flow. Systolic blood pressure can be maintained at 60 to 80 mm Hg when compressions are done correctly.
9. The ratio of compressions to breaths in one-rescuer CPR is 15:2. The ratio for two-rescuer CPR is 5:1.
10. Periodically the victim should be assessed for return of pulse and breathing. Allow enough time to perform the assessment adequately.
11. If vomiting occurs during CPR, stop compressions. Roll the victim to the side and sweep out the mouth. Return to CPR as soon as possible.
12. If gastric distention occurs, do not apply manual pressure to the gastric area, since vomiting may occur. Reassess ventilations and chest movement.
13. Cardiopulmonary resuscitation should not be stopped for more than 15 to 20 seconds for any reason.
14. There are three types of cardiopulmonary arrests: asystole, ventricular fibrillation, and cardiovascular collapse.
15. The effects of cardiopulmonary arrest include myocardial hypotonicity, acidosis, vasodilatation, and hypoxemia.
16. Definitive treatment should be instituted as quickly as possible to treat the arrest as well as correct the effects of the arrest. Equipment and medications that should be available include:

Equipment

a. External defibrillator unit with a cardioscope
b. Suction unit
c. Back board
d. Wall oxygen set-up or oxygen tank
e. Endotracheal tube
f. Bag-valve mask with adaptor or mechanical respirator
g. External pacemaker
h. Intravenous equipment

Medications
  a. Epinephrine
  b. Calcium chloride
  c. Sodium bicarbonate
  d. Digoxin
  e. Aminophylline
  f. Aramine or dopamine
  g. Procainamide hydrochloride (Pronestyl)
  h. Lidocaine hydrochloride
  i. Dilantin
  j. Isoproterenol hydrochloride (Isuprel)
17. To maintain competency in cardiopulmonary resuscitation techniques, it is necessary to practice them and to review them frequently.

NURSING ACTION/RATIONALE
One-Rescuer CPR
  1. Upon finding an unconscious victim, turn the victim as a single unit onto his/her back and note the time.
  2. Establish unresponsiveness:
     a. Shake the victim's shoulders.
     b. Shout "Are you OK?"
     c. Elicit a response by rubbing your knuckles on the sternum or pinching the trapezius muscle.
  3. Shout for help.
  4. Kneel at the victim's side.
  5. Place your hand that is nearest the victim's feet under the victim's neck and your other hand on the victim's forehead.
  6. Open the airway by tilting the head back and extending the neck (Figure 4-1).
  7. Establish breathlessness by looking at the victim's chest, keeping your ear directly over and close to the victim's mouth.
  8. Observe for respiratory effort and listen and feel for breathing.
  9. Maintain an open airway if the victim is breathing. Wait for help to arrive.
  10. If the victim is not breathing, pinch off the victim's nostrils with the thumb and index finger of the hand on the victim's forehead.
  11. Open your mouth widely and make a tight seal over the victim's mouth.
  12. Give four ventilations. Continue to maintain an open airway.
  13. Establish pulselessness:
     a. Place the fingers of your hand, nearest the victim's feet, on the trachea just below the chin.

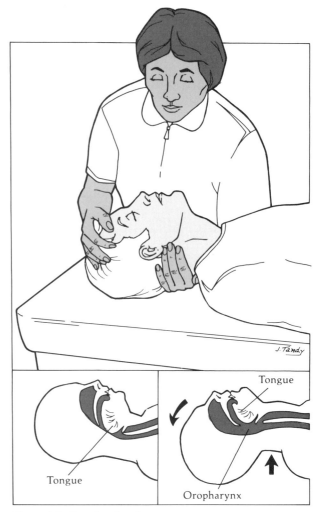

Figure 4-1. Opening the airway.

     b. Slide your fingers into the groove between the trachea and the neck muscle on the side nearer to you.
     c. Palpate for a carotid pulse (Figure 4-2).

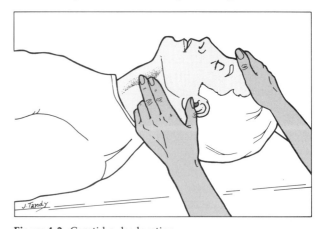

Figure 4-2. Carotid pulse location.

14. Continue to perform rescue breathing at a rate of one ventilation every 5 seconds if a pulse is present. Recheck the pulse every minute.
15. If no pulse is present, activate your emergency medical system, then move toward the victim's chest with your shoulders directly over the victim's sternum.
16. Establish chest landmarks by running the index and middle fingers of your hand, closest to the victim's feet, up the margin of the rib cage until your middle finger fits into the substernal notch.
17. Place the heel of your hand, closest to the victim's head, on the midline of the sternum so that the base of the thumb touches the index finger of your other hand.
18. Place your other hand directly over the heel of the hand already on the sternum. Keep the heels of both hands parallel, with the fingers and palms off the chest wall (Figure 4-3).

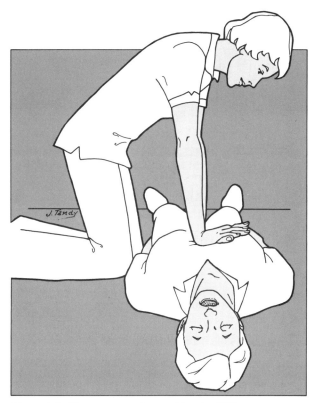

Figure 4-4. Chest compression position for CPR.

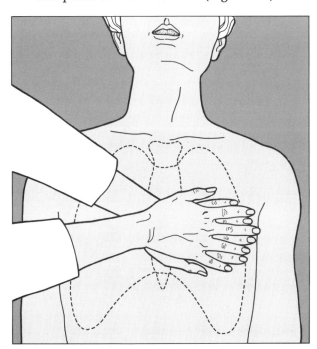

Figure 4-3. Proper hand position for chest compression.

19. Compress the chest by pushing straight down approximately 1½ to 2 inches, using your body weight and keeping your elbows locked (Figure 4-4).

20. Compress the chest at a rate of 80 compressions per minute. Count aloud, saying "one and two and three." Keep your hands resting lightly on the victim's sternum between compressions.
21. Compress the chest 15 times, then move to the victim's head, reestablish the airway, and ventilate the victim twice.
22. Return to the chest compressions and complete four cycles of compressions and ventilations at a 15:2 ratio, ending with two ventilations.
23. Stop CPR and assess for spontaneous return of pulse and/or breathing. If no pulse or breathing is present, continue CPR by giving 2 ventilations followed by 15 compressions. Reassess for pulse and breathing every 5 minutes:
    a. If pulse is present but no breathing, continue ventilations, assessing the pulse frequently.
    b. If both pulse and breathing have returned, maintain an open airway and continue assessing the pulse until help arrives.

Two-Rescuer CPR

1. Continue one-rescuer CPR until the second rescuer arrives.
2. Identify your ability to perform CPR (Rescuer 2).
3. Kneel opposite Rescuer 1 in the rescue breathing position.
4. Assess for a carotid pulse while Rescuer 1 continues compressions.
   a. Direct Rescuer 1 to reassess his/her hand position if no pulse is palpated.
   b. Reassess for a pulse with each compression.
5. Stop CPR (Rescuer 1) and assess for the return of pulse and breathing.
6. If none, give one ventilation (Rescuer 2) and resume chest compressions (Rescuer 1). Establish a compression and ventilation ratio of 5:1 with a compression rate of 60 per minute. Count aloud.
7. Change positions in two-rescuer CPR every few minutes.
   a. Change after the fifth compression by saying (Rescuer 1) "Four one-thousand, change one-thousand."
   b. Give two ventilations (Rescuer 2), and change positions.
   c. Establish the airway and assess for pulse and breathing.
   d. If none, give one ventilation followed by five compressions and continue CPR until the next change.
8. Assist with resuscitation and definitive treatment when help arrives.

PATIENT AND/OR FAMILY TEACHING

1. Reinforce and clarify the physician's explanation of the cardiopulmonary arrest following a successful resuscitation, if appropriate.
2. Provide explanations and support to the family as necessary.

DOCUMENTATION

1. Time of the arrest and names of persons performing CPR.
2. All medications given.
3. All treatments performed.
4. Results of the resuscitation.
5. All assessment parameters, including vital signs.
6. All patient or family teaching done and the level of understanding.

 # Obstructed Airway Rescue

PURPOSE

1. Provide a clear airway by repositioning the patient's head and neck or by removing a foreign body.

REQUISITES

None

GUIDELINES

1. An airway obstruction requiring rescue assistance may occur for a variety of reasons, including:
   a. Unconsciousness causing the tongue to fall back, obstructing the airway.
   b. Inhaled foreign bodies.
   c. Ingested substances such as large pieces of food.

2. Foreign body obstruction of the airway usually occurs during eating, and in adults is most often caused by meat.

3. A victim with a completely blocked airway cannot breathe, cough, or speak and needs assistance immediately.

4. If the victim can speak or cough, a partial airway obstruction should be suspected and rescue measures should not be implemented.

5. If a foreign body is seen in the mouth at any time during the rescue, attempt to remove it by sweeping your finger in a hooked motion behind the foreign body.

6. Vomiting may occur during this procedure. Turn the victim to the side and sweep out the mouth. Assess for return of breathing. If none, resume the rescue procedure.

7. Victims, with an airway obstruction that has been removed, may not begin breathing spontaneously. If a pulse is present, most victims will breathe spontaneously in a few minutes. Continue to ventilate the patient until spontaneous breathing resumes.

8. Following an airway obstruction that has been successfully removed, the victim should be seen by a physician.

9. The rescue procedure for an obstructed airway is usually performed in a standing position for a conscious victim. If the victim becomes unconscious, the rescuer must assume a kneeling position next to the lying victim.

NURSING ACTION/RATIONALE
Airway Obstruction: Conscious Victim

1. Identify complete airway obstruction by asking the victim, "Can you speak?" Observe, listen, and feel for breathing. Note the time.

2. If no breathing is assessed, stand just behind and to the side of the victim.

3. Support the victim's chest with your non-dominant hand while bending the victim forward, keeping the victim's head lower than the chest, if possible (Figure 4-5).

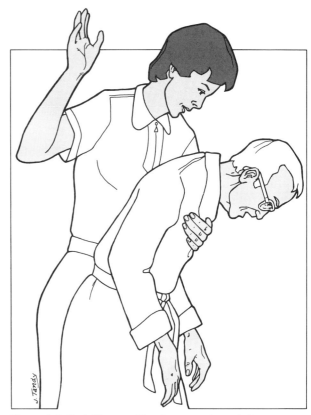

Figure 4-5. Back blow position for a conscious victim.

4. Deliver four sharp back blows rapidly and forcefully between the shoulder blades.

5. Assess for dislodgement of the foreign body.

6. If unsuccessful, wrap your arms around the victim's abdomen.

7. Place the fist of your non-dominant hand, thumb side inward, against the abdomen between the xyphoid process and the navel.

8. Grasp your fist with your other hand and give four abdominal thrusts by pressing into the victim's abdomen with a quick upward motion (Figure 4-6).

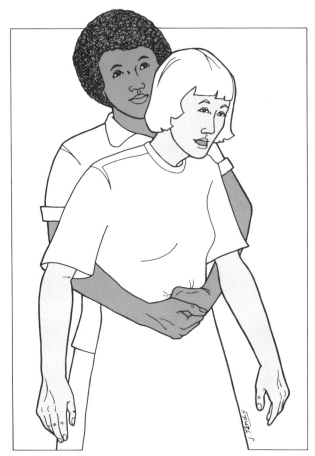

Figure 4-6. Abdominal thrust position for a conscious victim.

9. Assess for dislodgement of the foreign body.
10. If unsuccessful, repeat the series of four back blows and four abdominal thrusts until the obstruction is relieved or the victim becomes unconscious.
11. Continue supporting the patient throughout the procedure to prevent injury in case the victim becomes unconscious.
12. Arrange for a physician to assess the victim, if removal of the airway obstruction is successful.

Airway Obstruction: Unconscious Victim
1. Lower an unconscious victim to the floor.
2. Place the victim in a supine position and call for help.

3. Open the airway by placing your hand, nearest the victim's feet, under the victim's neck and your other hand on the victim's forehead. Tilt the head back, extending the neck.
4. Attempt to ventilate the victim by pinching off the victim's nostrils with the thumb and index finger of your hand on the victim's forehead. Place your mouth tightly over the victim's mouth and attempt to give ventilations.
5. If unable to ventilate, roll the victim toward you, using your thigh for support.
6. Deliver four sharp back blows rapidly and forcefully between the shoulder blades (Figure 4-7).

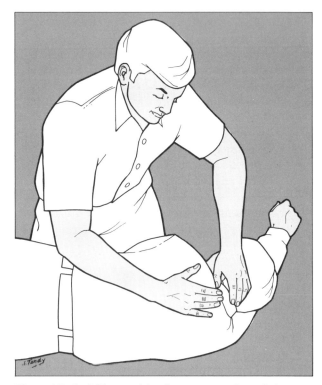

Figure 4-7. Back blow position for an unconscious victim.

7. Assess for dislodgement of the foreign body.
8. If unsuccessful, return the victim to the supine position.
9. Position yourself close to the victim with your knees parallel to the victim's hips.

10. Place the heel of your hand in the midline of the victim's abdomen between the xyphoid process and the navel.
11. Place your other hand on top of the first hand with your shoulders directly over the victim's abdomen.
12. Give four abdominal thrusts by pressing into the victim's abdomen with a quick upward motion (Figure 4-8).

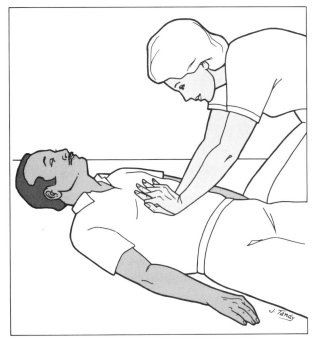

Figure 4-8. Abdominal thrust position for an unconscious victim.

13. Assess for dislodgement of the obstruction:
    a. Grasp the tongue and lower jaw between your thumb and fingers.
    b. Pull the jaw upward.
    c. Sweep deeply into the victim's mouth with the index finger of your other hand.
    d. Sweep along the cheek with a hooking action toward the other cheek.
    e. Remove the obstruction, if possible.
14. Position the head and neck and attempt to ventilate.

15. If unsuccessful, continue repeating back blows, abdominal thrusts, probing, and ventilations.
16. If successful, ventilate the patient as necessary and arrange for follow-up medical treatment.

PATIENT AND/OR FAMILY TEACHING
1. Explain the follow-up care to the patient or family, including the need to be examined by a physician.
2. Explain the importance of chewing food well and the danger of talking and laughing with food in the mouth, if appropriate.
3. Caution the patient regarding the effect of heavy alcohol intake and the potential for choking during eating, if appropriate.

DOCUMENTATION
1. Time the airway obstruction was noted and when it was relieved.
2. Type of procedure used.
3. Type of obstruction.
4. The patient's reaction to the procedure, if successful.
5. Any arrangements made for follow-up care.
6. All patient teaching done and the patient's level of understanding.

Telemetry Application

PURPOSE
1. Apply a cardiac monitoring system to detect arrhythmias.

REQUISITES
1. Telemetry transmitter unit with central console
2. 9 volt battery
3. Two lead wires
4. Carrying pouch
5. Disposable electrode pads—2
6. Defatting compound
7. Cotton balls

GUIDELINES
1. Telemetry cardiac monitoring units are used for patients with cardiac dysfunction where early detection of arrhythmias is imperative.
2. A physician's order is required to place a patient on a telemetry unit.
3. For the male patient with chest hair, a 4 to 5 inch area should be shaved for electrode placement in order to provide maximum contact.
4. Electrodes should be placed in the right subclavicular area and in the left midclavicular area below the nipple line for Lead II monitoring.
5. Patients should be instructed to avoid getting the telemetry unit wet.
6. Telemetry electrodes should be relocated to prevent skin irritation. Electrode wires should be detached and the electrode pads peeled off gently. New pads should be applied near the same area after cleansing the skin with a defatting compound. Previously used skin sites should be cleaned with soap and water and assessed for redness, irritation, or skin breakdown. The frequency of electrode changes is based on the type of electrode pad used and your health care facility's policy.
7. Telemetry transmitters should be assessed daily with a voltage meter for battery function. Batteries should be replaced when voltage is low.
8. When telemetry is discontinued, the battery should be removed from the transmitter, assessed for voltage level, and recharged or discarded if low.

9. When the patient temporarily leaves the nursing unit, program the monitoring unit according to the manufacturer's instructions and remove the telemetry transmitting unit.
10. The use of electrical devices such as razors or hair dryers is contraindicated when wearing the telemetry unit.

NURSING ACTION/RATIONALE
1. Assemble all equipment.
2. Insert a fresh battery into the transmitter unit and attach the lead wires according to the manufacturer's instructions.
3. Identify the patient.
4. Explain the procedure to the patient and display the transmitter unit.
5. Provide privacy.
6. Assist the patient to a supine position.
7. Wash your hands.
8. Expose the chest and upper abdomen. Drape the patient as necessary.
9. Select electrode sites in the right subclavicular area and the left midclavicular area below the nipple (Figure 4-9).

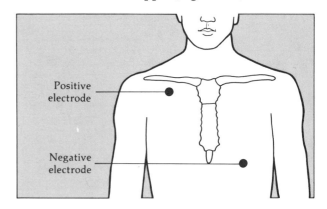

Figure 4-9. Electrode sites for telemetry monitoring.

10. Prep a 3 inch diameter area of skin at each electrode site with a cotton ball saturated with a defatting compound.
11. Remove the electrodes from the packaging and press firmly into place in each area.

12. Clip the lead wires from the transmitter onto the electrodes:
    a. Clip the lead wire plugged into the white socket, the negative electrode, to the right electrode pad.
    b. Clip the lead wire plugged into the red socket, the positive electrode, to the left electrode pad.
13. Insert the telemetry unit into a pouch and secure it at the midsternal area of the patient's chest by tying it around the neck and waist.
14. Assist the patient to a comfortable position.
15. Turn the monitoring unit on according to the manufacturer's instructions, set alarm rates as ordered, and assess for proper functioning.
16. Discard equipment or return it to the appropriate location.

PATIENT AND/OR FAMILY TEACHING
1. Explain the procedure and its purpose to the patient.
2. Instruct the patient to avoid getting the telemetry unit wet.
3. Instruct the patient to notify the nurse if the lead wires become disconnected or there is any change in activity level.
4. Instruct the patient to notify the nurse of any symptoms of chest pain or discomfort.

DOCUMENTATION
1. Time and date of the procedure.
2. Location of the electrode pads.
3. Description of the cardiac pattern on the monitor.
4. All patient teaching done and the patient's level of understanding.

Central Venous Pressure Measurement

PURPOSE
1. Assess intermittent or continuous central venous pressure readings.
2. Assess fluid balance.
3. Assess the relationship between circulating blood volume and the pumping action of the heart.

REQUISITES
1. Established central venous catheter connected to an intravenous therapy system
2. Central venous pressure water manometer kit with 18 gauge needle and mounting strips
3. IV standard
4. Carpenter's level
5. Alcohol wipes

GUIDELINES
1. A central venous pressure line provides the physician with hemodynamic measurements useful in the management of shock states and heart failure.
2. The patient is usually placed flat and supine for central venous pressure readings. If the patient is unable to tolerate this position, note the position that the patient can tolerate and record this position. For subsequent readings the patient should be placed in the same position.
3. Mark an X on the patient's chest at the right atrium level. The level of the right atrium must correspond to zero on the manometer. The X should be placed in the right midaxillary region at the fourth intercostal space.

4. If significant changes occur in the results of a reading, reassess the entire system and the patient's status. The following factors may affect the reading and should be assessed along with reading changes:
   a. Patient's level of discomfort.
   b. Baseline positioning of the patient.
   c. Level of the right atrium in relationship to zero on the manometer.
   d. The use of a ventilator. Ventilators may affect the central venous pressure readings.
5. If changes still occur beyond the established readings, notify the physician; report the readings and a total patient assessment.
6. Fluctuation of fluid in the manometer indicates patency of the entire intravenous line and ensures that the system is functioning properly.
7. Assess the system frequently to avoid complications. Assessment areas include:
   a. Patency of the tubing.
   b. Absence of air bubbles and/or blood clots.
   c. Secured connections.
   d. Adequately filled intravenous solution bottle.
   e. Secure, taut manometer tube.
   f. Proper positioning of tubing, avoiding kinking and/or entanglement.
   g. A dry filter at the end of the manometer.
8. Always read and follow the manufacturer's recommendations on the manometer package to assure patient safety.
9. Normal central venous pressure readings range from 5 to 12 cm water. Readings above 12 cm water may indicate fluid overload, heart failure, or pulmonary artery blockage. A low reading may indicate a fluid volume deficit.

NURSING ACTION/RATIONALE
1. Assemble all equipment.
2. Verify the physician's order.
3. Identify the patient.
4. Explain the procedure to the patient including the position required during the measurement.

5. Provide privacy.
6. Provide adequate lighting.
7. Mark an X on the patient's chest at the right midaxillary line in the fourth intercostal space (Figure 4-10).

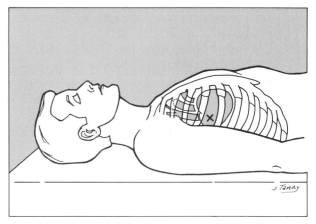

Figure 4-10. Level of right atrium.

8. Place the patient in a flat supine position.
9. Align the manometer's zero marking with the X on the patient's chest, using a level.
10. Secure the manometer to the IV standard with the mounting strips.
11. Remove the adapter cover from the central venous pressure tubing and attach the 18 gauge needle.
12. Cleanse the Y injection port with an alcohol wipe and allow it to dry.
13. Insert the needle into the Y injection port of the administration set (Figure 4-11).
14. Obtain a central venous pressure reading:
    a. Clamp off the administration tubing between the patient and the Y port with the slide clamp.
    b. Open the slide clamp on the central venous pressure tubing and the flow control clamp on the administration set. Allow the intravenous fluid to rise in the manometer to 18 to 20 cm of water above the anticipated reading.
    c. Close the flow control clamp on the administration set between the intravenous solution bottle and the Y injection port.
    d. Unclamp the slide clamp between the patient and the Y injection port.

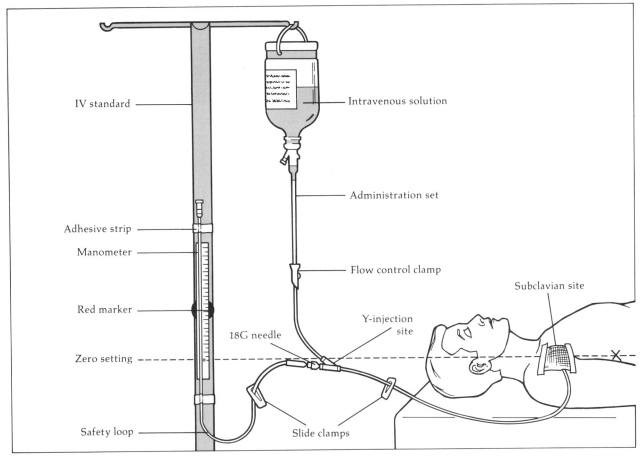

Figure 4-11. Diagram of a central venous pressure set-up.

e. Allow the intravenous solution to descend in the manometer until the meniscus (Figure 4-12) has stabilized. Read at eye level.

f. Move the red marker to the meniscus level.

g. Close the slide clamp on the central venous pressure tubing.

h. Open the flow control clamp on the intravenous solution tubing and adjust the flow as prescribed.

15. Assist the patient to a comfortable position.

16. Discard equipment or return it to the appropriate location.

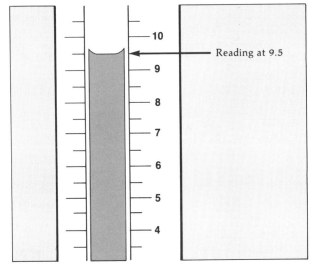

Figure 4-12. Meniscus reading at 9.5.

PATIENT AND/OR FAMILY TEACHING

1. Reinforce and clarify the physician's explanation for the procedure.
2. Instruct the patient on the necessary positioning for the reading.
3. Explain to the patient how often the readings will be taken.
4. Instruct the patient to avoid manipulating the tubing.
5. Reinforce the need to call the nurse immediately if:
   a. The tubing becomes disconnected.
   b. There is a backflow of blood into the tubing.
   c. Any unusual symptoms are experienced.

DOCUMENTATION

1. Date, time, and results of the baseline reading, and position of the patient.
2. Date, time, and results of all readings.
3. All assessment parameters.
4. Notification of the physician of specific readings.
5. All patient teaching done and the patient's level of understanding.

 # Rotating Tourniquets

PURPOSE

1. Decrease venous blood return and right cardiac output in acute pulmonary edema.
2. Provide temporary support therapy until additional definitive treatment is initiated.

REQUISITES

1. Three wide tourniquets of sufficient length to circle the upper and lower extremities or three blood pressure cuffs
2. Three small towels
3. Rotation documentation record

GUIDELINES

1. Rotating tourniquets are generally ordered by the physician as an emergency measure in conjunction with other supportive treatment to decrease the circulating blood volume and thus the work of the heart in cases of congestive heart failure or severe pulmonary edema.
2. Rotating tourniquets applied to three extremities are capable of reducing circulating blood volume by approximately 1000 mL.
3. The patient requiring this procedure will usually be exhibiting signs of extreme respiratory difficulty and consequently will be very apprehensive and will need continual reassurance.
4. Patients are normally placed in a semi- to high-Fowler's position to facilitate breathing. Oxygen therapy will be ordered by the physician to coincide with this treatment.
5. Emergency life support equipment should be available during this procedure.
6. Intravenous lines should be placed centrally so all extremities may be used during the procedure.
7. The time interval for the rotation schedule should be dictated by the physician's order. Time interval for rotating the tourniquets may range from 5 to 15 minutes. The maximum time for a tourniquet to remain in place is 45 minutes.
8. One extremity must be free of tourniquets at all times.
9. Tourniquets should not obliterate arterial pulses distal to the tourniquet.
10. Extremities should be assessed during and after tourniquet removal for color, warmth, and pulses.
11. Upon completion of this procedure, tourniquets should be removed one at a time at 15-minute intervals or as ordered by the physician to prevent pulmonary overload and recurrence of symptoms.
12. Rotating tourniquets are contraindicated in shock states.

NURSING ACTION/RATIONALE

1. Assemble all equipment.
2. Identify the patient.
3. Explain the procedure and purpose if patient condition permits. Explain that extremities may become slightly blue and may feel tingly and numb.
4. Obtain baseline vital signs, including an apical pulse, and breath sounds.
5. Mark peripheral pulse sites if possible.
6. Apply tourniquets to three extremities (Figure 4-13).

   a. Position tourniquet over a small towel.
   b. Apply tourniquet tightly to occlude venous circulation but not arterial circulation.
   c. Place tourniquets on upper extremities between the shoulder and elbow.
   d. Place tourniquets on lower extremities in the upper thigh area.
   e. Maintain one free extremity during each time interval.

7. Release one tourniquet every 15 minutes or as ordered by the physician. Reapply tourniquet to free extremity.
8. Rotate tourniquets in a clockwise pattern. Place a rotation schedule at the bedside (Figure 4-14).
9. Assess vital signs and peripheral circulation every 15 minutes. Assess urinary output every 30 minutes, since reduced circulating volume may cause decreased renal perfusion and oliguria.
10. Upon physician's order, remove tourniquets one at a time at 15-minute intervals or as ordered by physician.
11. Reassess vital signs, breath sounds, urinary output, and peripheral circulation every 15 to 30 minutes after tourniquet removal for at least 2 hours and then as the patient's condition warrants.
12. Assist the patient to a comfortable position.
13. Clean all equipment and return it to the appropriate location.

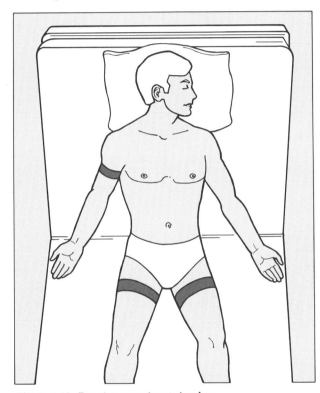

Figure 4-13. Rotating tourniquets in place.

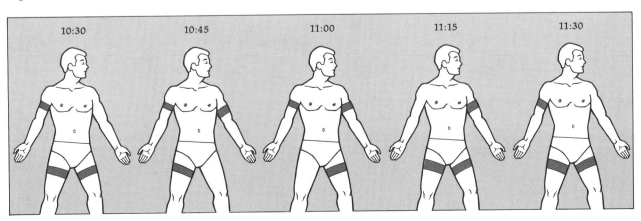

Figure 4-14. Sample rotation schedule.

PATIENT AND/OR FAMILY TEACHING

1. Instruct the patient before the procedure.
2. Instruct the patient to notify the nurse if experiencing any pain or paresthesia in the extremities.
3. Reinforce the physician's explanation regarding the patient's disease process.
4. Explain other therapeutic measures used for treatment including:
   a. Medications.
   b. Oxygen therapy.
5. Plan further teaching when the patient's condition permits, regarding prevention of recurrence by:
   a. Restricting dietary sodium as prescribed.
   b. Taking prescribed medications.
   c. Avoiding overexertion.
   d. Weighing daily to monitor fluid accumulation.
   e. Sleeping with head elevated.
   f. Seeking early medical attention if symptoms of breathing difficulty occur.

DOCUMENTATION

1. Baseline assessment data prior to the procedure.
2. Procedure with rotating times.
3. Duration of procedure.
4. Condition of extremities including color, temperature, sensation, movement, and pulses.
5. Vital signs including breath sounds and respiratory status.
6. Urine output.

 # Teaching the Patient to Measure Blood Pressure

PURPOSE

1. Teach the patient the steps for measuring blood pressure for the purpose of monitoring illness or therapy.

REQUISITES

1. Sphygmomanometer
2. Stethoscope

GUIDELINES

1. The patient should be encouraged to use the same arm, the same position, and to take the blood pressure at the same time each day.
2. The patient should be aware that the blood pressure reading is not a fixed number; it will vary from day to day.
3. Vocabulary and style of teaching must be appropriate for the patient's level of understanding.
4. The nurse and the patient must be aware of what the physician wants to do regarding readings and any follow-up medical care.
5. A quiet environment and a readiness to learn are essential.
6. Written instructions reinforce learning.

NURSING ACTION/RATIONALE

1. Assess the patient's ability to assume responsibility for taking his/her own blood pressure. If he/she is unable, instruct a family member in the procedure.
2. Assess the patient's understanding regarding his/her condition and the need for home blood pressure monitoring.

3. Demonstrate the procedure on self, repeating the instructions aloud:
   a. Push up the sleeve and palpate the brachial artery in the inner aspect of the elbow.
   b. Wrap the cuff around the upper arm, placing the center of the bladder over the artery.
   c. Rest the arm on a table or on the arm of the chair.
   d. Place the stethoscope in your ears and place the diaphragm on the inner aspect of the elbow below the cuff, using one hand.
   e. With the other hand, grasp the bulb of the blood pressure cuff, tighten the screw on the bulb and squeeze the bulb to inflate the blood pressure cuff 20 to 30 mm Hg above the last systolic reading.
   f. Place the gauge so that it can be seen (Figure 4-15).

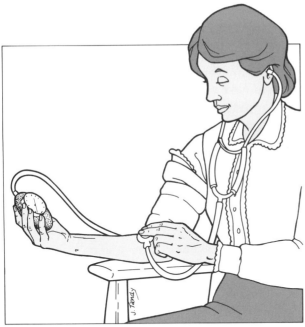

Figure 4-15. Proper set-up for taking one's own blood pressure.

   g. With eyes on the gauge, release the screw on the bulb slightly so that air pressure in the cuff is released gradually.
   h. Note the reading on the gauge when the pulse beat is first heard. This is the systolic blood pressure.

   i. Release the pressure slowly until the beat can no longer be heard. Note the reading on the gauge where the last beat was heard. This is the diastolic blood pressure.
   j. Release the remainder of the air from the cuff and unwrap the cuff.
   k. Record the reading as systolic/diastolic (*Example:* 120/80).
4. Have the patient or family member repeat the demonstration on self until able to perform the procedure successfully.
5. Evaluate the retention of information and reinforce as necessary.

PATIENT AND/OR FAMILY TEACHING
1. Reinforce the physician's explanation of the disease process and therapy pertaining to home blood pressure monitoring.
2. Teach the patient the signs and symptoms associated with elevated blood pressure.
3. Give the patient guidelines concerning when to notify the physician regarding elevated blood pressure readings or other related symptoms.
4. Instruct the patient on the importance of continuing the medication even though the blood pressure readings may be normal.
5. Arrange a dietary consultation for special dietary restrictions if prescribed.

DOCUMENTATION
1. All patient teaching done and the methods used.
2. The patient's ability to demonstrate the procedure.
3. The patient's reaction to performing the procedure.
4. All written instructions and visual aids given to the patient.
5. Further learning needs of the patient.
6. Blood pressure measurements obtained.

Oxygen Administration

PURPOSE

Provide adequate tissue oxygenation for problems associated with:

1. Reduced oxygen-carrying capacity of blood.
2. Decreased cardiac output.
3. Hypoventilation.
4. Increased metabolism.

REQUISITES

Oxygen set-up including:

1. Disposable single-patient oxygen humidifier
2. Flowmeter
3. Oxygen delivery device—nasal cannula, nasal catheter, mask
4. Sterile water
5. Water-soluble lubricant (catheter only)
6. Sign: "No Smoking, Oxygen in Use"

GUIDELINES

1. Prolonged hypoxemia causes damage to all body tissues including the vital organs. Classic signs of oxygen deprivation are tachycardia, dyspnea, and decreased mental alertness.
2. Oxygen must be administered carefully to patients with chronic obstructive pulmonary disease (COPD). High oxygen concentrations may decrease the respiratory drive, causing hypoventilation and bradypnea, since the respiratory drive in patients with COPD is sensitive to low oxygen levels rather than high carbon dioxide levels.
3. Oxygen equipment must be handled carefully because oxygen supports combustion. "No Smoking" signs must be displayed prominently in the area.
4. Patients receiving oxygen therapy must be assessed frequently for changes in vital signs, skin color, and level of consciousness. Physician-ordered arterial blood gas measurements provide a valuable assessment for respiratory function.
5. Oxygen administration to infants requires special considerations that are not included in this procedure.

6. Oxygen may be administered by nasal cannula, nasal catheter, or a variety of oxygen masks. The type of oxygen delivery device chosen is based on physician order and/or the patient's condition. Types of oxygen masks include:
   a. Simple mask.
   b. Partial rebreather mask.
   c. Nonrebreather mask.
   d. Venturi mask.
7. If oxygen mask therapy is continuous, a nasal cannula may be used during eating periods.
8. Since oxygen administration equipment is a potential source for bacterial invasion, equipment should be changed every 3 days.
9. Water in the humidifier should be kept at the correct level and not allowed to run dry. Oxygen tubing should be kept free of kinks.
10. Arrangements for portable equipment should be made when it is necessary to transport a patient requiring oxygen therapy.
11. Certain hospitals and health care facilities will have a respiratory care department that may be responsible for performing the major portion of this procedure.

NURSING ACTION/RATIONALE

1. Assemble all equipment.
2. Identify the patient.
3. Explain the procedure to the patient, emphasizing that no smoking will be allowed in the area.
4. Wash your hands.
5. Assemble the oxygen unit and flowmeter, making sure all connections are secure.
6. Fill the humidifier container to the correct level with distilled water and attach to the oxygen unit.
7. Attach the oxygen delivery device ordered by the physician to the oxygen unit.
8. Insert the oxygen unit into the wall oxygen outlet or attach it to an alternative oxygen source.
9. Turn the unit on to the desired flow rate and assess equipment for proper functioning:
   a. Air flow should be felt through the oxygen delivery device.
   b. Bubbles should be seen diffusing through the humidifier reservoir.

10. Place the oxygen delivery device on the patient, adjusting it to achieve patient comfort:

  a. Nasal cannula (Figure 4-16):

  (1) Place oxygen outlet tips in patient's nostils.

  (2) Adjust head strap or alternative chin strap for comfort, making sure cannula is secure.

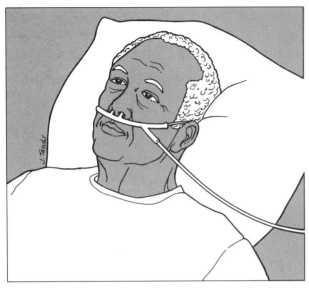

Figure 4-16. Oxygen nasal cannula in correct position.

  b. Nasal catheter (Figure 4-17):

  (1) Measure the catheter from the earlobe to the tip of the nose and mark.

  (2) Lubricate the catheter.

  (3) Insert gently into one nostril to marked point.

  (4) Check catheter for position by depressing patient's tongue with a tongue blade and examining for catheter tip correctly positioned directly behind the uvula.

  (5) Tape catheter to nose.

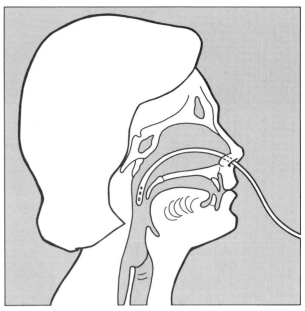

Figure 4-17. Oxygen nasal catheter in correct position.

  c. Oxygen mask (Figure 4-18):

  (1) Place mask over patient's mouth and nose.

  (2) Adjust elastic strap around patient's head comfortably but securely.

  (3) Adjust metal nose strap on mask to prevent oxygen from leaking around the nose.

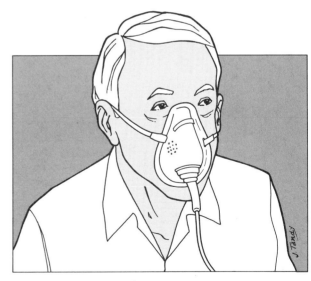

Figure 4-18. Oxygen mask in correct position.

11. Reassess oxygen flowmeter for correct liter flow.
12. Assist the patient to a comfortable position.
13. Place the "No Smoking, Oxygen in Use" warning sign on the patient's room door or in other appropriate locations.
14. Discard equipment or return it to the appropriate location.

PATIENT AND/OR FAMILY TEACHING

1. Instruct the patient prior to the procedure about the nature and purpose of oxygen therapy.
2. Instruct the patient and family regarding the hazards of smoking and open flames when oxygen is in use. Include other patients in the room as well as visitors.
3. Instruct the patient to call the nurse if experiencing any breathing difficulty.
4. Instruct the patient to call for assistance with ambulation if permitted.

DOCUMENTATION

1. Time of procedure and person performing the procedure.
2. Type of oxygen delivery device used.
3. Oxygen liter flow.
4. The patient's reaction to the procedure.
5. Specific assessment areas including vital signs, skin color, and level of consciousness.
6. All patient teaching done and the patient's level of understanding.

 # Arterial Puncture

PURPOSE

1. Obtain a sample of arterial blood for accurate blood gas analysis.

REQUISITES

1. Arterial blood sampling kit
   a. Plastic bag
   b. Rubber stopper or syringe cap
   c. 10 cc syringe
   d. Antiseptic prep
   e. Anticoagulant (usually heparin 1000 U/mL)
   f. 2 × 2 sterile gauze sponge
   g. 20 gauge needle, 1½ inch
2. Identification label
3. Lab requisition
4. Ice
5. Bed protector
6. Tape—1 inch

GUIDELINES

1. Arterial blood gases are generally ordered to evaluate oxygenation, ventilation, and acid-base status of a patient.
2. Persons performing the procedure should be properly instructed. Health care facility policies should determine those qualified to perform the procedure.
3. Contraindications to performing an arterial puncture include:
   a. Anticoagulant therapy.
   b. History of clotting disorders.
   c. History of arterial spasms following previous punctures.
   d. Severe peripheral vascular disease.
   e. Abnormal or infectious skin processes at or near the puncture sites.
   The patient and the medical record should be assessed carefully for any of the above and the physician notified.

4. Arterial punctures are usually performed in the radial, brachial, or femoral arteries. Since arterial puncture may cause vessel spasm or clotting, collateral blood flow should be considered prior to puncture site selection. The radial artery has the best collateral blood flow and is the site of choice if possible.

5. Superficial arteries such as the radial artery are more easily palpated, stabilized, and punctured than deeper arteries such as the brachial and femoral.

6. Allen's test should be performed to assess collateral circulation prior to an arterial puncture in the radial artery. A positive Allen's test indicates adequate collateral circulation.

7. Selection of an arterial puncture site should include consideration of adequate tissue since bone periosteum, nerves, and veins must be avoided during the puncture:
   a. The radial artery is not in close proximity to nerves or veins but is close to bone periosteum.
   b. The brachial artery is close to both nerves and veins.
   c. The femoral artery is close to both nerves and veins.

8. In most hospitals and institutions, only physicians may perform arterial punctures in the femoral artery, since the danger of bleeding is greater.

9. Arterial blood gas studies may be affected by recent changes in the patient's respiratory status or by increased activity levels. If possible, allow 20 minutes following suctioning, changes in oxygen or ventilator settings, respiratory therapy treatments, or increased activity levels before drawing an arterial blood gas sample.

10. Arterial blood gases should be drawn with the assistance of a second person.

11. If repeated arterial punctures are required, an arterial line should be suggested.

NURSING ACTION/RATIONALE

1. Assemble all equipment.
2. Identify the patient.
3. Explain the procedure and its purpose. Instruct the patient to report excessive pain during the procedure. Explain the importance of breathing normally for accurate test results.
4. Select an appropriate puncture site:
   a. Inspect the skin condition.
   b. Ascertain the presence of a palpable pulse.
5. Explain and perform the Allen's test:
   a. Position the patient's arm on a flat surface with the wrist supported on a rolled towel.
   b. Ask the patient to make a fist while you simultaneously occlude both the radial and ulnar arteries with the index and middle fingers of both your hands for several seconds (Figure 4-19).
   c. Ask the patient to unclench his or her fist.
   d. Release only the ulnar artery and assess for the return of a good blood supply to the hand. A good blood return signifies a positive Allen's test.

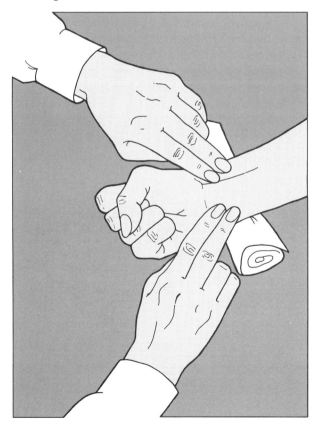

Figure 4-19. Hand position for Allen's test.

e. If the test is negative, select an alternative site and notify the physician of inadequate circulation in the extremity.

f. If the test is positive, you may proceed with the arterial puncture.

6. Prepare for performing the procedure:

a. Notify the laboratory that the arterial blood gases are being drawn.

b. Fill the plastic bag with ice and attach the patient identification label.

c. Establish adequate lighting.

7. Wash your hands.

8. Prepare the syringe.

a. Anticoagulate the syringe, including the puncture needle.

b. Expel *all* air and return the needle sheath to its position.

c. Place the syringe on a flat surface to prevent plunger withdrawal.

9. Place a bed protector and a rolled towel under the patient's wrist (elbow).

10. Cleanse the puncture site and your fingers to be used for palpation with an antiseptic prep.

11. Locate the artery between your index and middle fingers.

12. Inform the patient that you will be puncturing the skin. Caution the patient regarding sudden movement.

13. Puncture the skin with the needle bevel up at a 45 to 90 degree angle to the artery and parallel to the arm, keeping fingers in position (Figure 4-20).

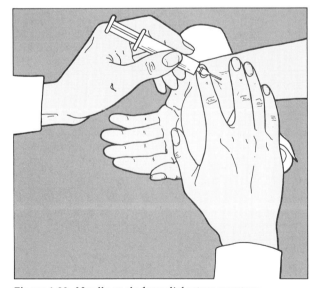

Figure 4-20. Needle angle for radial artery puncture.

14. Advance the needle into the artery, observing for a flashback of blood. Spontaneous filling of the syringe indicates artery filling. Never apply traction to the plunger to withdraw the blood sample.

15. Withdraw the needle slowly if syringe does not fill spontaneously. Make sure your needle is withdrawn as far as possible before changing the angle of penetration, or nerve, vessel, or tissue damage can occur.

16. Collect approximately 3 to 5 cc of arterial blood. Using less than 3 cc may distort the study results.

17. Withdraw the syringe and immediately apply firm pressure to the puncture site while palpating the pulse. Avoid extreme pressure, which could occlude the artery.

18. Instruct your assistant to carefully place the needle into the rubber stopper or remove the needle and cap the syringe, making sure no air enters the syringe.

19. Instruct your assistant to rotate the syringe to facilitate the mixing of the anticoagulant and blood.

20. Instruct your assistant to place the syringe into the container of ice, making sure the blood sample is completely surrounded by ice.

21. Instruct your assistant to take the labeled sample to the laboratory with a requisition immediately.

22. Continue to apply pressure to the puncture site for approximately 5 minutes or until bleeding has stopped.

23. Place a sterile 2 × 2 inch gauze dressing over the puncture site and secure firmly with adhesive tape.

24. Assess the pulse distal to the puncture site and assess circulation every 15 minutes for 1 hour or as ordered.

25. Discard equipment or return it to the appropriate area.

26. Communicate results of arterial gas analysis to the physician if indicated.

PATIENT AND/OR FAMILY TEACHING

1. Explain the procedure to the patient as stated in nursing rationale.
2. Instruct the patient to avoid rubbing the puncture site.
3. Reinforce the physician's explanation regarding the patient's disease process.
4. Instruct the patient to notify the nurse immediately if any pain or numbness occurs in the extremity.
5. Explain activity restrictions if ordered.

DOCUMENTATION

1. Time of the procedure.
2. Artery used for the procedure.
3. Results of Allen's test.
4. Quality of the pulse and circulation distal to the puncture site before and after the arterial puncture.
5. Length of time pressure was applied to the puncture site.
6. Disposition of the specimen.
7. The patient's tolerance of the procedure.
8. Adverse side effects of the procedure.
9. Notification of the physician.
10. All patient teaching done and the patient's level of understanding.

 # Assisting the Physician with a Thoracentesis

PURPOSE

1. Assist the physician in removing fluid and/or air from the pleural space.
2. Assist the physician with a diagnostic aspiration of pleural fluid.

REQUISITES

1. Thoracentesis tray including:
   a. Aspirating needle (16 gauge, 3½ inch with adjustable clamp)
   b. 5 cc and 50 cc syringes
   c. 21 and 25 gauge needles
   d. Local anesthetic
   e. Specimen tubes with caps—3
   f. Drain tube and collection bag
   g. Antiseptic prep
   h. Fenestrated drape
   i. Gauze sponges
   j. Adhesive bandage
2. Sterile gloves

GUIDELINES

1. A thoracentesis may be performed on patients with a variety of clinical problems including pleural effusions from infection, neoplastic disease, traumatic injury, cardiac disease, and kidney disease.
2. The requirement for a signed consent form for invasive procedures varies among health care facilities. Refer to your hospital's policy manual.
3. Placing the patient in an upright sitting position facilitates the removal of fluid that usually localizes at the base of the pleural cavity.
4. The patient should be given specific instructions regarding the procedure to alleviate as much tension as possible.
5. Sudden movement or coughing should be avoided during the procedure to prevent trauma to the pleura and lung.
6. Pneumothorax is a possible complication following a thoracentesis. The patient should be watched carefully for vital sign changes, dyspnea, chest pain, or diminished breath sounds on the affected side. If these symptoms occur, notify the physician and prepare for possible insertion of chest tubes.

7. Patient allergies should be determined prior to implementing the procedure.

NURSING ACTION/RATIONALE

1. Assemble all equipment.
2. Identify the patient.
3. Reinforce the physician's explanation of the procedure to the patient:
   a. Reason for the procedure.
   b. Position required and importance of remaining immobile.
   c. Sensations of pressure and cold experienced during injection of local anesthetic.
4. Obtain an informed consent for the procedure, if necessary.
5. Provide privacy.
6. Dress the patient in a clean hospital gown.
7. Obtain baseline vital signs and assess breath sounds.
8. Administer sedation if indicated.
9. Wash your hands.
10. Assist the physician by opening the thoracentesis tray and sterile gloves, using aseptic technique.
11. Position the patient comfortably with adequate support in one of the following positions:
    a. Sitting upright supported by an overbed table with a pillow to lean on (Figure 4-21a).
    b. Sitting on the side of the bed with the feet placed on a chair (Figure 4-21b).
    c. Lying on the unaffected side with a small pillow placed under the chest (Figure 4-21c).
12. Elevate the arm on the affected side by placing the patient's hand on the opposite shoulder to expose the puncture area.
13. Reassure and support the patient during the procedure.
14. Assist the physician as necessary.
15. Observe the patient for any changes in color, pulse, and respirations throughout the procedure and inform the physician of any changes.
16. Assist the physician with applying an occlusive dressing following removal of the aspirating needle.

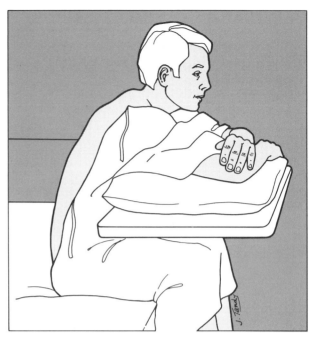

Figure 4-21. Alternative positions for thoracentesis. (a) Supported by an overbed table.

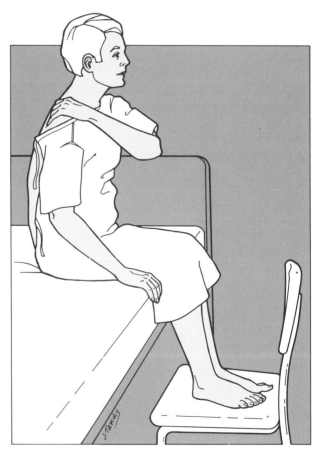

Figure 4-21(b). Sitting on the side of the bed.

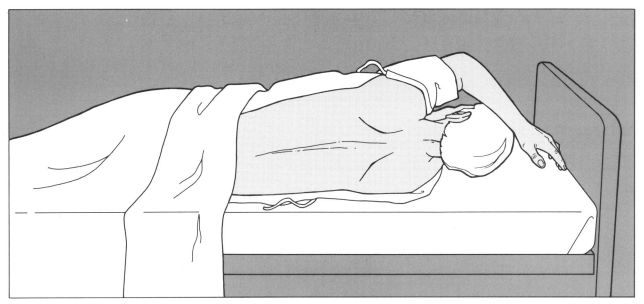

Figure 4-21(c). Lying on the unaffected side.

17. Position the patient on the unaffected side for approximately 1 hour to permit the puncture site to seal.
18. Assess vital signs every 30 minutes for 2 hours, then every hour for 4 hours, then every 4 hours for 24 hours, or as ordered.
19. Assess the patient at the same time intervals for signs and symptoms as stated in guideline 6.
20. Inspect the dressing over the puncture site and the surrounding skin area for drainage or inflammation when assessing other parameters.
21. Measure the amount of fluid if fluid was removed.
22. Send labeled specimen to the laboratory if diagnostic studies are ordered.
23. Discard any remaining thoracentesis drainage according to your health care facility's disposal policy.
24. Discard equipment or return it to the appropriate location.

PATIENT AND/OR FAMILY TEACHING

1. Instruct the patient prior to the procedure as described in the "Nursing Action" section.
2. Reinforce the physician's explanation regarding the patient's disease process.

3. Instruct the patient to call the nurse if difficulty in breathing is experienced.
4. Instruct the patient to call for assistance with ambulation if permitted.

DOCUMENTATION

1. Time and type of procedure and name of physician performing the procedure.
2. Amount, color, and consistency of the fluid obtained.
3. Disposition of the specimen.
4. Type and amount of medication used.
5. Nursing assessments of the patient during the procedure and the patient's tolerance of the procedure, including vital signs and breath sounds.
6. All patient teaching done and the patient's level of understanding.

Assisting the Physician with Insertion or Removal of Chest Tubes _____

PURPOSE

1. Assist the physician with the insertion of chest tubes attached to a closed drainage system.
2. Assist the physician with chest tube removal.

REQUISITES

Insertion

1. Sterile thoracotomy tray (usually a standard tray is available, or consult with the physician regarding specific equipment desired)
2. Sterile gloves
3. Sterile closed drainage system with optional holder
4. Sterile water—pour bottle
5. Two straight 6 to 7 inch hemostats
6. Sign: "Do Not Empty"
7. Suction source (optional)

Removal

1. Sterile suture removal kit including:
   a. Forceps
   b. Suture scissors
   c. 2 × 2 inch gauze sponges
   d. Antiseptic prep
2. Sterile 4 × 4 inch gauze sponges
3. Adhesive tape—3 inch
4. Waste receptacle

GUIDELINES

1. Chest tubes with a closed drainage system are inserted into the pleural space to reestablish negative pressure lost due to chest trauma, surgery, or pleural effusion.
2. Closed drainage is established by inserting a chest tube into the pleural space, attaching it to a closed drainage system, and placing the

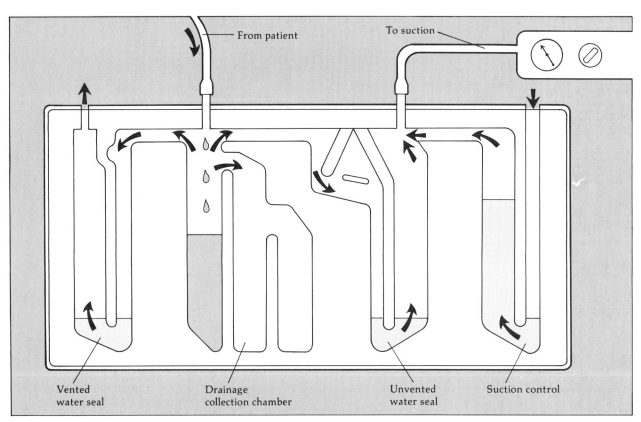

Figure 4-22. Types of closed water-seal chest drainage systems. (a) Disposable drainage unit.

distal end of the system under water to prevent air from being drawn into the pleural space.

3. The purposes for chest tube insertion include:
   a. Removal of air or fluid from the pleural space.
   b. Reexpansion of the lung.
4. Two chest tubes may be placed in one side of the thoracic cavity. They may be connected to

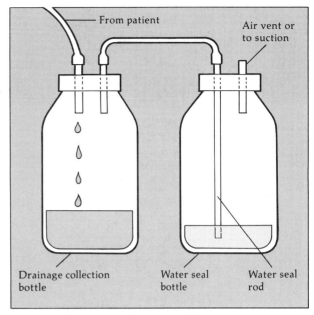

Figure 4-22(c). Two-bottle water-seal drainage.

a Y connector and one closed drainage system or to two closed drainage systems.

5. When two chest tubes are in place, less drainage is expected from the upper chest tube, with the greater amount of drainage occurring from the lower chest tube.
6. There are several types of closed drainage systems available, including disposable water-seal drainage units as well as standard glass one, two, or three bottle water-seal drainage systems (Figures 4-22 **a** through **d**).

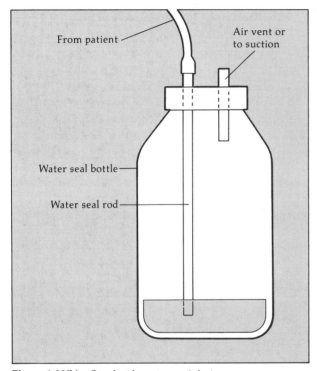

Figure 4-22(b). One-bottle water-seal drainage.

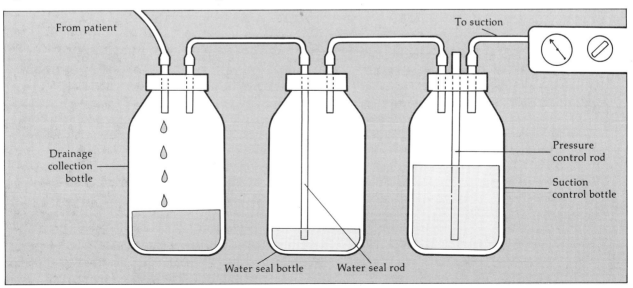

Figure 4-22(d). Three-bottle water-seal drainage.

7. Closed drainage systems may drain by gravity, or a suction system may be attached to facilitate lung reexpansion. Additional suction also assists in keeping the drainage system patent.

8. The requirement for a signed consent form for invasive procedures varies among health care facilities. Refer to your hospital's policy manual.

9. Patient allergies should be determined prior to implementing the procedure.

10. Chest tube removal is determined by the physician. Lung reexpansion may be confirmed by chest auscultation and a chest x-ray.

NURSING ACTION/RATIONALE

Insertion

1. Assemble all equipment.
2. Identify the patient.
3. Reinforce the physician's explanation, including:
   a. Reason for the procedure.
   b. Position required and importance of remaining immobile during the procedure.
   c. Sensations of pressure that may be experienced during the procedure.
4. Obtain an informed consent for the procedure, if necessary.
5. Provide privacy.
6. Dress the patient in a clean hospital gown.
7. Obtain baseline vital signs and assess breath sounds.
8. Administer sedation, if indicated.
9. Wash your hands.
10. Assist the physician in preparing the closed water-seal drainage glass bottle system by pouring sterile water into the water-seal bottle so that the tip of the glass rod is approximately 1 inch below the water line. (See Figure 4-22 for various types of water-seal drainage set-ups.) If a plastic disposable unit is used, follow manufacturer's instructions.
11. Place the cover with the glass rod system on the bottle and secure tightly, using aseptic technique.

12. Attach a piece of 1 inch adhesive tape vertically to the bottle and mark the original level of fluid in the bottle, including the date and time.
13. Assist the physician by opening the thoracotomy tray and sterile gloves, using aseptic technique.
14. Position the patient as directed by the physician.
15. Reassure and support the patient during the procedure.
16. Assist the physician as necessary during the chest tube insertion procedure.
17. Observe the patient for changes in color, pulse, and respirations as well as signs of discomfort throughout the procedure, and inform the physician of any changes.
18. Assist the physician with attaching the closed drainage system to the chest tube. (Refer to Figure 4-22 for proper system set-up.)
19. Tape the tubing connections to ensure an airtight system. Be sure that the weight of the tubing does not kink at the connection to the glass rod, if using a bottle system.
20. Assist the physician with attaching additional suction if ordered. The physician should specify the amount of suction to be used. Only continuous suction should be used.
21. Assist the patient to a comfortable position.
22. Place the "Do Not Empty" sign on the chest bottle.
23. Discard equipment or return it to the appropriate location.
24. Refer to "Nursing Management of Chest Tubes" procedure for nursing care following insertion.

Removal

1. Assemble all equipment.
2. Identify the patient.
3. Explain the procedure to the patient. Instruct the patient to exhale as the chest tube is withdrawn.
4. Provide privacy.
5. Obtain baseline vital signs and assess breath sounds.
6. Administer sedation, if indicated.
7. Wash your hands.
8. Assist the physician by opening suture set and dressings, using aseptic technique.
9. Position the patient as directed by the physician.

10. Assist the physician as necessary during the chest tube removal procedure and dressing application.
11. Observe the patient closely for any signs of respiratory difficulty following chest tube removal.
12. Assist the patient to a comfortable position.
13. Discard equipment or return it to the appropriate location.
14. Assess chest tube removal site for drainage.

PATIENT AND/OR FAMILY TEACHING
1. Instruct the patient before the procedure as described in the "Nursing Action" section.
2. Instruct the patient to call the nurse if breathing difficulty is experienced.
3. Instruct the patient and family regarding the importance of maintaining the water-seal drainage system in an upright position and below chest level.
4. Instruct the patient regarding activity orders, coughing and deep breathing schedules, and analgesic needs.
5. Instruct the patient to call for assistance with repositioning or ambulation, if permitted.

DOCUMENTATION
Insertion
1. Time and type of procedure and name of physician performing the procedure.
2. Nursing assessment of baseline vital signs and breath sounds.
3. Size and location of the chest tube(s).
4. Type of closed drainage system used.
5. Pressure setting for additional suction unit, if applicable.
6. Amount, color, and consistency of initial drainage.
7. The patient's reaction to the procedure.
8. Type and amount of medication used.
9. Nursing assessments of the patient during the procedure.
10. All patient teaching done and the patient's level of understanding.

Removal
1. Time of the procedure and name of physician performing the procedure.
2. Total amount, color, and consistency of drainage in drainage unit.
3. Condition of the skin at the insertion site and type of dressing used.
4. The patient's reaction to the procedure.
5. Nursing assessment of the patient's respiratory status during and after the procedure.
6. All patient teaching done and the patient's level of understanding.

Nursing Management of Chest Tubes

PURPOSE

1. Provide nursing care for a patient with a chest tube attached to a closed water—seal drainage system.

REQUISITES

1. Two straight 6 to 7 inch hemostats
2. Sterile water—pour bottle

GUIDELINES

1. Nursing management of patients with chest tubes requires knowledge of the principles of pulmonary physiology and familiarity with closed chest drainage systems and suction equipment.
2. An extra closed chest drainage system should be available in the patient care area for emergency use in case of malfunction or breakage in the system.
3. Drainage systems are never emptied unless specifically ordered by the physician.
4. Chest tubes must remain patent in order to function properly. Fluid in the water-seal glass rod will rise on inspiration and fall on expiration if chest tubes are patent.
5. Closed chest drainage systems must remain below chest level at all times unless chest tubes are clamped.
6. Chest tubes should not be clamped unless there is a leak in the system or the closed chest drainage system must be raised above chest level. Prolonged clamping may cause air and fluid to accumulate in the pleural space, causing further lung collapse.
7. Bubbling in the water-seal bottle may indicate an air leak, which is normal following certain thoracic procedures. It is produced by air moving out of the pleural space and into the closed chest drainage system.
8. In most health care facilities the physician is responsible for changing a closed chest drainage unit except in emergency situations such as malfunction or breakage.

9. Following thoracic procedures, patients are susceptible to pulmonary complications such as atelectasis and pneumonia, making effective nursing management imperative.
10. The patient with a chest tube may be positioned on either side or on the back unless contraindicated.
11. "Milking" of a chest tube should only be done with a physician's order.

NURSING ACTION/RATIONALE
Closed Chest Drainage System

1. Assess amount, color, and consistency of chest drainage at ordered time intervals. Notify the physician if chest drainage exceeds 100 cc/hour or if the color of the drainage changes to indicate an active bleeding problem.
2. Assess the fluid fluctuation in the long glass rod in the water-seal bottle. Fluctuation should continue until the lung has expanded.
3. Assess chest drainage tubing for any kinking. Do not allow drainage tubing to loop below drainage system entry level.
4. Assess for bubbling in the water-seal bottle. Any change from an established pattern may indicate a break in the system.
5. Mark the level of drainage on a piece of adhesive tape affixed to the side of the drainage system every shift, or as ordered. Include date, time, and your initials.
6. Do not empty the drainage bottle unless ordered to do so by the physician with specific instructions. Disposable plastic drainage units cannot be emptied.
7. "Milk" the chest tube at prescribed intervals in the direction of chest drainage to promote chest tube patency:
   a. Lubricate the drainage tubing with lubricant or soap for approximately 12 inches.
   b. Pinch the tubing above the lubrication with one hand. With the other hand compress the tubing, allowing the fingers to slide over the lubrication toward the drainage bottle. Release both hands.
   c. Use designated areas on certain drainage units for milking tubing.

8. Do not clamp chest tubes unless absolutely necessary. If necessary to clamp chest tubes, use two 6 to 7 inch hemostats clamped in opposite directions as close to the chest wall as possible.

Patient Observations and Nursing Care
1. Assess patient carefully for any signs of respiratory difficulty, cyanosis, chest pressure, crepitation, and/or hemorrhage.
2. Assess vital signs and breath sounds every 4 hours or as ordered.
3. Observe the dressing at the chest tube insertion site for excessive drainage. Assess skin condition during dressing changes.
4. Assist the patient to cough and deep breathe at least every 2 hours or as ordered. The patient should be assisted to a sitting position if possible to promote effective deep breathing and coughing. A pillow or blanket should be used to splint the affected area.
5. Assist the patient to change position at least every 2 hours to promote drainage and prevent complications. Make sure the tubing remains free of kinks and is in proper position.
6. Assist the patient with range of motion for the affected upper extremity to maintain joint mobility.
7. Maintain patient comfort by giving analgesics as required, especially prior to deep breathing and coughing.

Transporting and Ambulating
1. Transport or ambulate a patient with a chest tube(s), keeping the water-seal unit below chest level and upright at all times unless the chest tube is clamped. Clamps should be removed as soon as possible.
2. Assist and instruct personnel from other departments in transporting or ambulating the patient. Nursing staff should accompany the patient.
3. Disconnect the closed chest drainage system from additional suction for transportation or ambulation. Make sure the air vent rod is open.
4. Attach hemostats to the patient's hospital gown during transportation or ambulation for emergency use.

Emergency Troubleshooting
1. Water-seal unit broken or emptied:
   a. Clamp the chest tube(s) unless there has been a large air leak. Chest tube(s) with a large air leak should be left open, since clamping may cause a rapid pneumothorax.
   b. Reestablish a closed drainage system.
   c. Remove the clamps if applied.
   d. Notify the physician.
   e. Assess the patient for respiratory distress.
2. Tubing disconnected:
   a. Clamp the chest tube(s).
   b. Cleanse the ends of the tubing with an antiseptic solution and reconnect.
   c. Remove the clamps.
   d. Tape the connection.
   e. Notify the physician.
   f. Assess the patient for respiratory distress.
3. Water-seal unit tipped over:
   a. Return unit to upright position.
   b. Assist the patient to deep breathe to force air out of the pleural space.
   c. Notify the physician.
   d. Assess the patient for respiratory distress.
4. Chest tube pulled out of chest wall:
   a. Cover the site with sterile 4 × 4 gauze sponges and tape occlusively.
   b. Notify the physician.
   c. Assess the patient for respiratory distress.

PATIENT AND/OR FAMILY TEACHING
1. Explain the purpose and function of the chest tube(s) to the patient.
2. Instruct the patient regarding activity orders, coughing and deep breathing schedules, and analgesic needs.
3. Instruct the patient to call for assistance with repositioning or ambulation if permitted.
4. Instruct the patient to call the nurse if breathing difficulty is experienced.
5. Explain other therapeutic measures utilized including:
   a. Oxygen therapy.
   b. Range of motion to the affected upper extremity.
   c. Fluids.
6. Instruct the patient and family regarding the importance of maintaining the water-seal unit in an upright position and below chest level.

DOCUMENTATION

1. Amount, color, and consistency of chest drainage.
2. Presence or absence of air leaks or bubbling in the water-seal unit.
3. Presence or absence of fluid fluctuation in the glass rod of the water-seal unit.
4. Time and results of chest tube "milking."
5. Specific patient assessment areas including vital signs, breath sounds, and skin color.
6. Results of deep breathing and coughing.
7. Position changes or activity, including range of motion.
8. Condition of chest tube insertion site and dressing.

 # Tracheostomy Care

PURPOSE

1. Maintain a patent airway.
2. Minimize respiratory infections.

REQUISITES

1. Tracheostomy dressing—precut sterile 4 × 4 gauze sponges
2. Tracheostomy ties—sterile precut
3. Antiseptic swabs
4. Clean scissors
5. Sterile applicators
6. Sterile basins—2
7. Hydrogen peroxide
8. Sterile saline—pour bottle
9. Sterile test tube brush
10. Sterile 4 × 4 gauze sponges
11. Sterile gloves—2 pairs
12. Exam gloves—2
13. Waste receptacle

GUIDELINES

1. A tracheostomy is performed to:
   a. Provide an airway because upper airway is obstructed.
   b. Facilitate the removal of tracheobronchial secretions.
   c. Prevent aspiration of secretions, food, and/or fluids into the lungs.
   d. Replace an endotracheal tube for long-term airway management.
   e. Facilitate the use of an artificial ventilator.
   f. Provide a permanent airway.
2. Emergency tracheostomy reinsertion supplies should be available at the bedside at all times.
3. The tracheostomy cuff should remain deflated at all times unless ordered to be inflated by the physician. Inflate only with air.
4. The tracheostomy dressing and ties should be changed whenever necessary to keep the dressing and ties dry. The dressing should be changed at least every 8 hours and the ties at least every 24 hours.
5. Tracheostomy ties should be changed with the assistance of another person to prevent dislodgement.

6. Tracheostomy tubes with inner cannulas should have the cannula removed and cleaned at least every 8 hours.
7. Tracheal secretions should be considered contaminated and handled according to wound isolation procedure.
8. The tracheostomy care procedure should be performed as aseptically as possible.
9. The patient may become very apprehensive during this procedure and must be reassured frequently.
10. A method of communication should be established with the patient prior to implementing the procedure.
11. If an artificial ventilator is in use, this procedure may be performed without disrupting its use.

NURSING ACTION/RATIONALE

1. Assemble all equipment.
2. Identify the patient.
3. Explain the procedure to the patient and establish a method of communication.
4. Position the patient in a semi-Fowler's position unless contraindicated.
5. Wash your hands.
6. Suction the tracheostomy, following the "Endotracheal/Tracheostomy Suctioning" procedure.
7. Wash your hands.
8. Open dressings, sterile basins, and other supplies, using aseptic technique.
9. Pour hydrogen peroxide into one sterile basin and sterile saline into the other sterile basin, using aseptic technique.
10. Apply exam gloves and remove soiled tracheostomy dressing. Discard in waste receptacle.
11. Cut and remove soiled ties with a second person continually holding the tracheostomy tube with a sterile gloved hand until new ties are securely in place. Discard the ties in the waste receptacle.
12. Remove exam gloves.
13. Put on sterile gloves.

14. Clean inner cannula if present:
    a. Unlock the inner cannula and remove.
    b. Place the inner cannula in the hydrogen peroxide, allowing it to soak for a few minutes.
    c. Clean the inner cannula with the test tube brush.
    d. Rinse the inner cannula in the sterile saline.
    e. Remove the inner cannula from the saline and allow it to drain on a sterile 4 × 4 gauze sponge.
15. Cleanse the tracheostomy incision and surrounding area with antiseptic swabs. If crusting occurs, remove with sterile swabs soaked with hydrogen peroxide. Do not allow cleansing solutions to enter the tracheostomy opening.
16. Reinsert the inner cannula and lock.
17. Reapply sterile precut ties to each side of the tracheostomy tube. Secure ties around the patient's neck with a knot at the side of the neck. Never tie bows. Trim off any excess tie. Ties should be tight enough to allow only one finger to slide underneath.
18. Apply a sterile tracheostomy dressing (Figure 4-23).

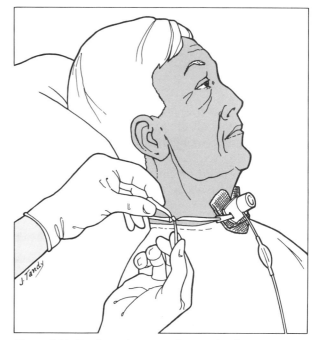

Figure 4-23. Sterile tracheostomy dressing in place.

19. Remove gloves and discard. Wash your hands.
20. Assist the patient to a comfortable position.
21. Discard or return all equipment to the appropriate location.

PATIENT AND/OR FAMILY TEACHING

1. Explain tracheostomy care to the patient prior to performing the procedure.
2. Reinforce the need to cough and deep breathe every hour.
3. Instruct the patient to notify the nurse if experiencing any breathing difficulty. Provide a call signal or bell for this purpose.

DOCUMENTATION

1. Time of the procedure and name of person performing the procedure.
2. The patient's reaction to the procedure.

3. Specific assessment parameters including:
   a. Color, amount, and consistency of tracheal secretions.
   b. Respirations.
   c. Breath sounds.
   d. Condition of tracheal incision.
4. All patient teaching done and the patient's level of understanding.

Endotracheal/Tracheostomy Suctioning

PURPOSE

1. Maintain airway patency by the removal of secretions from the tracheobronchial tree.
2. Decrease the potential for infection that may result from accumulated secretions.
3. Stimulate an effective cough.

REQUISITES

1. Portable continuous suction machine or gauge to attach to wall suction
2. Sterile suction kit containing:
   a. Sterile suction catheter (14 to 18 Fr)
   b. Sterile solution container
   c. Sterile gloves
3. Sterile saline—pour bottle
4. 2 × 2 gauze sponges—2
5. Sterile normal saline, 5 cc packets for tracheal instillation
6. Oxygen flowmeter with a ventilator or manual resuscitator
7. Waste receptacle

GUIDELINES

1. Aseptic technique must be used in performing the endotracheal/tracheostomy suctioning procedure.
2. Suctioning should be performed as often as necessary to maintain a patent airway.
3. Prior to initiating the procedure, oropharyngeal suctioning should be completed as described in "Oropharyngeal/Nasopharyngeal Suctioning." Always use a new sterile catheter and sterile equipment for endotracheal or tracheostomy suctioning.
4. Continuous suction should be limited to 10 seconds, since hypoxia may result.
5. Patients should be hyperoxygenated prior to suctioning and between suction attempts by means of a ventilator or a manual resuscitator attached to an oxygen flowmeter set at 100% oxygen. This step limits the hypoxia caused by the suctioning.
6. The suction catheter should be introduced gently into the endotracheal or tracheostomy tube. Suction should not be applied during catheter insertion to prevent injury to the mucous membranes.

7. Secretions trapped near inflated endotracheal or tracheostomy cuffs should be removed at least every 8 hours by deflating the cuff and performing both oropharyngeal and tracheal suctioning, using appropriate techniques. Reinflate the cuff to the minimum occluding volume or according to physician's order.

8. Thick secretions may be controlled by instilling 5 cc of sterile normal saline into the endotracheal or tracheostomy tube immediately prior to suctioning. Increasing airway humidity will also assist in liquifying secretions.

9. Although only one sterile glove on the dominant hand is necessary for the suctioning procedure, a second glove on the non-dominant hand is recommended to protect both the nurse and the patient.

10. Suction catheters should be inserted until resistance is felt, then withdrawn slightly before suction is applied. The depth of suctioning may be determined by physician order or by health care facility policy.

11. A patient with an endotracheal or tracheostomy tube should be given meticulous oral hygiene at least three times per day to reduce the potential for respiratory infections.

12. Suction collection bottles should be emptied and rinsed every 8 hours and cleaned with soap and water every 24 hours. Connecting tubing should be rinsed after each suctioning and should be changed every 3 days, or more often if secretions are thick or infected.

NURSING ACTION/RATIONALE

1. Assemble all equipment.
2. Identify the patient.
3. Explain the suction procedure to the patient including:
   a. Hyperoxygenation procedure.
   b. Instillation of normal saline.
   c. Coughing during the procedure.
4. Provide privacy.
5. Assess breath sounds and vital signs including respirations.
6. Position the patient in a semi-Fowler's position.
7. Provide a clean work area.
8. Wash your hands.

9. Open the suction kit and sterile 2 × 2 sponges, using the wrapper to create a sterile field.
10. Pour 30 to 50 cc of sterile normal saline into the sterile solution container, using aseptic technique.
11. Turn on the suction unit. Set the desired pressure according to equipment specifications or the physician's order.
12. Put on the sterile gloves.
13. Attach the sterile suction catheter to the connecting tubing by holding the catheter in your dominant hand (sterile hand) and the connecting tube in your non-dominant hand (non-sterile hand) (Figure 4-24).

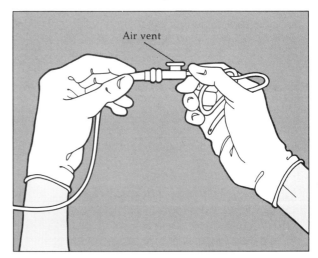

Figure 4-24. Attaching the suction catheter.

14. Moisten the suction catheter tip with the sterile normal saline solution.
15. Instruct an assistant to hyperoxygenate the patient and remove the ventilator, if present.
16. Insert the sterile suction catheter gently into the endotracheal or tracheostomy tube until resistance is felt. Pull back slightly.
17. Place the thumb of your non-dominant (non-sterile) hand over the suction control.

18. Rotate the catheter between the thumb and index finger of your sterile hand while applying intermittent suction and withdrawing the catheter (Figure 4-25). Do not suction for longer than 10 seconds.

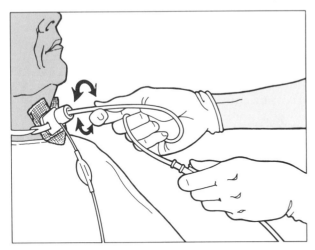

Figure 4-25. Suctioning a tracheostomy.

19. Rinse the suction catheter. Wipe off excess secretions on the outside of the catheter by wiping with a sterile 2 × 2 gauze sponge toward the catheter tip with your sterile hand.
20. Instruct an assistant to reapply the ventilator, if present, and hyperoxygenate the patient between suction attempts.
21. Instill 5 cc of sterile normal saline into the trachea if secretions are thick. Wait 5 seconds and suction the patient again.
22. Repeat the suction procedure until the airway is clear, rinsing the catheter and hyperoxygenating the patient.
23. Reconnect the patient to the ventilator, if appropriate.
24. Perform oropharyngeal suctioning, if appropriate.
25. Shut off the suction machine.
26. Remove your gloves and place them in the waste receptacle.
27. Assess the patient's breath sounds and vital signs.
28. Assist the patient to a comfortable position.
29. Discard the suction kit equipment and return all equipment to the appropriate area.
30. Wash your hands.

PATIENT AND/OR FAMILY TEACHING
1. Explain the procedure to the patient regardless of mental alertness.
2. Explain to the patient that the catheter may elicit a cough reflex. Encourage the patient to cough and expectorate secretions, if possible.
3. Instruct the patient and/or family to notify the nurse if any breathing difficulty is experienced.
4. Explain and demonstrate the suctioning procedure to the family if suctioning will be necessary following discharge.

DOCUMENTATION
1. Time and frequency of procedure and name of person performing the procedure.
2. Hyperoxygenation procedure and the equipment used.
3. Specific assessment parameters including:
   a. Color, amount, consistency, and odor of secretions.
   b. Vital signs.
   c. Breath sounds.
4. Instillation of normal saline during the procedure, if appropriate.
5. The patient's reaction to the procedure.
6. The patient's position in bed, if appropriate.
7. The type of respiratory care equipment attached to the endotracheal or tracheostomy tube following the procedure.
8. Any patient teaching done and the patient's level of understanding.

Oropharyngeal/Nasopharyngeal Suctioning

PURPOSE
1. Provide oral hygiene.
2. Maintain airway patency by the removal of secretions from the pharynx, mouth, and nose.
3. Prevent the potential for infection that may result from accumulated secretions.
4. Stimulate an effective cough.

REQUISITES
1. Portable continuous suction machine or gauge to attach to wall suction
2. Connecting tubing
3. Sterile whistle-tip straight catheter (14 to 18 Fr) with a valve or Y connector
4. Exam gloves
5. Disposable cup with tap water
6. Towel
7. Waste receptacle

GUIDELINES
1. Oropharyngeal/nasopharyngeal suctioning is a clean procedure provided suctioning is limited to the oral, nasal, or pharyngeal areas. Asepsis must be observed if performing endotracheal or tracheostomy suctioning.
2. The patient should be positioned on one side with the head elevated to facilitate airway patency and drainage of secretions.
3. Protective gloves should be worn during the suctioning procedure to prevent the transmission of infection.
4. Continuous suction should be limited to 15 seconds, since hypoxia may result.
5. The suction catheter may be inserted gently into the mouth or nose. During insertion the catheter should not be forced, nor should suction be applied, in order to prevent injury to the mucous membranes.
6. Suction catheters should be replaced at least every 8 hours and may be stored in a clean towel after rinsing. Cost generally precludes changing the catheter more frequently, but protocols may vary.

7. Suction collection bottles should be emptied and rinsed every 8 hours and cleaned with soap and water every 24 hours. Connecting tubing should be rinsed after each suctioning and should be changed every 3 days or more often if secretions are thick or infected.
8. Caution must be used when suctioning patients who have had oral or nasal surgery.

NURSING ACTION/RATIONALE
1. Assemble all equipment.
2. Identify the patient.
3. Explain the suctioning procedure to the patient. Explain that it may stimulate the cough reflex.
4. Provide privacy.
5. Assess breath sounds and respirations.
6. Position the patient on one side in a semi-Fowler's position.
7. Provide a clean working area.
8. Wash your hands.
9. Open the suction catheter package and attach the end to the connecting tubing from the machine. Place on a clean towel.
10. Put tap water in a clean paper cup.
11. Turn on the suction unit. Set the desired pressure according to equipment specifications or the physician's order.
12. Apply the exam gloves.
13. Moisten the suction catheter tip in the cup of water to reduce friction.
14. Insert the catheter tip gently into the nose or mouth. Do not apply suction during insertion.
15. Advance the catheter to the posterior oral/nasal pharynx. Stimulate a cough reflex if the patient is unable to cough effectively.
16. Begin suctioning by placing the thumb of your non-dominant hand over the catheter valve or Y connector. Rotate the catheter while withdrawing to prevent irritation to the oral/nasal mucosa. Suction all secretions from the mouth.
17. Suction for no more than 15 seconds. Allow the patient to rest for 2 to 3 minutes between catheter insertions.

18. Rinse the catheter in the cup of water.
19. Repeat the suctioning procedure as necessary until the airway is clear.
20. Rinse the catheter and tubing thoroughly with clean water by applying suction with the catheter control valve.
21. Turn off the suction unit and detach the catheter from the connecting tubing.
22. Rinse the catheter thoroughly with tap water, dry, and store in a clean towel until the next use.
23. Remove your gloves and discard them in the waste receptacle.
24. Reassess breath sounds and respirations.
25. Assist the patient to a comfortable position while maintaining a patent airway.
26. Discard equipment or return it to the appropriate area.
27. Wash your hands.

PATIENT AND/OR FAMILY TEACHING

1. Explain the procedure to the patient regardless of mental alertness.
2. Explain to the patient that the catheter may elicit a cough reflex. Encourage the patient to cough and expectorate secretions if possible.
3. Instruct the patient and/or family to notify the nurse if any breathing difficulty is experienced.
4. Explain and demonstrate the suctioning procedure to the family if suctioning will be necessary following discharge.

DOCUMENTATION

1. Time and frequency of procedure and name of person performing procedure.
2. Specific assessment parameters including:
   a. Color, amount, consistency, and odor of secretions.
   b. Respirations.
   c. Breath sounds.
3. The patient's reaction to the procedure.
4. The patient's position in bed if appropriate.
5. Any suction catheter or equipment changes.
6. All patient teaching done and the patient's level of understanding.

Sputum
Specimen Collection

PURPOSE
1. Obtain sputum for diagnostic analysis.
2. Collect sputum specimens according to laboratory protocol.

REQUISITES
Expectorated or Induced Specimen
1. Sterile sputum collection container according to laboratory protocol
2. Plastic bag
3. Disposable tissue

Oropharyngeal/Nasopharyngeal or Tracheal Aspiration
1. Sterile aspirating collection tube
2. Sterile suction kit including:
   a. Suction catheter
   b. Solution container
   c. Gloves
3. Sterile saline—pour bottle
4. Sterile 2 × 2 gauze sponges
5. Portable continuous suction unit or gauge to attach to wall suction
6. Plastic bag
7. Waste receptacle

GUIDELINES
1. Sputum specimens are collected as diagnostic aids for a variety of respiratory problems including tuberculosis, respiratory malignancies, and respiratory infections.
2. Sputum specimens should be collected early in the morning, since secretions tend to accumulate in the lungs during sleep.
3. Sputum specimens must originate from the lower respiratory tract. If the patient is not able to produce a deep cough, the physician may order respiratory therapy treatments to facilitate expectoration (induced specimen).
4. Sputum specimens must be fresh and at least 3 to 5 cc in volume. They should be transported to the laboratory immediately unless a quantitative specimen is ordered.

5. The teeth should not be brushed nor mouthwash used prior to obtaining a sputum specimen. The patient's mouth should be rinsed with water, and any dentures should be removed.
6. Sputum specimens for culture should be obtained prior to the administration of any antimicrobial agents.
7. If a sputum culture is ordered, the sputum container must be sterile. The patient must be instructed to expectorate into the container without touching the inside of the container. Sputum containers should always be kept covered.
8. Medical asepsis should be maintained during collection of sputum specimens; this includes proper disposal of tissues, conscientious handwashing technique, and careful handling of the sputum container. The use of a mask and gloves may be appropriate in some situations.
9. For sputum specimens collected by aspiration, refer to the procedures "Oropharyngeal/ Nasopharyngeal Suctioning" and "Endotracheal/Tracheostomy Suctioning" for proper suctioning techniques.
10. For some diagnostic sputum tests the sputum may need to be collected in a container with a preservative. For example, a sputum specimen for cytology is collected in a container of 70% alcohol. Consult with the facility's microbiologist for answers to specific questions.

NURSING ACTION/RATIONALE
Expectorated or Induced Method
1. Assemble all equipment.
2. Identify the patient.
3. Explain the procedure to the patient including:
   a. Use of the specimen container.
   b. Proper deep breathng and coughing technique.
4. Provide privacy.
5. Assist the patient to a sitting position.
6. Wash your hands.

7. Instruct the patient to rinse his/her mouth with water.
8. Open the sputum collection container, using aseptic technique.
9. Instruct the patient to inhale and exhale deeply three times. Instruct the patient to cough deeply on the last exhalation.
10. Instruct the patient to expectorate into the center of the container.
11. Contact the respiratory care department for assistance if the patient is unable to produce sputum.
12. Place the lid on the sputum container.
13. Label the specimen and place it in a plastic bag. Send it to the laboratory immediately.
14. Assist the patient to a comfortable position.
15. Wash your hands.

Aspiration Method
1. Assemble all equipment.
2. Identify the patient.
3. Explain the procedure to the patient.
4. Provide privacy.
5. Position the patient in a semi- to high-Fowler's position.
6. Wash your hands.
7. Open the sterile suction kit, using aseptic technique, and create a sterile field with the wrapper.
8. Open the sterile aspirating collection tube and place it on the sterile field, using aseptic technique.
9. Pour 30 to 50 cc of sterile saline into the solution container.
10. Turn on the suction unit. Set the desired pressure according to equipment specifications or the physician's order.
11. Put on the sterile gloves.
12. Attach the aspirating collection tube to the suction unit connecting tubing, maintaining asepsis of the dominant hand (Figure 4-26).

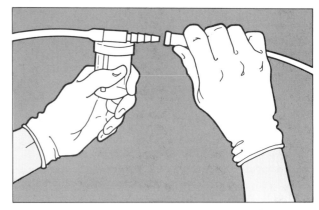

Figure 4-26. Attaching suction unit to aspirating collection tube.

13. Attach the sterile suction catheter to the aspirating tip of the aspirating collection tube, maintaining asepsis of the dominant hand (Figure 4-27).

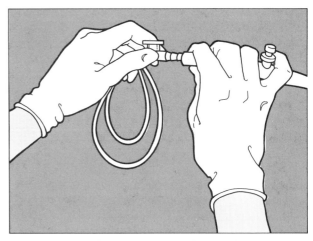

Figure 4-27. Attaching the suction catheter to the aspirating collection container.

14. Assure that the top of the aspirating tube is firmly in place and tight.
15. Suction the patient. Refer to the procedures "Oropharyngeal/Nasopharyngeal Suctioning" and "Endotracheal/Tracheostomy Suctioning."
16. Clear the mucus from the catheter by placing it in the normal saline and applying suction. Mucus and normal saline will collect in the aspirating tube.

17. Disconnect the aspirating collection tube from the suction catheter and connecting tube. Seal according to manufacturer's instructions.
18. Remove your gloves.
19. Turn off the suction unit.
20. Label the specimen and place it in a plastic bag. Send it to the laboratory immediately.
21. Assist the patient to a comfortable position.
22. Discard equipment or return it to the appropriate location.

PATIENT AND/OR FAMILY TEACHING

1. Explain the procedure to the patient, including the deep breathing and coughing processes.
2. Instruct the patient regarding the proper disposal of secretions and proper handwashing technique.
3. Explain the purpose of any medications ordered.

DOCUMENTATION

1. Time specimen was obtained and method used for collecting specimen.
2. Amount, color, consistency, and odor of the sputum.
3. The patient's ability to cough deeply.
4. Any respiratory therapy treatments given.
5. Disposition of the specimen.
6. All patient teaching done and the patient's level of understanding.

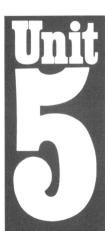

Unit 5

Gastrointestinal/ Metabolic Procedures

Assisting the Physician with a Liver Biopsy

PURPOSE

1. Assist the physician with obtaining a sample of liver tissue for diagnostic analysis.
2. Provide nursing care and support for the patient during and following the procedure.

REQUISITES

1. Liver biopsy tray including:
   a. Biopsy needle—type and size as requested
   b. 5 cc syringe
   c. 21 and 25 gauge needles
   d. Local anesthetic
   e. Scalpel blade with handle
   f. Fenestrated drape
   g. Gauze sponges
   h. Injectable normal saline—5 cc vial
   i. Adhesive bandage
   j. Antiseptic solution
2. Sterile gloves
3. Specimen bottles containing 10% formalin
4. Sandbag

GUIDELINES

1. A liver biopsy is performed on patients with liver dysfunction to determine the precise type of hepatic disorder.
2. The requirements for a signed consent form for invasive procedures vary among health care facilities. Refer to your policy manual.
3. Serum coagulation and hematology studies should be completed prior to performing a liver biopsy since patients with hepatic dysfunction are prone to clotting disorders.
4. Blood type and crossmatch testing should be performed prior to performing a liver biopsy, and several donor units should be available.
5. The patient should be given specific instructions regarding the procedure to alleviate as much anxiety as possible.
6. Placing the patient in a flat supine position with the right arm above the head facilitates access to the liver biopsy site.
7. Sudden movement or coughing should be avoided during the procedure to prevent trauma to the liver or thoracic area.

8. Vital signs and the patient's biopsy dressing must be assessed frequently following a liver biopsy, since hepatic bleeding, bile peritonitis, and pneumothorax are possible complications.
9. Prior to the biopsy needle insertion and during the biopsy (approximately 5 to 10 seconds) the patient must be able to exhale and hold his/her breath.
10. Patient allergies should be determined prior to implementing the procedure.

NURSING ACTION/RATIONALE

1. Assemble all equipment.
2. Identify the patient.
3. Explain the procedure to the patient including:
   a. Clarification of the physician's explanation.
   b. The position required and the importance of remaining immobile.
   c. Sensations of pressure and cold experienced during injection of the local anesthetic.
4. Obtain an informed consent for the procedure, if required.
5. Instruct the patient to void if no urinary catheter is in place.
6. Provide privacy.
7. Assist the patient into a clean hospital gown.
8. Obtain baseline vital signs.
9. Provide adequate lighting.
10. Assist the patient to a supine position close to the side of the bed with the right arm over the head or as requested by the physician (Figure 5-1).
11. Expose the upper abdomen and drape the patient as necessary.
12. Wash your hands.
13. Assist the physician by opening the liver biopsy tray and sterile gloves, using aseptic technique.

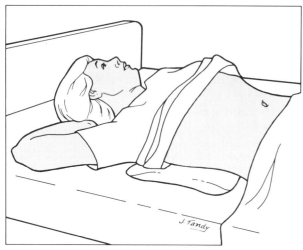

Figure 5-1. Position for a liver biopsy.

14. Assist the physician as requested.
15. Instruct the patient regarding the breathing technique when the physician performs the biopsy:
    a. Instruct the patient to inhale and exhale deeply several times.
    b. Instruct the patient to exhale deeply and hold his/her breath during the biopsy (5 to 10 seconds).
    c. Instruct the patient to breathe normally.
16. Reassure and support the patient during the procedure.
17. Assist the physician with the specimen collection.
18. Assess the patient's vital signs, color, and level of consciousness during the procedure and inform the physician of any changes.
19. Assist the physician with applying a dressing over the biopsy site.
20. Position the patient on the right side with a sandbag between the lateral chest wall and the bed to add additional pressure to the biopsy site. Place the call signal within reach.
21. Instruct the patient to remain in the right lateral position and to remain immobile for at least 2 hours or as ordered by the physician.
22. Send labeled specimens to the laboratory.

23. Assess vital signs and the biopsy dressing site every 15 minutes for 1 hour, then every 30 minutes for 2 hours, then hourly for 6 hours, then every 4 hours for 24 hours.
24. Report to the physician any significant decrease in blood pressure, increase in pulse, bleeding at the biopsy site, increase in temperature, or severe pain at the biopsy site.
25. Discard equipment or return it to the appropriate location.

PATIENT AND/OR FAMILY TEACHING

1. Explain the procedure and its purpose to the patient.
2. Reinforce and clarify the physician's explanation of the disease process.
3. Instruct the patient about how to breathe during the biopsy.
4. Explain the activity restrictions required following the biopsy.
5. Instruct the patient to inform the nurse if experiencing any pain or unusual sensations in the biopsy area.
6. Explain that frequent patient assessments will be made, including vital signs and biopsy site inspections.

DOCUMENTATION

1. Time of the procedure, type of procedure, and name of physician performing procedure.
2. Type and amount of medication used.
3. Disposition of the tissue specimen.
4. An assessment of the patient during and after the procedure, including vital signs and biopsy site inspections.
5. The patient's tolerance of the procedure, any untoward reactions, and actions taken.
6. All patient teaching done and the patient's level of understanding.

Assisting the Physician with a Paracentesis

PURPOSE

1. Assist the physician in removing fluid from the peritoneal cavity for diagnostic or treatment purposes.
2. Provide nursing care and support for the patient during and following the procedure.

REQUISITES

1. Thoracentesis or paracentesis tray including:
   a. Aspirating needle (16 gauge, 3½ inch with adjustable clamp) or trochar and cannula
   b. 5 cc and 50 cc syringes
   c. 21 and 25 gauge needles
   d. Local anesthetic
   e. Specimen tubes with caps—3
   f. Drain tube and collection bag
   g. Antiseptic prep
   h. Fenestrated drape
   i. Gauze sponges
   j. Adhesive bandage
2. Sterile gloves

GUIDELINES

1. A paracentesis may be performed on patients with a variety of clinical problems including liver disease, carcinoma, abdominal trauma, and abdominal infection.
2. The requirements for a signed consent form for invasive procedures vary among health care facilities. Refer to your policy manual.
3. Patients should be instructed to void immediately prior to the paracentesis procedure to avoid the possibility of any bladder damage.
4. Placing the patient in an upright position facilitates the removal of fluid, since the fluid will localize in the base of the peritoneal cavity.
5. The patient should be given specific instructions regarding the procedure to alleviate as much anxiety as possible.
6. Sudden movement or coughing should be avoided during the procedure to prevent trauma to the peritoneal organs.

7. Vital signs and urinary output must be assessed frequently following paracentesis, since shifts in circulating volume may cause hypotension or reduced urine output.
8. Patient allergies should be determined prior to implementing the procedure.

NURSING ACTION/RATIONALE

1. Assemble all equipment.
2. Identify the patient.
3. Explain the procedure to the patient, including:
   a. Clarification of the physician's explanation.
   b. The position required and the importance of remaining immobile.
   c. Sensations of pressure and cold experienced during injection of the local anesthetic.
4. Obtain an informed consent for the procedure, if required.
5. Instruct the patient to void if no urinary catheter is in place.
6. Provide privacy.
7. Assist the patient into a clean hospital gown.
8. Obtain baseline vital signs and an abdominal girth measurement.
9. Provide adequate lighting.
10. Wash your hands.
11. Assist the physician by opening the paracentesis tray and sterile gloves, using aseptic technique.
12. Position the patient comfortably with adequate support in one of the following positions:
    a. Sitting upright on the side of the bed with the feet on a stool.
    b. Lying in bed in a semi- to high-Fowler's position.
13. Expose the abdomen and drape the patient as necessary.
14. Reassure and support the patient during the procedure.
15. Assist the physician with specimen collection or drainage collection as necessary.

16. Assess the patient's color, vital signs, and level of consciousness throughout the procedure and inform the physician of any changes.
17. Assist the physician with applying an occlusive dressing following removal of the aspirating needle.
18. Assist the patient to a comfortable position.
19. Measure the amount of drainage and the patient's abdominal girth.
20. Send labeled specimens to the laboratory if diagnostic studies are ordered.
21. Discard any remaining paracentesis drainage according to your health care facility's disposal policy.
22. Assess vital signs every 30 minutes for 2 hours, then every hour for 4 hours, then every 4 hours for 24 hours, or more frequently, if necessary.
23. Inspect the dressing over the puncture site and the surrounding skin area for drainage or inflammation when assessing other parameters.
24. Assess urinary output at least every 2 hours.
25. Discard equipment or return it to the appropriate location.

PATIENT AND/OR FAMILY TEACHING

1. Explain the procedure and its purpose to the patient.
2. Reinforce the physician's explanation regarding the patient's disease process.
3. Explain any activity restrictions, if appropriate.
4. Instruct the patient to notify the nurse if experiencing any unusual symptoms.
5. Reinforce any dietary restrictions that may be prescribed.
6. Reinforce the importance of measuring fluid intake and output.

DOCUMENTATION

1. Time of the procedure, type of procedure, and name of physician performing the procedure.
2. Amount, color, odor, and consistency of the fluid obtained.
3. Disposition of the specimens.
4. Type and amount of medication used.
5. Any assessment of the patient during and after the procedure including vital signs, urinary output, and dressings.
6. The patient's tolerance of the procedure, any untoward reactions, and actions taken.
7. All patient teaching done and the patient's level of understanding.

Insertion and Removal of Gastrointestinal Tubes

PURPOSE

1. Provide a route for removal of fluid and/or gas from the gastrointestinal tract.
2. Establish a route for the administration of medications, fluids, or nutrients into the gastrointestinal tract.
3. Provide a route for performing diagnostic testing.
4. Remove the gastrointestinal tube with minimal irritation and discomfort to the patient.

REQUISITES

Insertion

1. Gastrointestinal tube (type and size as ordered by the physician)
2. Water-soluble lubricant
3. Disposable irrigation kit containing:
   a. 50 cc Asepto or barrel syringe with catheter tip
   b. Graduated solution container
   c. Bed protector
   d. Solution collection container
4. Tape or nasogastric tube holder
5. Glass of water
6. Straw
7. Emesis basin
8. Towel
9. Safety pin
10. Stethoscope

Removal

1. Paper towel
2. Exam gloves
3. Waste receptacle
4. Washcloth and towel
5. Bed protector

GUIDELINES

1. A variety of gastrointestinal tubes and sizes are available. The tube selected and the size will depend upon the purpose for the tube, the physician's order, the availability of the tube, and the size of the patient.

2. In general, tubes that are inserted for suctioning purposes are larger in diameter and have an air vent.
3. Tubes that are inserted for the administration of nutrients, fluids, or medication are smaller in diameter and have no air vent.
4. Tubes are available with a weighted tip. The weighted tip allows the tube to pass by gravity through the stomach and into the proximal end of the small intestine. These tubes are usually used for administering nutrients.
5. Intestinal tubes with a mercury-weighted balloon on the tip are used for relieving bowel obstructions and should be inserted and removed by a physician.
6. Refer to the specific procedures "Gastrointestinal Tube Irrigation," "Gastrointestinal Suctioning," "Gastric Lavage," "Gastric Gavage," "Ice Lavage," and "Tube Feeding" for the steps in performing each procedure.
7. Prior to the procedure the tube can be made more or less pliable as desired:
   a. For a soft rubber tube, place it in a container of ice.
   b. For a hard plastic tube, place it under warm running water or in a container of warm water.
8. A very small nasogastric tube (6 to 8 Fr.) can be passed more easily by placing the tip in half of a gelatin capsule, along with the tip of a larger nasogastric tube. The tubes are passed together, following the steps in the procedure. The larger nasogastric tube is removed after the gelatin capsule has dissolved.
9. Stylets are available for insertion of some pliable tubes. After the tube is inserted, the stylet is removed.
10. Patients with gastrointestinal tubes should have frequent oral hygiene to keep the oral mucosa clean and moist.
11. Verification of the correct placement of a nasogastric tube in the stomach of a comatose patient should be assessed carefully. (See Nursing Action 17.)

NURSING ACTION/RATIONALE
Insertion
1. Assemble all equipment.
2. Verify the physician's order.
3. Identify the patient.
4. Explain the procedure and its purpose. Instruct the patient that he/she will need to swallow as the tube is passed and reassure the patient that you will coach him/her through the procedure.
5. Provide privacy.
6. Assist the patient into a hospital gown.
7. Assess bowel sounds and vital signs as appropriate.
8. Assist the patient to a sitting or high-Fowler's position.
9. Select the most patent nostril by having the patient block one side and breathe through the other, alternately.
10. Place a towel over the patient's chest.
11. Wash your hands.
12. Estimate the length of tubing necessary to enter the patient's stomach (Figure 5-2).
    a. Using the tube, measure the distance from the patient's ear lobe to the tip of the nose.
    b. Starting at the last measurement, use the tube to measure the distance from the tip of the nose to the xyphoid process.
    c. Mark the spot of the combined measurements with a piece of tape.
13. Lubricate the tip of the tubing for 6 to 8 inches to reduce friction and irritation.
14. Place the emesis basin close to the patient or allow the patient to hold it.
15. Insert the tube gently through the selected nostril, aiming back and down. Do not force the tube. If an obstruction is met, withdraw the tube slightly and advance again. As the tube reaches the pharnyx, instruct the patient to swallow. The patient can take sips of water through a straw to help the swallowing reflex.
16. Continue to advance the tube each time the patient swallows, until the tape mark on the tube is at the patient's nostril. If there are signs of distress such as gasping, coughing, or cyanosis, immediately withdraw the tube, as this can indicate placement in the trachea.

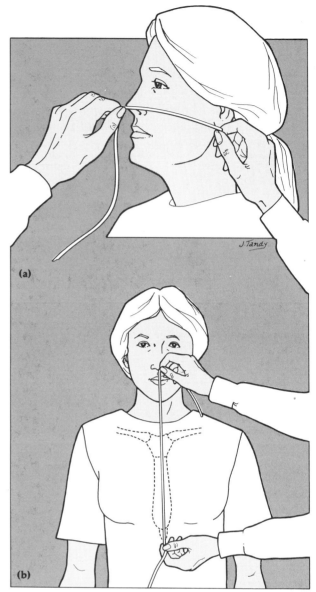

Figure 5-2. Measure (a) from the earlobe to the tip of the nose and (b) from the tip of the nose to the xyphoid process.

17. Assess for tube placement:
    a. Connect a barrel syringe to the end of the tube and aspirate stomach contents, or
    b. Connect a syringe with 30 cc of air to the end of the tube. Place the stethoscope over the epigastrium and inject the air. Listen for sounds of air entering the stomach, or
    c. Assess tube placement by x-ray if prescribed by the physician.

18. Tape the tubing securely to the nose or apply a tube holder to secure the tube in place. Be sure the tape is not obstructing the patient's vision or pressing against the nares. Weighted intestinal tubes should not be taped. Consult with the physician.

19. Apply a piece of flagged tape to the tube close to the distal end and pin the tape to the patient's gown. Allow enough slack so the patient can move freely (Figure 5-3).

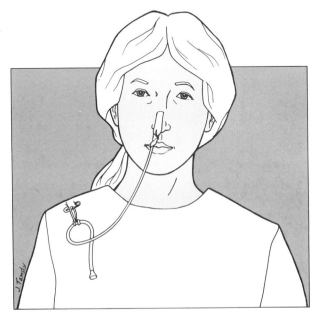

Figure 5-3. Nasogastric tube taped and secured appropriately.

20. If the tubing will not be used immediately, place a catheter plug in the end of the tube.

21. Reposition the patient comfortably. Reassure the patient, since this can be a frightening procedure.

22. Discard equipment or return it to the appropriate location. Save the disposable irrigation kit at the patient's bedside.

Removal

1. Assemble all equipment.
2. Verify the physician's order.
3. Identify the patient.
4. Explain the procedure to the patient.
5. Assist the patient to a high-Fowler's position.
6. Place a bed protector over the patient's chest.
7. Wash your hands.
8. Turn off the suction unit, if appropriate.
9. Remove the tape from the nose.

10. Apply exam gloves.
11. Instruct the patient to take a deep breath and hold it during removal.
12. Grasp the tubing with one hand and pinch, while gently withdrawing in one easy motion.
13. Guide the tubing with a paper towel in your other hand, catching the tip in the paper towel as it is withdrawn.
14. Instruct the patient to breathe normally.
15. Remove the exam gloves.
16. Cleanse the nares with a washcloth and towel and assess for irritation.
17. Assist the patient to a comfortable position.
18. Measure the gastric drainage, if appropriate.
19. Discard equipment or return it to the appropriate area.

PATIENT AND/OR FAMILY TEACHING

1. Explain the procedure and its purpose to the patient.
2. Explain the patient's role in swallowing as the tube is being advanced.
3. Instruct the patient not to pull on or manipulate the tube.
4. Instruct the patient to notify the nurse if irritation develops at the nares.

DOCUMENTATION

1. Time of procedure, type of procedure, and size of the nasogastric tube inserted.
2. The patient's tolerance of the procedure.
3. Method used to verify correct tube placement.
4. Amount, color, consistency, and odor of gastric drainage, if appropriate.
5. All patient teaching and the patient's level of understanding.

Management of Gastrointestinal Suction

PURPOSE

1. Establish gastrointestinal suction to remove fluid or air from the stomach.
2. Provide nursing care for patients with gastrointestinal suction.

REQUISITES

1. Gastrointestinal tube in place in the patient
2. Continuous or intermittent portable suction machine or a continuous or intermittent suction regulator for wall vacuum
3. Barrel connector
4. Connecting tube
5. 50 cc Asepto or barrel syringe with catheter tip
6. Collection container
7. Bed protector
8. Stethoscope
9. Cotton-tipped applicators
10. Lubricant or ointment as prescribed by the physician for nares

GUIDELINES

1. Gastrointestinal suctioning is ordered to remove fluid and/or air from the stomach for many reasons, including to:
   a. Relieve nausea and vomiting.
   b. Prepare a patient for surgery or diagnostic testing.
   c. Maintain gastric decompression postoperatively.
   d. Remove irritants from the stomach.
   e. Treat bleeding of the upper gastrointestinal tract.
   f. Treat a patient with a bowel obstruction.
2. The physician's order for suctioning should include the type of suction (continuous or intermittent) and the amount of pressure to be used for suctioning.
3. One of the major problems with gastrointestinal suctioning is damage to the mucosa if the catheter suctions against it. Gastrointestinal tubes with air vents decrease the possibility of this occurring. Intermittent suctioning or continuous suctioning with an interrupting device (interrupts at a specified pressure) also decreases the possibility of damage to the mucosa.

4. In some situations, such as postoperative gastric resections, bleeding from the stomach is expected. If the blood in the gastric drainage increases in intensity or amount from the baseline, the physician must be notified immediately.
5. Low gastrointestinal suction is usually 80 to 100 mm Hg pressure and high gastrointestinal suction is usually 100 to 120 mm Hg pressure.
6. Refer to the operator's manual for the proper setup and troubleshooting of the specific suction apparatus to be used.

NURSING ACTION/RATIONALE

1. Assemble all equipment.
2. Identify the patient.
3. Explain the procedure and its purpose to the patient.
4. Provide privacy.
5. Assess bowel sounds and vital signs, as appropriate.
6. Assist the patient to a semi-Fowler's position. This is the ideal position for suctioning.
7. Wash your hands.
8. Verify the placement of the tube by aspirating stomach contents with a syringe, or by instilling 30 cc of air into the tube and listening over the epigastrium with a stethoscope for the rush of air into the stomach.
9. Connect the gastrointestinal tube to the suction connecting tubing, using a barrel connector.
10. Turn the suction machine on.
11. Set the machine to the desired pressure.
12. Observe the tubing for a few minutes to ensure that suctioning is occurring.
13. Coil any extra connecting tubing on the bed. Tubing should not remain in a dependent position because suctioning will not be as effective.
14. Place the air vent on the gastrointestinal tube so that it is not in a dependent position. If stomach contents drain through the air vent, inject 10 cc of air into the air vent to clear it. Never cap or clamp the air vent.

15. Irrigate the gastrointestinal tube as necessary to maintain patency of the system. Refer to the procedure "Gastrointestinal Tube Irrigation" for the correct steps for irrigating.
16. Assess the system for correct functioning at least every hour at first and every 3 hours after the patient and system are stable. Assess for:
    a. Patency of the tubing.
    b. Kinking or bending of the tubing.
    c. Correct pressure setting of the machine.
    d. Amount, color, and consistency of returns.
17. Assess the patient every hour or more frequently until stable. Assess for:
    a. Bowel sounds.
    b. Vital signs.
    c. Abdominal distention and/or discomfort.
    d. Irritation to the nares.
    e. Dry mouth discomfort.
18. Empty the suction drainage container every 8 hours, or when two-thirds full. To empty:
    a. Turn the suction off.
    b. Disconnect the container.
    c. Empty the contents and measure.
    d. Rinse the container.
    e. Replace the container on the suction machine.
    f. Turn the suction on.
    g. Assess the system for proper function.
19. Cleanse the nares every 4 hours using water and cotton-tipped applicators. Apply lubricant or ointment, as prescribed by the physician, with a cotton-tipped applicator. Replace the tape on the nose as it becomes soiled or loosened.
20. Offer oral hygiene every 4 hours or oftener as necessary. Refer to the "Special Mouth Care" procedure. Patients are usually allowed to chew gum or suck on candy to keep oral mucosa moist. Consult with the physician.
21. Ambulate patients, if allowed:
    a. Turn the suction off.
    b. Disconnect the gastrointestinal tube from the connecting tubing.
    c. Insert a catheter plug into the lumen of the gastrointestinal tubing.
    d. Reverse the procedure when finished ambulating.
22. Rinse reuseable equipment after each use. Discard all other equipment or return it to the appropriate location.

PATIENT AND/OR FAMILY TEACHING

1. Explain each procedure and its purpose to the patient before starting.
2. Instruct the patient to notify the nurse of any:
   a. Abdominal discomfort.
   b. Nausea or vomiting.
   c. Oral or nares discomfort.
   d. Leakage from the tubing.
3. Encourage the patient to ask questions as necessary.
4. Explain activity restrictions.
5. Instruct the patient not to manipulate the tubing or suction equipment.
6. Reinforce the physician's explanation of the disease process.
7. Explain any other therapeutic or diagnostic orders as appropriate.

DOCUMENTATION

1. Type of procedure and time the suction was applied.
2. Amount, color, and consistency of gastric drainage.
3. Regular assessments of the patency of the system.
4. All parameters of assessment of the patient.
5. Any irrigations performed and the results.
6. All supportive care given to the patient, including oral and nares care as well as positioning.
7. Any problems encountered, interventions, and results.
8. All patient teaching done and the patient's level of understanding.

Gastrointestinal Tube Irrigation

PURPOSE
1. Assess for patency of the gastrointestinal tube.
2. Restore patency of the gastrointestinal tube.

REQUISITES
1. Disposable irrigation kit containing:
   a. 50 cc Asepto or barrel syringe with a cathether tip
   b. Graduated solution container
   c. Bed protector
   d. Solution collection container
2. 500 cc bottle of sterile normal saline for irrigation
3. Stethoscope

GUIDELINES
1. Irrigation of a gastrointestinal tube is indicated when the tube is connected to suction and the suctioned material is not returning as anticipated or when a drip tube feeding will not infuse.
2. When a gastrointestinal tube is not patent, generally either the lumen is blocked by a solid particle or the tip of the tube is against the gastric mucosa. Irrigation should resolve either of these problems.
3. Never instill liquid into a gastrointestinal tube before checking for correct placement. Refer to "Insertion and Removal of Gastrointestinal Tubes."
4. Disposable irrigation kits should be rinsed well between irrigations, and replaced daily.

NURSING ACTION/RATIONALE
1. Assemble all equipment.
2. Identify the patient.
3. Explain the procedure to the patient.
4. Provide privacy.
5. Assist the patient to a semi-Fowler's position.
6. Wash your hands.
7. Place the bed protector under the end of the tube.
8. Turn off the suction or tube feeding as appropriate, and disconnect.
9. Assess for tube placement by either instilling 30 cc of air while listening over the epigastrium with a stethoscope for air entering the stomach or by aspirating with a syringe for the return of stomach contents.
10. Pour 50 to 100 cc of solution into the solution container.
11. Draw up 20 cc of solution into the syringe.
12. Instill the solution into the tube.
13. Withdraw the 20 cc of solution and empty the syringe into the collection container.
14. Repeat the irrigation again.
15. Reconnect the tube to the suction or to the tube feeding setup as appropriate. Observe for patency and function.
16. Rinse the irrigation kit as necessary and return it to the patient's bedside.
17. Wash your hands.

PATIENT AND/OR FAMILY TEACHING
1. Explain the procedure and its purpose to the patient. Assure the patient that there will be no discomfort.
2. Instruct the patient to call the nurse if any unusual symptoms occur.

DOCUMENTATION
1. Method used to verify tube placement.
2. Time of the procedure and type and amount of solution instilled.
3. The amount, color, consistency, and odor of solution returned.
4. An assessment of the patency of the tube following irrigation.
5. All patient teaching done and the patient's level of understanding.

Gastric Lavage

PURPOSE

1. Remove irritating substances from the stomach.
2. Prepare the patient for gastric surgery or diagnostic tests.

REQUISITES

1. Nasogastric tube, type and size as ordered by physician
2. Water-soluble lubricant
3. Emesis basin
4. Tape
5. Disposable irrigation tray, including:
   a. Asepto or barrel syringe with catheter tip—50 cc
   b. Graduated solution container
   c. Bed protector
   d. Solution collection container
6. Irrigating solution as ordered by the physician
7. Towels
8. Gastric suction equipment available (see "Management of Gastrointestinal Suction")
9. Oral suction equipment (see "Oropharyngeal/ Nasopharyngeal Suctioning")

GUIDELINES

1. Gastric lavage is generally performed as an emergency treatment after a patient has ingested poisons or an overdose of medications. It can be ordered to cleanse the stomach before gastric surgery; this is generally a non-emergency procedure.
2. Gastric lavage should not be performed if a patient has ingested flammable liquids such as petroleum or corrosive liquids such as acids. In these cases the proper antidote must be administered first. Consult with the physician immediately.
3. A team approach may be needed to attend the patient since other emergency treatment may need to be administered simultaneously with the gastric lavage.
4. Irrigation solution must never be forced into the stomach during gastric lavage, since this may cause stomach contents to enter the small intestine.

5. In suspected poisonings or overdoses it may be necessary to save all stomach contents and irrigation returns. Check your hospital policy before discarding.
6. Stop the procedure immediately and notify the physician if the patient experiences severe pain or the gastric contents return bloody.
7. Patients who have ingested overdoses of medications should be observed closely for changes in level of consciousness. If blood levels of the ingested substance are high, a dialysis procedure may be considered by the physician.
8. Psychiatric counseling may be necessary for patients with intentional overdoses.

NURSING ACTION/RATIONALE

1. Assemble all equipment.
2. Identify the patient.
3. Explain the procedure to the patient.
4. Assist the patient to a high-Fowler's position for the nasogastric tube insertion.
5. Wash your hands.
6. Insert the nasogastric tube and verify placement as described in "Insertion and Removal of Gastrointestinal Tubes."
7. Place the patient on the left side with the head elevated 15 degrees. This will allow the tip of the tube to lie in the greater curvature of the stomach. Place towels around the patient's head to contain any drainage.
8. Gently aspirate all stomach contents, using a barrel syringe.
9. Instruct your assistant to put the stomach contents into a labeled specimen container and send it to the laboratory for analysis.
10. Remove the plunger from the syringe.
11. Attach the barrel of the syringe to the nasogastric tube.
12. Raise the barrel of the syringe about 12 inches above the patient's head.
13. Pour approximately 500 cc of the irrigating solution into the syringe. Allow the solution to flow in slowly by gravity. Assess the patient carefully for abdominal distention. Do not overdistend the stomach.

14. Remove the syringe and lower the end of the nasogastric tube below the level of the patient. Allow the stomach contents to drain by gravity into the collection container. It may be necessary to connect the syringe and aspirate gently to get the flow to start.
15. Repeat the procedure at least ten times, or as ordered by the physician.
16. Follow the physician's orders for further treatment following the gastric lavage.
17. Cleanse the patient as necessary and reposition comfortably.
18. Discard equipment or return it to the appropriate location.

PATIENT AND/OR FAMILY TEACHING

1. Explain the procedure and purpose to the patient and/or family.
2. Explain other emergency treatment as appropriate.
3. In the case of accidental poisonings, after the patient stabilizes, discuss safety precautions to prevent recurrence.

DOCUMENTATION

1. Procedure and time started and stopped.
2. Amount, color, and consistency of stomach contents initially aspirated.
3. Type and amount of irrigating solution instilled.
4. The amount, color, and consistency of gastric return.
5. All parameters of assessment, including level of consciousness and vital signs.
6. The amount, color, and consistency of any vomitus.
7. All emergency procedures performed.
8. Notification or presence of the physician.
9. Disposition of the stomach contents specimen and all gastric returns.
10. All patient teaching done and the patient's level of understanding.

Iced Gastric Lavage

PURPOSE
1. Control upper gastrointestinal bleeding.

REQUISITES
1. Large gastrointestinal tube (20 to 40 Fr.) or as ordered by the physician
2. Water-soluble lubricant
3. Tape
4. Emesis basin
5. Disposable irrigation tray including:
   a. Asepto or barrel syringe with catheter tip—50 cc
   b. Graduated solution container
   c. Bed protector
   d. Collection container
6. Irrigating solution as ordered by the physician—usually normal saline or Ringer's lactate
7. Large container full of clean ice
8. Towels
9. Gastric suction equipment available (see "Management of Gastric Suction")
10. Oral suction equipment (see "Oropharyngeal/ Nasopharyngeal Suctioning")

GUIDELINES
1. Upper gastrointestinal bleeding is a critical situation, and measures to control the bleeding must be instituted immediately.
2. Patients requiring iced gastric lavage require a nursing team approach. One nurse should perform the lavage, while other team members monitor vital signs and perform other emergency procedures as necessary.
3. A number of therapeutic procedures may need to be performed simultaneously during the ice lavage. They include:
   a. Oxygen therapy.
   b. Monitoring vital signs closely.
   c. Blood transfusions.
   d. Intravenous therapy.
   e. Foley catheter insertion.
   f. Drawing blood for diagnostic studies.
   g. Preparing the patient for an endoscopy or for surgery.

4. If a large-lumen gastrointestinal tube is used, it may need to be inserted through the mouth. The procedure is the same as for "Insertion and Removal of Gastrointestinal Tubes," except that entry is through the mouth.
5. If someone qualified to insert an endotracheal tube is available, the endotracheal tube can be inserted first to prevent the patient from aspirating stomach contents. Oral suction equipment should be available for immediate use in the event the patient vomits.
6. Vital signs including temperature should be taken every 5 to 30 minutes, depending on the amount of bleeding and the condition of the patient.

NURSING ACTION/RATIONALE
1. Assemble all equipment.
2. Identify the patient.
3. Explain the procedure to the patient. Provide reassurance if the patient is alert, since this is a very frightening situation.
4. Assist the patient to a high-Fowler's position for the nasogastric tube insertion.
5. Wash your hands.
6. Insert the nasogastric tube and verify placement as described in "Insertion and Removal of Gastrointestinal Tubes."
7. Before starting the lavage, place the patient on the left side with the head elevated 15 degrees. Place towels around the patient's head to contain drainage.
8. Aspirate stomach contents, using the barrel syringe, until no contents return. Place the aspirated contents in the collection container for measuring.
9. Pour the irrigating solution over the clean ice in the container.
10. Draw up 50 cc of iced solution into the barrel syringe.
11. Inject the iced solution slowly into the nasogastric tube.
12. Wait 30 seconds.
13. Use the barrel syringe and aspirate all stomach contents.
14. Repeat the procedure of administering iced solution and aspirating until the solution returns clear, or as ordered by the physician.

15. Reposition the patient and/or advance or withdraw the tube slightly if the iced solution will not return. Never force aspiration, since the tip of the tube may be against the mucosa, and damage to the mucosa could occur.
16. Maintain an accurate account of the amount of iced solution administered and the amount of drainage returned. If more drainage returns than the amount of solution administered, the difference should be added to the estimated blood loss.
17. Follow the physician's orders for further treatment following the iced lavage.
18. Cleanse the patient as necessary and reposition as appropriate following the iced lavage.
19. Discard equipment or return it to the appropriate location.

PATIENT AND/OR FAMILY TEACHING

1. Explain the procedure before starting, as appropriate.
2. Explain other emergency treatments as appropriate.
3. Reinforce the physician's explanation of the medical problem.

DOCUMENTATION

1. Type and size of nasogastric tube and time inserted.
2. Time gastric lavage started, type of solution used, and time lavage was stopped.
3. Amount, color, consistency, and odor of stomach contents originally aspirated from the stomach.
4. Amount of irrigating solution administered and amount of solution returned, along with the color, consistency, and odor.
5. An estimate of the amount of any vomitus that may have occurred, including the color, consistency, and odor.
6. All parameters of assessment, including the patient's level of consciousness and vital signs.
7. All emergency procedures performed.
8. Presence of the physician, or notification of the physician.
9. All patient teaching done and the patient's level of understanding.

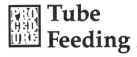 **Tube Feeding**

PURPOSE

1. Administer an intermittent or continuous feeding into the stomach or small intestines by means of a tube when the oral route cannot be used.

REQUISITES

1. All equipment for inserting a nasogastric tube, if necessary
2. Tube feeding (amount and type as ordered by the physician)
3. Water (amount as ordered by the physician)
4. 50 cc barrel or Asepto syringe
5. Stethoscope
6. Tape
7. Clamp or plug
8. IV standard
9. Feeding bag, gavage feeding set, or infusion pump with tubing (type as ordered by the physician)

GUIDELINES

1. Tube feedings are administered to provide a means of nutrition for a variety of medical problems including:
   a. Nutritional depletion from debilitation.
   b. Anorexia.
   c. An impairment in swallowing.
   d. Oral surgery.
2. Tube feeding formulas have the necessary nutrients to sustain normal body weight and maintain fluid and electrolyte balance.
3. Commercially prepared tube feedings can be purchased, or a specific formula can be made in the hospital by using a blender.
4. Patient sensitivity to a particular formula is manifested by abdominal cramping, vomiting, or diarrhea.
5. Possible complications related to tube feedings are:
   a. Nausea, vomiting, or gastric distention related to administering too much formula too rapidly.
   b. Diarrhea related to a formula that is contaminated, too cold, or administered too rapidly.
   c. Aspiration of the formula from an improperly placed nasogastric tube, or from vomiting.
   d. Dehydration from an insufficient fluid intake.
   e. Electrolyte imbalance from an improperly balanced diet.
6. Complications from a contaminated tube feeding can be prevented by:
   a. Thoroughly cleaning the equipment with soap and water and rinsing it between feedings.
   b. Replacing the tube feeding equipment every 24 hours.
   c. Never allowing tube feeding formula to remain at room temperature for more than 8 hours.
7. Patients receiving tube feedings should have an intake and output assessment done every 8 hours.
8. The physician should prescribe the type of formula to be used, the method of administration, the amount of formula to be administered, the rate of administration, the amount of supplemental water to be administered, and all laboratory work to monitor electrolytes.
9. Prior to administering a tube feeding, the patient should be given good oral hygiene, and the environment should be free of annoying odors or sights.
10. When oral medications are to be given by nasogastric tube, consult with your pharmacist. Liquid medications are available, some tablets can be crushed, and some capsules can be opened for administration through the nasogastric tube. Always give medications by the Asepto syringe method, with water.
11. If the tube feeding is to be done through a gastrostomy tube:
    a. Drape the patient to expose the tube.
    b. Administer the feeding using the Asepto syringe method.

12. When the patient has a tracheostomy tube and a nasogastric tube:
    a. Always administer the feeding by the Asepto syringe method and assess the patient closely during the feeding.
    b. Perform tracheostomy care and suctioning before the feeding to prevent gagging and vomiting.
    c. If the tracheostomy tube has an inflatable cuff, inflate it with enough air to make a gentle seal before initiating the feeding. Deflate the cuff 30 minutes after the feeding, or follow the physician's orders. Pediatric cuffs are never inflated.
13. Before a tube feeding is administered, the stomach contents should be aspirated completely to assess for residual formula in the stomach. Large amounts of residual formula in the stomach can indicate that:
    a. Too much volume of formula is being administered too frequently for the patient to digest adequately.
    b. The patient has a decrease in gastrointestinal absorption ability.
    c. The patient has decreased peristalsis.
14. The amount of residual formula in the patient's stomach may affect the volume of formula to be administered. Consult with the physician regarding orders for a specific patient, but general guidelines are:
    a. If less than 50 cc of residual formula is aspirated, return the formula to the stomach and administer the prescribed volume of formula for the feeding.
    b. If between 50 to 100 cc of residual formula is aspirated, return the residual to the stomach, and subtract the volume of residual from the prescribed amount for the feeding.
    c. If more than 100 cc of residual formula is aspirated, return the residual to the stomach, hold the tube feeding, and notify the physician.
15. Returning the residual to the stomach after measuring is essential, since the residual feeding from the stomach is mixed with the patient's own fluid and electrolytes. The residual must be returned to assist the patient to maintain a fluid and electrolyte balance.

NURSING ACTION/RATIONALE
1. Assemble all equipment.
2. Verify the physician's order.
3. Prepare the tube feeding formula. Warm to room temperature.
4. Identify the patient.
5. Explain the tube feeding procedure to the patient.
6. Provide adequate lighting.
7. Provide privacy.
8. Assist the patient to a semi- to high-Fowler's position as tolerated.
9. Wash your hands.
10. Insert the feeding tube, if necessary. Refer to the procedure "Insertion and Management of Nasogastric Tubes."
11. Assess the feeding tube for placement and assess for the amount of residual gastric contents in the stomach:
    a. Unclamp the tube. Use a barrel syringe to aspirate all of the stomach contents.
    b. If unable to aspirate any stomach contents, inject 5 to 10 cc of air into the feeding tube while listening over the left upper quadrant of the abdomen with a stethoscope. The sound of air gurgling in the stomach verifies placement of the tube.
    c. If residual stomach contents are aspirated, measure the total amount and return the residual to the patient's stomach, using the Asepto syringe tube feeding method. Calculate any changes in the volume of the impending tube feeding.
12. Administer the feeding by one of the following methods:

Asepto Syringe
    a. Remove the bulb from the syringe and attach the syringe to the feeding tube.
    b. Hold the Asepto syringe 6 inches above the patient's head. The flow can be regulated by raising or lowering the syringe.
    c. Clear the feeding tube with 30 to 50 cc of water.
    d. Pour part of the feeding into the syringe and allow it to flow by gravity. Refill the syringe until the feeding is completed. Do not allow air to enter the feeding tube.
    e. Flush the tube with approximately 30 cc of water.

Feeding Bag: Drip Infusion

a. Hang the bag from the IV standard and clamp the tubing.

b. Pour 50 cc of water into the feeding bag. Fill the drip chamber half full, and clear the tubing of air.

c. Connect the feeding bag and tubing to the feeding tube. Secure the connection with tape.

d. Open the clamp and allow the water to slowly clear the feeding tube.

e. Pour the feeding into the bag. Do not allow air to enter the tubing.

f. Regulate the drip with the clamp as ordered.

g. Flush the tube with approximately 50 cc of water after the tube feeding has infused.

Gavage Feeding Set: Drip Infusion

a. Remove the screw cap from the formula and screw on the cap with the attached tubing.

b. Hang the bottle from the IV standard. Fill the drip chamber half full and clear the tubing of air.

c. Connect the tubing to the feeding tube. Secure the connection with tape.

d. Regulate the drips with the clamp as ordered.

e. When the feeding is completed, remove the gavage feeding set and attach an Asepto syringe.

f. Flush the tube with approximately 30 cc of water using the Asepto syringe method.

Infusion Pump

a. Connect the tubing to the feeding container. Fill the feeding container with the solution to be infused.

b. Hang the container from the IV standard. Fill the drip chamber.

c. Attach the tubing to the infusion pump and flush the solution through the tubing according to the manufacturer's directions.

d. Connect the tubing to the feeding tube. Secure the connection with tape.

e. Set the rate as ordered and begin the infusion.

f. Change the solution in the container every 8 hours to reduce the possibility of contamination.

g. If the feeding is temporarily discontinued, flush the tubing with 60 cc of water after discontinuing and before restarting the feeding, using the Asepto syringe method.

13. Instruct the patient to notify the nurse of any discomfort during or after the feeding.

14. Clamp or plug the feeding tube when the feeding is completed. Secure the tube as necessary to prevent dislodging.

15. Keep the patient in a semi-Fowler's position for about 30 minutes. Make certain that the patient is comfortable. If the patient is unconscious, position the head to one side to prevent aspiration should vomiting occur.

16. Discard equipment or return it to the appropriate area. The tube feeding equipment can be washed, dried, and reused, but it should be discarded after 24 hours.

PATIENT AND/OR FAMILY TEACHING

1. Explain the nature and purpose of the tube feeding to the patient.

2. Reinforce and clarify the physician's explanation of the disease process.

3. Explain any additional therapeutic orders.

4. Remind the patient to call the nurse should any discomfort be experienced during or after the tube feeding.

5. Explain that the patient must remain in a semi-Fowler's position during and after the feeding to aid digestion.

6. Teach the patient appropriate aspects of nutrition and the nutritional value of the tube feeding.

7. Teach the patient and/or a family member to administer the feedings if the tube feedings are to be continued after discharge.

DOCUMENTATION

1. Insertion of the tube including the date, time, type, and size as appropriate.

2. Feeding, amount given, method used, rate at which administered, and amount of water given.

3. The patient's reaction to the tube feeding, especially any discomfort.

4. All patient teaching done and the patient's level of understanding.

Disposable Ileostomy Appliance Change

PURPOSE

1. Permit visualization of the stoma and the surrounding skin.
2. Prevent stool leakage and skin excoriation.
3. Control odor.

REQUISITES

1. Drainable ileostomy appliance with karaya ring
2. Stoma measuring guide
3. Skin protectant
4. Skin barrier
5. Appliance clamp
6. Appliance deodorant
7. Scissors
8. 3 × 3 gauze sponges
9. Graduated collection container
10. Bulb syringe
11. Disposable tissue
12. Washbasin
13. Soap
14. Washcloth
15. Towel
16. Waste receptacle

GUIDELINES

1. The most important concern in ileostomy care is skin protection. Ileostomy drainage is rich in enzymes that will break down the parastomal skin, causing skin irritation.
2. A well-fitting, properly applied appliance will prevent leakage by providing a good seal to keep drainage away from the skin. Adjust the size of the appliance as the stoma shrinks. It may take 6 months for the swelling to subside after surgery.
3. Most ileostomy appliances are drainable. The small bowel is active most of the time, and the fecal drainage is usually liquid or pastelike. Therefore, the appliance should be emptied frequently or when the bag becomes one-third full.
4. Ileostomies are never irrigated, except by a physician to clear an obstruction. Continent ileostomies are drained at regular intervals with a catheter, but this procedure will not include that technique. Refer to the references for additional information.
5. The ileostomy appliance change is a clean, non-sterile procedure.
6. The appliance can stay in place as long as the seal protecting the skin remains intact. This may vary from 1 to 7 days, depending on the product. The appliance should be changed every other day on a new surgical patient so that the stoma can be assessed.
7. The best time to change the appliance is the first thing in the morning or 2 to 4 hours after a meal when the bowel is relatively inactive. However, the appliance should be changed immediately if the patient complains of burning or itching around the stoma underneath the appliance.
8. Do not use cream, ointment, or oil on the parastomal skin. Always remove all soap. These products may leave a residue that prevents adherence of the appliance to the skin.
9. The patient should be encouraged to look at the stoma and participate in the care, but should never be forced.
10. Encourage and allow the patient to express feelings regarding the stoma and the change in body image that has occurred.
11. A positive, accepting attitude on the part of the nurse can help the ostomy patient to adjust. Adjustment will follow the grieving process as the patient integrates the stoma into his/her body image.
12. There are many ostomy appliances available. The patient may need to experiment with a variety of equipment to find the system that works best.

NURSING ACTION/RATIONALE

1. Assembly all equipment.
2. Identify the patient.
3. Explain the procedure to the patient.
4. Provide privacy.
5. Provide adequate lighting.
6. Position the patient in a semi-Fowler's position to facilitate participation.
7. Wash your hands.
8. Gently remove the old appliance. Measure the drainage if indicated. Discard the old appliance in a waste receptacle but save the clamp.
9. Wipe excess stool from around the stoma with a disposable tissue.
10. Wash the skin around the stoma with soap and warm water. Rinse well and pat dry with a towel.
11. Place a gauze over the stoma to protect the skin from additional drainage while working.
12. Wash your hands.
13. Measure the stoma, using the measuring guide (Figure 5-4). The smallest size that fits without touching the stoma is the correct size.
14. Apply the skin protectant or skin barrier.
    a. Skin protectant—for normal skin.
       (1) Skin gel—spread a thin layer on the skin with your finger. Allow it to dry.
       (2) Skin prep—spray or wipe a thin layer on the skin. Allow it to dry.
    b. Skin barrier—for irritated skin.
       (1) Using the selected hole from the measuring guide, cut the correct size hole in the center of the skin barrier.
       (2) Peel off the backing, center the barrier over the stoma, and press firmly onto the skin.
15. Peel off the cellophane on the karaya ring and the paper backing on the adhesive of the drainable appliance.
16. Moisten the ring with water. Wait a few minutes until it becomes tacky.

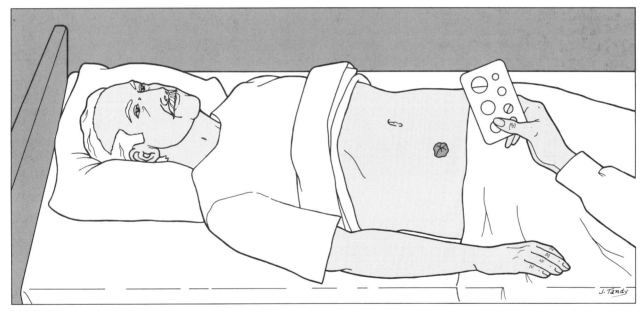

Figure 5-4. Use of the stoma measuring guide.

17. Center the karaya ring over the stoma and press down (Figure 5-5).
18. Place 8 to 10 drops of appliance deodorant into the appliance through the bottom opening.
19. Apply the clamp to the open end of the appliance after folding the end up twice.
20. Assist the patient to a comfortable position.
21. Instruct the patient to notify the nurse of any discomfort at the stoma site.
22. Discard equipment or return it to the appropriate location.
23. Wash your hands.
24. Empty the appliance when it is one-third full:
    a. Remove the clamp and unroll the end.
    b. Allow the contents to drain into the toilet or a suitable container.
    c. Rinse the bag with warm water, using a bulb syringe.
    d. Wipe the bottom of the appliance with tissue.
    e. Fold the end up twice and replace the clamp.

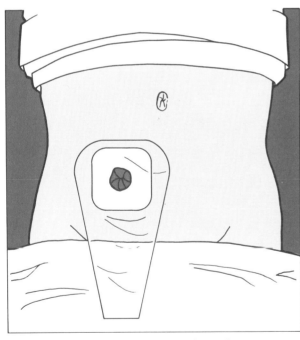

Figure 5-5. Ileostomy appliance applied over the stoma.

PATIENT AND/OR FAMILY TEACHING
1. Explain the procedure to the patient.
2. Reinforce and clarify the physician's explanation of the disease process.
3. Explain any additional therapeutic orders.

4. Instruct the patient to notify the nurse of any discomfort at the stoma site.
5. Teach the procedure step by step to the patient and/or a family member. Have the patient do a return demonstration and practice as much as possible prior to discharge. Give the patient written instructions and any other available literature.
6. Explain ostomy equipment, the types available to the patient, and where the supplies can be purchased in the community.
7. Teach the patient how to control odor by the use of appliance deodorant and avoidance of gas-producing foods.
8. Instruct the patient to follow the diet prescribed by the physician. Reinforce foods allowed and restricted.
9. Teach the patient how to cope with skin problems and when to seek help.
10. Inform the patient about the local ostomy support group. Give him/her the name and number of the enterostomal therapist.

DOCUMENTATION
1. The ileostomy appliance change, date and time of change, and type and size of appliance used.
2. An assessment of the stoma and surrounding skin.
3. As assessment of the fecal drainage.
4. The patient's reaction to the procedure.
5. All patient and family teaching done and the level of understanding.

Colostomy Care and Irrigation

PURPOSE

1. Cleanse the colon and stimulate peristalsis.
2. Establish a regular pattern of evacuation.
3. Prevent intestinal obstruction.
4. Prevent skin excoriation due to irritating fecal contents.
5. Permit visualization of the stoma and the surrounding skin.

REQUISITES

1. Drainable colostomy appliance
2. Cone/tube irrigation set
3. Skin prep or gel
4. Appliance deodorant
5. Graduated collection container
6. Water-soluble lubricant
7. Exam gloves
8. Bedpan
9. Washcloth
10. Towel
11. Soap
12. Waste receptacle

GUIDELINES

1. Irrigation of a colostomy is an enema given through a colon stoma.
2. The irrigating technique is most effective for sigmoid and descending colon colostomies because a regular pattern of evacuation can usually be established. Irrigation of transverse or ascending colon colostomies is usually not successful since the stool is liquid or semi-liquid.
3. Age, manual dexterity, ability to learn, and previous bowel pattern habits all influence the degree of success an irrigation may achieve.
4. The initial irrigation is usually performed 7 to 10 days after surgery. It is a clean, non-sterile procedure.
5. If possible, stoma care should be done in the bathroom. If the patient is unable to ambulate to the bathroom, the irrigation can be done in bed using a bedpan to collect the drainage.

6. Performing the colostomy irrigation at the same time every day assists in developing bowel control. Emptying the bowel regularly discourages stoma activity between irrigations.
7. Difficulty inserting the catheter could be due to anxiety or a firm stool. Never force the catheter, since the lining of the colon contains no sensory nerves and injury may result.
8. Never place the irrigator bag higher than the patient's shoulder level to prevent backflow of water from the colon due to increased pressure.
9. Water retention after irrigation may be due to:
   a. Bowel spasm.
   b. Dehydration.
   c. Insertion of the catheter too far into the bowel.
10. The patient should be encouraged to look at the stoma and participate in the care, but should never be forced.
11. Encourage and allow the patient to express feelings regarding the stoma and the change in his/her body image.
12. A positive, accepting attitude on the part of the nurse can help the ostomy patient to adjust. Adjustment will follow the grieving process as the patient integrates the stoma into his/her body image.
13. There are many ostomy appliances available. The patient may need to experiment until he/she finds the system that works best.
14. Irrigator sleeves can be used several times. Irrigator bags last 6 months to 1 year.

NURSING ACTION/RATIONALE

1. Assemble all equipment.
2. Identify the patient.
3. Explain the procedure to the patient.
4. Wash your hands.
5. Assist the patient to the bathroom.
6. Seat the patient on the toilet or on a chair next to the toilet.
7. Fill the irrigator bag with tap water warmed to 37.7 to 43.3°C (100 to 110°F). The amount of solution ranges from 500 cc to 1000 cc or as prescribed by the physician.

8. Hang the irrigator bag so that the bottom is no higher than the shoulder level of the seated patient.
9. Clear the tubing of air by allowing the water to flow to the tip of the cone or catheter.
10. Remove the old appliance. Measure the stool if indicated. Discard the drainable appliance, but save the clamp.
11. Cleanse the skin gently around the stoma with a washcloth using soap and warm water. Rinse well.
12. Dilate the stoma to help prevent strictures if ordered by the physician.
    a. Apply an exam glove and lubricate the finger closest in size to the stoma.
    b. Gently insert your finger into the stoma approximately 2 inches.
    c. Rotate your finger gently to dilate the stoma (Figure 5-6). Never force the finger.
13. Apply the irrigator sleeve over the stoma site, centering the face plate over the stoma and securing it with a belt (Figure 5-7). The irrigator sleeve is long enough to reach the toilet and is open on both ends.
14. Lubricate the end of the tube or cone with lubricant.
15. Insert the tube or cone through the open top of the irrigator sleeve and insert it gently into the stoma. Insert the tube 4 to 6 inches into the stoma, but do not force it (Figure 5-8). The cone can be inserted $\frac{1}{2}$ to 1 inch and acts like a dam, preventing backflow (Figure 5-9). There is less danger of perforating the colon with a cone.
16. Open the clamp on the irrigator bag, allowing the water to flow slowly into the colon (Figure 5-10). If it is instilled too quickly, cramping may occur. If this happens, stop the flow for a short time, and then proceed slowly.
17. Remove the tube or cone after the water has been instilled.
18. Fold over the top of the irrigator sleeve and secure.
19. Allow the returns to drain into the toilet through the lower end of the irrigator sleeve.
20. Once the initial returns have passed, cleanse the lower end of the sleeve, fold it up, and apply a clamp.

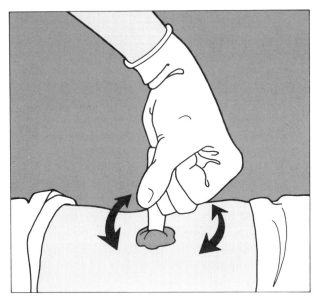

Figure 5-6. Gloved finger dilating the stoma.

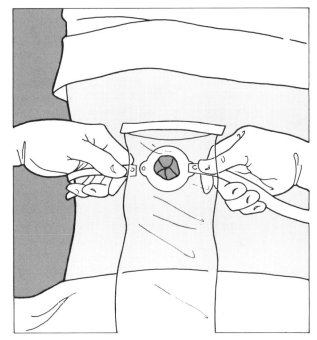

Figure 5-7. Irrigator sleeve applied to the patient.

21. Wash your hands.
22. Assist the patient to ambulate as desired. This can hasten complete evacuation.
23. Assist the patient to the bathroom and remove the irrigator sleeve and belt after the evacuation is completed, approximately 40 minutes.
24. Cleanse the skin and dry thoroughly.
25. Apply skin prep or gel to the site.

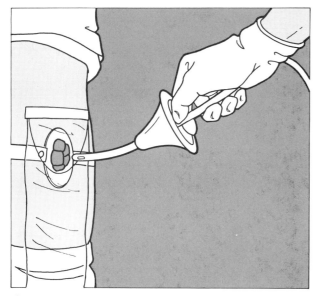

Figure 5-8. Inserting the tube.

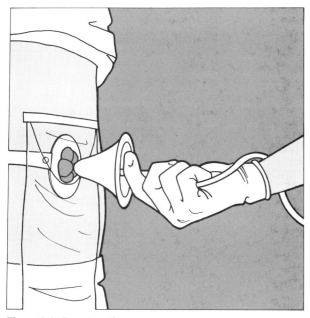

Figure 5-9. Inserting the cone.

26. Measure the stoma according to the measuring guide in the irrigation kit or the appliance box.
27. Select the correct size appliance.
28. Place 6 to 8 drops of appliance deodorant into the appliance through the bottom opening. Apply the clamp to the open end of the appliance after folding the end up twice.

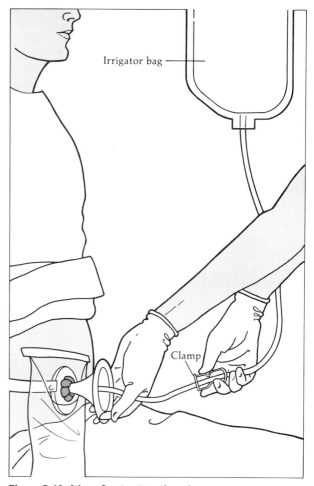

Figure 5-10. Water flowing into the colon.

29. Adhere the new appliance according to the manufacturer's directions.
30. Wash your hands.
31. Assist the patient back to the bed.
32. Instruct the patient to notify the nurse of any stoma discomfort.
33. Wash the irrigator sleeve with soap and water and allow it to dry.
34. Discard equipment or return it to the appropriate area.

PATIENT AND/OR FAMILY TEACHING

1. Explain the procedure to the patient.
2. Reinforce and clarify the physician's explanation of the disease process.
3. Explain any additional therapeutic orders.
4. Remind the patient to notify the nurse of any stoma discomfort.
5. Teach the procedure step by step to the patient and/or a family member. Have the patient do a return demonstration and practice as much as possible prior to discharge. Give the patient written instructions and any other available literature.
6. Explain ostomy equipment, the types available, and where the supplies can be purchased in the community.
7. Teach the patient how to control odor by use of appliance deodorant and avoidance of gas-producing foods.
8. Teach the patient how to cope with skin problems and when to seek help.
9. Inform the patient about the local ostomy support group. Give the patient the name and number of the enterostomal therapist.

DOCUMENTATION

1. Time of irrigation and amount of solution used for irrigation.
2. An assessment of the stoma and surrounding area.
3. An assessment of the irrigation returns.
4. The patient's reaction to the procedure.
5. All patient and family teaching and the level of understanding.

Examination for and/or Removal of a Fecal Impaction

PURPOSE
1. Assess for impacted fecal material in the rectum.
2. Remove impacted fecal material from the rectum.

REQUISITES
1. Exam gloves
2. Water-soluble lubricant
3. Bath blanket
4. Bed protector
5. Bedpan and toilet tissue
6. Washcloth and towel
7. Waste receptacle

GUIDELINES
1. Removal of a fecal impaction by a nurse should ordinarily not be done on patients with cardiac problems, bleeding tendencies, perianal surgery, or irradiation to the pelvis— or on pregnant women. Consult with the physician.
2. An oil retention enema may be ordered prior to the removal of a fecal impaction. A physician's order should be obtained for both procedures.
3. Vagal nerve stimulation can occur when performing this procedure, causing cardiac arrhythmias.
4. The procedure should be stopped immediately if the patient experiences pain or bleeding.

NURSING ACTION/RATIONALE
1. Assemble all equipment.
2. Identify the patient.
3. Explain the procedure. Be sure to inform the patient that the procedure may be uncomfortable.
4. Provide privacy.
5. Assess baseline vital signs.
6. Position the patient in a Sim's (lateral) position and raise the siderail on the side of the bed the patient will face.
7. Place a bath blanket over the patient and a bed protector under the patient's buttocks.
8. Place the bedpan and toilet tissue next to the patient on the bed.
9. Wash your hands.
10. Apply exam gloves and generously lubricate the index finger of your dominant hand.
11. Instruct the patient to take steady even breaths of air through the mouth. This will help the patient relax.
12. Gently insert the lubricated finger into the rectum as far as you can reach, following the wall of the rectum. If the procedure is being done to assess for an impaction, stop at this step. The exam is positive for an impaction if hard stool is found in the rectum.
13. Proceed with the following steps if the physician's order is to manually remove the impaction.
14. Inform the patient of the presence of the impaction and clarify the procedure for removal.
15. Move the index finger into the lower portion of the mass. Gently dislodge small amounts of fecal material and place it in the bedpan. Stop the procedure at intervals to allow the patient to rest.
16. Reassess vital signs if the patient is not tolerating the procedure.
17. Remove as much of the fecal material as can be reached. Reapply lubricant as necessary for patient comfort.
18. Remove the exam gloves.
19. Wash and dry the anal area with a washcloth and towel.
20. Remove the bed protector and bath blanket.
21. Reposition the patient comfortably.
22. Discard equipment or return it to the appropriate location.
23. Wash your hands.

PATIENT AND/OR FAMILY TEACHING
1. Explain the procedure to the patient, including relaxation techniques.
2. With the patient, assess factors that may be contributing to constipation, and plan corrective action. Factors may be:
   a. Limited fluid intake.
   b. Diet low in fiber and roughage.
   c. Lack of exercise.
   d. Lack of a regular pattern of daily living.
   e. Medications being taken.

DOCUMENTATION

1. Time of procedure and type of procedure performed.
2. Results of the procedure.
3. Color, consistency, amount, and odor of fecal material removed.
4. The patient's tolerance of the procedure, including vital signs as appropriate.
5. All patient teaching done and the patient's level of understanding.

▦ Enema Administration

PURPOSE

1. Administer prescribed solutions into the colon.

REQUISITES

1. Enema administration set:
   a. Container with tubing and clamp, or
   b. 50 cc syringe barrel with tubing and a clamp, used for retention enemas
2. Water-soluble lubricant
3. Prescribed solution, warmed to correct temperature
4. Bath blanket
5. Bedpan (optional)
6. Waterproof bed protector
7. Towel and washcloth
8. Exam gloves
9. Toilet tissue
10. IV standard

GUIDELINES

1. There are basically two types of enemas: retention enema and nonretention enema.
   a. A retention enema is a relatively small amount of solution (100 to 300 cc), retained for 20 to 30 minutes and given for the purpose of promoting flatulence, administering medication, softening fecal material, or lubricating the rectal mucosa (Table 5-1).
   b. A nonretention or cleansing enema is a greater volume of solution (usually 1000 cc), retained for approximately 10 minutes and given for the purpose of stimulating peristalsis and evacuating fecal material from the colon (Table 5-1).
2. Nonretention enemas may be ordered preoperatively or prediagnostically to prevent complications to the colon and to provide better visualization of the colon. The results of the enemas are important and should be reported.
3. If enemas are to be given until the solution returns clear, it is important to remember that fluid and electrolyte imbalances can occur with repeated enemas. Consult with the physician if returns are not clear after the third enema.
4. Repeated enemas are very tiring for the patient and are very irritating to the bowel mucosa. The patient will require supportive care.
5. Hemorrhoids may make enema administration painful for the patient. Extra lubricant and extra gentleness can decrease discomfort.
6. The cardiac patient must be closely assessed during enema administration, because the procedure may cause vagal nerve stimulation and cardiac arrhythmias.
7. Abdominal cramping during enema administration may be decreased by:
   a. Lowering the solution container to decrease the pressure or flow of solution.
   b. Stopping the flow of solution by clamping the tubing and waiting for the cramping to subside.
   c. Instructing the patient to inhale through the nose and exhale through the mouth during the procedure.
8. A physician's order should be obtained before administering an enema.
9. For commercially prepared enemas, follow the directions on the package.

Table 5-1. Various Types of Retention and Nonretention Enemas

Kind	Prescription	Temperature	Solution	Purpose
Nonretention	Soap suds	37.7–43.3°C (100–110°F)	1000 cc water to one prepared enema soap packet	Cleanse the colon and rectum
	Tap water (hypotonic solution)	37.7–43.3°C (100–110°F)	1000 cc of tap or distilled water	Cleanse the colon and rectum
	Saline (hypertonic solution)	37.7–43.3°C (100–110°F)	1 T salt to 1000 cc water or 0.9% saline for irrigation	Cleanse the colon and rectum
Retention	Phosphate	36.6–37.7°C (98–100°F)	Prepackaged-disposable	Cause peristalsis and evacuation of feces
	Oil	36.6–37.7°C (98–100°F)	Prepackaged-disposable	Soften feces and lubricate mucosa
	Milk and molasses	37.7–43.3°C (100–110°F)	Equal parts of milk and molasses—amount as prescribed	Promote expulsion of flatus
	One, two, three	37.7–43.3°C (100–110°F)	1 oz magnesium sulfate, 2 oz glycerine, 3 oz water	Promote expulsion of flatus
	Neomycin	36.6–37.7°C (98–100°F)	Concentration as prescribed by the physician	Reduces bacterial count in bowel, thus lowers serum ammonia level
	Kayexalate with sorbitol	36.6–37.7°C (98–100°F)	Concentration as prescribed by the physician	Lowers serum potassium level

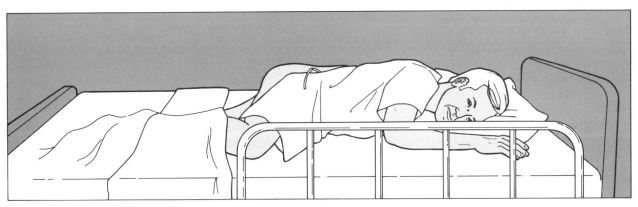

Figure 5-11. Left Sim's position for enema administration.

NURSING ACTION/RATIONALE

1. Assemble all equipment.
2. Verify the physician's order.
3. Identify the patient.
4. Explain the procedure and the purpose of the enema to the patient. Instruct the patient in the breathing technique described in the guidelines.
5. Provide privacy.
6. Assist the patient to a left Sim's (lateral) position and raise the siderail on the side of the bed that the patient will face (Figure 5-11).
7. Place the waterproof bed protector under the patient's buttocks and drape the patient with a bath blanket.
8. Wash your hands.
9. Assemble the enema equipment into a functional unit:
    a. Clamp off the enema tubing.
    b. Pour the prepared enema solution warmed to the correct temperature into the enema container (see Table 5-1).
    c. Unclamp the tubing to clear the air, and reclamp.
    d. Hang the container on the IV standard approximately 16 to 18 inches above the patient's buttocks.
10. Put on exam gloves.
11. Lubricate the tubing for 3 to 5 inches from the tip, using water-soluble lubricant.
12. Tell the patient that you are going to insert the tube. Instruct the patient to take a deep breath.

13. Separate the buttocks and gently insert the tube into the anus 3 to 5 inches beyond the anal sphincter. Never force the tube.
14. Unclamp the tube and allow the solution to flow:
   a. If this is a retention enema, administer the solution slowly so peristalsis will not occur. Lowering the solution container will allow the solution to flow more slowly.
   b. If the patient has the urge to defecate, stop the solution and hold the buttocks together until the urge subsides. Then resume the procedure.
   c. Refer to Guideline 7 for managing abdominal cramping.
15. Clamp the tubing and remove it gently when the appropriate amount of solution has been administered.
16. Remove the exam gloves. Wash your hands.
17. Instruct the patient to try to hold the enema for the appropriate period of time. Leave the nurse call signal within reach.
18. Assist the patient to a safe and comfortable position to defecate as necessary, either on the bedpan or the toilet. If the patient is using the toilet, instruct the patient not to flush the toilet until results are seen by a nurse.
19. If the patient is unable to expel the enema solution, the solution can be siphoned:
   a. Place the patient in a right side-lying position so the sigmoid colon is uppermost.
   b. Fill the enema bucket with approximately 50 cc of warm tap water and clear the enema tubing of air.
   c. Insert the tip of the enema tubing into the rectum.
   d. Elevate the enema bucket approximately 12 inches above the anus and open the clamp on the tubing.
   e. Lower the bucket below the level of the anus immediately after the fluid begins to flow. This will cause a siphoning effect and the fluid, along with fecal material, will flow back into the bucket.

20. Provide soap and water and a towel and washcloth for cleansing the perineum after defecation. Assist the patient as necessary.
21. Assess the results of the enema, if appropriate. Assess the patient's abdomen if the enema was given because of abdominal distention.
22. Discard equipment or return it to the appropriate area.
23. Wash your hands.

PATIENT AND/OR FAMILY TEACHING
1. Explain the procedure and its purpose to the patient. Instruct the patient on the proper breathing technique during the procedure.
2. Instruct the patient to notify the nurse if abdominal cramping occurs.
3. Instruct the patient to save the enema results, if using the toilet.
4. Explain additional therapeutic orders, as appropriate.

DOCUMENTATION
1. Time of procedure.
2. Type and amount of solution administered.
3. Results of enema, as appropriate, including amount of flatus passed.
4. The patient's tolerance of the procedure.
5. Other assessment parameters as appropriate including:
   a. Distention of the abdomen before and after the procedure.
   b. Condition of hemorrhoids, if present.
6. All patient teaching done and the patient's level of understanding.

Insertion
of a Rectal Tube

PURPOSE
1. Promote expulsion of flatus and/or fluid.

REQUISITES
1. Rectal tube with attached vented bag (22–24 Fr.)
2. Water-soluble lubricant
3. Bed protector
4. Exam gloves
5. Washcloth and towel

GUIDELINES
1. Rectal tubes are used to relieve abdominal distention from flatus or fluid in the lower digestive tract and to increase patient comfort.
2. A physician's order should be obtained before using a rectal tube.
3. Diets should be increased gradually from liquid to regular following surgery to prevent postoperative abdominal distention.

NURSING ACTION/RATIONALE
1. Assemble all equipment.
2. Verify the physician's order.
3. Identify the patient.
4. Provide privacy.
5. Explain the procedure to the patient.
6. Assess the abdomen for abdominal distention.
7. Assist the patient to a left side-lying position with knees slightly flexed.
8. Place the bed protector under the patient's buttocks.
9. Cover the patient with a bath blanket.
10. Wash your hands.
11. Put on exam gloves.
12. Lubricate the tip of the rectal tube with water-soluble lubricant.
13. Separate the patient's buttocks and gently insert the tip of the tube 3 to 5 inches into the rectum. DO NOT FORCE THE TUBE.

14. Place the bagged end of the tube on the bed protector.
15. Remove the exam gloves.
16. Leave the tube in place for 20 minutes or as ordered by the physician.
17. Remove the tube after the prescribed time.
18. Wash and dry the anal area.
19. Position the patient comfortably.
20. Reassess the abdomen for distention.
21. Discard equipment or return it to the appropriate location.
22. Wash your hands.

PATIENT AND/OR FAMILY TEACHING
1. Explain the procedure and its purpose to the patient.
2. Instruct the patient that smoking, chewing gum, and drinking liquids with a straw may cause air to be swallowed, increasing abdominal distention.
3. Encourage activity, if allowed, which will help pass flatus.
4. Instruct the patient to massage the abdomen, if appropriate, to move the flatus along the intestines.
5. Instruct the patient to avoid gas-producing foods.

DOCUMENTATION
1. Time the rectal tube was inserted and removed.
2. Assessment of the abdomen before and after the procedure.
3. The patient's reaction to the procedure.
4. All patient teaching done and the patient's level of understanding.

Collection of a Stool Specimen

PURPOSE

1. Obtain stool (feces) for diagnostic analysis.

REQUISITES

1. Bedpan or stool collection container
2. Tongue blades
3. Wax-coated stool specimen container
4. Identification label
5. Exam gloves
6. Toilet tissue
7. Small clear plastic bag

GUIDELINES

1. Stool specimens can be collected for a variety of tests. The nurse should know the test that is to be done and any necessary precautions for the stool collection. This information can be obtained from laboratory personnel.
2. In general, stool specimens collected for identification of parasites must be kept at body temperature and examined within 30 minutes after defecation.
3. Stools for bacteria should be examined by laboratory personnel immediately. If a delay in examination is anticipated, the specimen should be refrigerated.
4. For some tests, such as parasites, the entire stool must be used as a specimen. Other tests may require only a portion of the stool. The best specimen is that portion of the stool containing blood or mucus.
5. If an enema is required to obtain a stool specimen for examination, a tapwater or saline solution should be used. Refer to the procedure "Enema Administration."
6. If a rectal swab culture is ordered, follow the procedure "Breakstick Technique or Culturette Method for Specimen Collection." Insert the swab beyond the anal sphincter and rotate it, then withdraw.
7. Specimens collected from patients in enteric isolation should be double-bagged and labeled "Contaminated" before sending to the laboratory.
8. Urine on the stool may affect the results of the test. Every attempt should be made to avoid contamination of the stool specimen with urine.

NURSING ACTION/RATIONALE

1. Assemble all equipment.
2. Identify the patient.
3. Explain the procedure for collecting a stool specimen to the patient including:
   a. The use of the collection container provided.
   b. Instructions to urinate prior to the bowel movement so the urine does not touch the stool.
   c. Instructions to notify the nurse immediately after defecating.
4. Assist the patient as necessary when the urge to defecate occurs. Provide privacy while the patient is defecating, and assist the patient as necessary to cleanse the perineum following defecation.
5. Remove the bedpan or collection container to an appropriate location away from the patient.
6. Put on exam gloves.
7. Use a tongue blade to transfer the feces to the wax-coated specimen container.
8. Cover the container tightly.
9. Label the container.
10. Place the container inside a clear small pre-opened plastic bag and seal.
11. Remove the exam gloves.
12. Seal the plastic bag.
13. Send the specimen to the laboratory immediately.
14. Discard equipment or return it to the appropriate location.
15. Wash your hands thoroughly.

PATIENT AND/OR FAMILY TEACHING

1. Instruct the patient in the procedure as described in the nursing action.
2. Reinforce the physician's explanation of the disease process.

DOCUMENTATION

1. Specimen collection and time.
2. Amount, color, consistency, and odor of the stool.
3. Disposition of the specimen.
4. All patient teaching done and the patient's level of understanding.

Straining Stool

PURPOSE

1. Recover gallstones from feces following an endoscopic papillotomy.
2. Remove ingested foreign objects from feces.

REQUISITES

1. Bedpan or collection container
2. Clear plastic bags—3
3. Exam gloves
4. Sign: "Strain All Stool"
5. Paper towels
6. Toilet tissue
7. Tongue blade
8. Specimen container

GUIDELINES

1. This procedure is performed when ordered by the physician.
2. The physician may order the patient to be on a papillotomy diet in conjunction with ordering this procedure. A papillotomy diet restricts all nuts or seeds.

NURSING ACTION/RATIONALE

1. Assemble all equipment.
2. Identify the patient.
3. Explain the procedure and purpose to the patient. Instruct the patient to defecate in the bedpan or container provided, to save all stools, and to notify the nurse after defecating.
4. Place the "Strain All Stool" sign in an appropriate prominent location.
5. Line the patient's bedpan with a clear plastic bag. If the patient uses a toilet, provide a plastic collection container lined with a clear plastic bag.

6. After the patient defecates, remove the bedpan and assist the patient as necessary.
7. Take the bedpan to an appropriate location out of the patient's area to perform the procedure.
8. Put on exam gloves.
9. Remove the plastic bag from the bedpan.
10. Remove air from the bag and tie off the bag.
11. Place the bag on a hard surface, over paper toweling.
12. Mash the stool with your hands gently, feeling and observing for stones through the bag. Stones are very fragile, and care must be taken not to crush them.
13. Save any stone or questionable particle:
    a. Open the bag.
    b. Remove the stone with a tongue blade.
    c. Place the stone in a specimen container.
14. Turn the plastic bag inside out and discard all feces in the toilet.
15. Remove exam gloves.
16. Place the exam gloves and used plastic bag inside another plastic bag and seal before discarding.
17. Reline the bedpan or collection container and return it to the patient for the next defecation.
18. Label the specimen container if a stone or particle was recovered.
19. Wash your hands thoroughly.
20. Notify the physician if a stone or particle was recovered.

PATIENT AND/OR FAMILY TEACHING

1. Instruct the patient regarding the procedure as described in the nursing action.
2. Instruct the patient on the papillotomy diet as appropriate.
3. Reinforce the physician's explanation of the disease process.
4. Teach the patient the procedures, if straining stool will be done following discharge.

DOCUMENTATION

1. Procedure performed following each defecation.
2. Results of procedure.
3. Disposition of any specimen found.
4. Notification of the physician.
5. Any unusual observations regarding the stool.
6. All patient teaching done and the patient's level of understanding.

 # Hemoccult

PURPOSE

1. Test for the presence or absence of occult blood in the stool.

REQUISITES

1. Hemoccult test kit containing:
   a. Filter paper slides
   b. Developing solution
2. Exam gloves
3. Stool specimen container
4. Tongue blade
5. Tap water
6. Dropper
7. Bedpan or stool collection container
8. Toilet tissue

GUIDELINES

1. Hemoccult is a diagnostic tool to aid the physician in determining whether bleeding has occurred in the gastrointestinal tract.
2. Since bleeding in the gastrointestinal tract may be intermittent, it is recommended that the hemoccult test be done on three consecutive stool specimens.
3. A false positive test may occur if patients are bleeding from some other source such as hemorrhoids or menses.

4. Ascorbic acid consumed in large doses has caused false negative tests.
5. Hemoccult filter paper should not be used after the expiration date, or if the paper has turned blue or green.
6. The hemoccult developing solution should be stored away from extremes of heat or cold and away from light. The bottle should be kept tightly capped when not in use.

NURSING ACTION/RATIONALE

1. Assemble all equipment.
2. Identify the patient.
3. Explain the purpose of the procedure to the patient. Instruct the patient to use the collection container provided, or the bedpan, when defecating. Instruct the patient to save all stools and to notify the nurse after defecating.
4. Assist the patient as necessary after defecation to remove the bedpan and cleanse the perineum.
5. Put on the exam gloves.
6. Place a random sample of the stool specimen in the specimen container, using a tongue blade.

7. Clean the bedpan or collection container and return it to the appropriate location.
8. Apply a thin smear of stool to the inside circle of the slide kit, using the tongue blade, and close the cover.
9. Open the perforated window in the back of the slide.
10. Apply two drops of developing solution and wait 30 seconds.
11. Read the results. Any trace of blue on the filter paper indicates a positive test for occult blood.
12. Remove the exam gloves.
13. Discard equipment or return it to the appropriate location.
14. Wash your hands.

PATIENT AND/OR FAMILY TEACHING
1. Explain the procedure and purpose to the patient as outlined in the nursing action.
2. Reinforce the physician's explanation of the disease process.
3. Instruct the patient in the steps of the procedure if the procedure will need to be performed after discharge.

DOCUMENTATION
1. Procedure performed and results of test.
2. Assessment of the amount, color, consistency, and odor of the stool.
3. All patient teaching done and the patient's level of understanding.

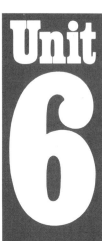

Unit

6

Renal/Urological Procedures

PROCEDURES

Urinary
Catheterization

PURPOSE
1. Empty the bladder when the patient is unable to void.
2. Obtain a sterile urine specimen.
3. Determine the amount of residual urine in the bladder after the patient voids.

REQUISITES
1. Sterile disposable catheter kit containing:
   a. Rubber catheter
   b. Graduated container
   c. Water-soluble lubricant
   d. Antiseptic solution
   e. Fenestrated drape
   f. Plastic-coated protector
   g. Gloves
   h. Forceps
   i. Cotton balls
2. Washcloth and towel
3. Bath blanket
4. Adequate lighting

GUIDELINES
1. Strict surgical asepsis should be employed during this procedure. If any break in technique occurs causing contamination, the procedure should be restarted with sterile equipment.
2. For a residual urine specimen, have the patient void immediately before the procedure and measure the output. Catheterize the patient. The amount of urine returned is the residual urine.
3. Assistance of a second person may be needed if the patient is obese, combative, or unable to cooperate.
4. The physician should be consulted regarding preference for the amount of urine to be drained from a distended bladder.
   a. Some physicians may wish to specify the amount of urine drained from the bladder at one time.

b. Some physicians may want the entire bladder drained completely. In this case, if more than 1000 cc is drained, certain precautions should be taken:
   (1) The patient should be kept in a supine position during and following the procedure to prevent shock symptoms, if the abdominal aorta has been compressed by the distended bladder.
   (2) A large lumen catheter should be used. Rapid decompression of the bladder may cause small blood vessels on the bladder mucosa to rupture, and some bleeding into the bladder may occur. The large lumen catheter will allow for small clots to be passed.
   (3) Fluids must be forced, or an intravenous infusion may be necessary to promote diuresis in the patient. This will help to flush the bladder of any small clots.
   (4) The patient should be assessed closely for hematuria and/or changes in vital signs.

NURSING ACTION/RATIONALE
1. Assemble all equipment.
2. Identify the patient.
3. Explain the procedure to the patient. Warn the patient that a burning sensation may be felt as the catheter is introduced.
4. Provide privacy.
5. Ensure adequate lighting.
6. Wash your hands.
7. Position the patient and cover the upper torso with a bath blanket:
   a. *Female*—Assist the patient to a dorsal recumbent position with the knees flexed (Figure 6-1).

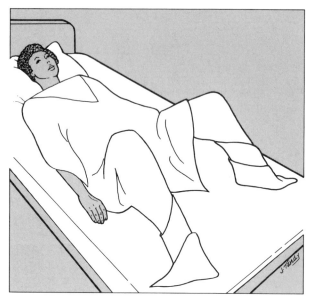

Figure 6-1. Dorsal recumbent position.

   b. *Male*—Assist the patient to a supine
      position with his legs flat.
8. Wash the perineal area or penis with soap and
   water.
9. Wash your hands.
10. Open sterile supplies, using aseptic
    technique.
11. Place the plastic-coated protector under the
    patient's buttocks.
12. Put on sterile gloves.
13. Place the fenestrated drape on the patient
    with the hole over the genitalia.
14. Apply sterile lubricant liberally to the
    catheter tip. Lubricate at least 3 inches for the
    female and 6 inches for the male. Leave the
    lubricated catheter on the sterile field.
15. Pour the antiseptic solution over the cotton
    balls.
16. Place the urine specimen container within
    reach.
17. Cleanse the urinary meatus:
    a. *Female*—Expose the meatus by separating
       the labia majora with the thumb and index
       finger of your non-dominant hand. Using
       the forceps and cotton balls, cleanse the
       labia majora from top to bottom, using one
       cotton ball for each stroke. Follow the
       same procedure to cleanse the labia minora
       and the meatus. Continue to hold the labia
       apart after cleansing (Figure 6-2).

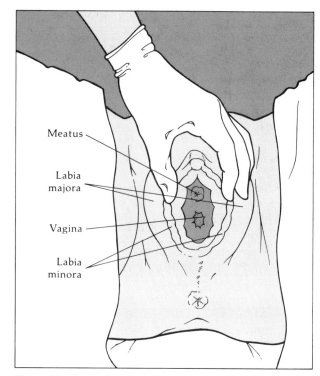

Figure 6-2. Separating the labia majora to expose the meatus.

    b. *Male*—Grasp the patient's penis and hold
       firmly but gently with your non-dominant
       hand. Retract the foreskin on an
       uncircumcised male (Figure 6-3). Using the
       forceps and cotton balls, cleanse around
       the meatus (the male meatus opens as a
       vertical slit at the tip of the glans) in a
       circular motion. Discard the cotton ball
       after each completed circle. Continue
       outward to clean the entire glans.
18. Grasp the lubricated catheter 3 inches from
    the tip.
19. Insert the catheter into the urinary meatus:
    a. *Female*—Angle the catheter slightly
       upward as it is advanced. Insert the
       catheter approximately 1 inch beyond the
       flow of urine. Do not force the catheter. If
       the catheter will not advance, instruct the
       patient to inhale and exhale slowly. This
       may relax the muscle sphincter so that the
       catheter can be advanced. If the catheter is
       inadvertently placed in the vagina, leave it
       in place temporarily. Insert another sterile
       catheter properly by repeating the entire
       procedure with sterile equipment. After a
       successful catheterization, the catheter in
       the vagina can be removed.

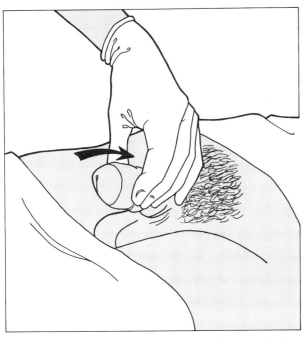

Figure 6-3. Retracting the foreskin of an uncircumcised male.

b. *Male*—Hold the penis at a 90 degree angle to the body and gently insert the catheter through the urinary meatus (Figure 6-**4a**). Gradually lower the penis to a 60 degree angle (Figure 6-**4b**). You may encounter resistance at the prostatic sphincter; pause and allow the sphincter to relax, and then continue to advance the catheter. Never force a catheter to advance. When the catheter has passed through the sphincter into the bladder, urine will flow. Advance the catheter 1½ inches further.

20. Hold the catheter in place while the urine drains into the graduated collection container.
21. Obtain a sterile urine specimen by placing the specimen container under the stream of flowing urine.
22. When the urine flow has ceased, remove the catheter gently by pinching the catheter and pulling with gentle steady pressure.
23. Wash the perineum or penis with soap and water to remove excess antiseptic on the skin. Reposition the foreskin on the uncircumcised male.

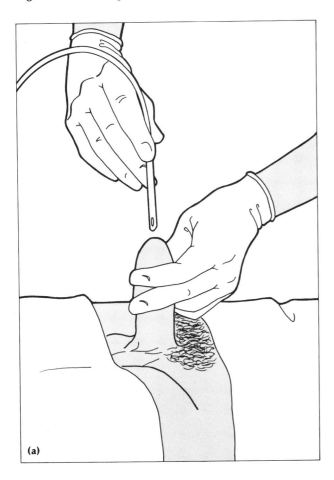

(a)

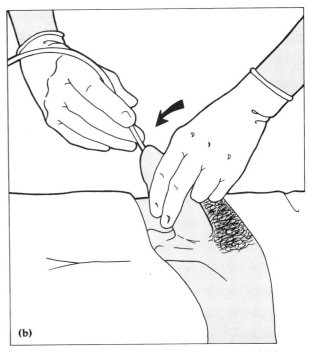

(b)

Figure 6-4. Inserting a catheter into the penis. (**a**) Hold the penis at a 90 degree angle. (**b**) Gradually lower the penis to a 60 degree angle.

24. Remove the sterile gloves.
25. Assist the patient to a comfortable position.
26. Measure the urine.
27. Discard equipment or return it to the appropriate location.
28. Label the urine specimen and send it to the laboratory as ordered.

PATIENT AND/OR FAMILY TEACHING

1. Instruct the patient about the procedure to be performed.
2. Instruct the patient to call the nurse for symptoms such as:
   a. Burning on urination.
   b. Blood in the urine.
   c. Any feeling of fullness or pressure in the bladder area.
   d. Inability to urinate.
3. Instruct on other therapeutic or diagnostic orders as appropriate, such as:
   a. Intake and output.
   b. Medications.
   c. Increasing fluids.

DOCUMENTATION

1. Time of procedure and name of person who performed procedure.
2. Disposition of specimen.
3. The patient's reaction to the procedure.
4. Specific parameters of assessment including:
   a. Amount, color, and clarity of the urine.
   b. Difficulties with the procedure.
   c. Presence of hematuria.
5. All patient teaching done and the patient's level of understanding.

Teaching the Patient
Intermittent Self-Catheterization _____

PURPOSE
1. Teach the patient to empty the bladder mechanically at regular intervals.

REQUISITES
Hospital Care
1. Sterile gloves
2. Sterile catheterization tray with straight french catheter, size as ordered by the physician
3. Adequate lighting
4. Portable mirror
5. Washcloth and towel
6. Soap and water
7. Plastic bag
8. Visual aids

Home Care
1. French catheter, size as ordered by the physician
2. Water-soluble lubricant
3. Plastic bags
4. Collection container
5. Pan for boiling equipment
6. Portable mirror
7. Washcloth and towel
8. Soap and water

GUIDELINES
1. Regular intermittent catheterization is an alternative treatment for patients who are unable to empty their bladders either partially or completely because of medical problems such as spinal injuries or tumors.
2. Regular intermittent catheterizations decrease the risk of urinary tract infections and urinary tract irritation often associated with indwelling catheters. Use of intermittent catheterization affords the outpatient greater independence and a more normal lifestyle.
3. Because of the danger of nosocomial infections, intermittent catheterizations should be done as a sterile procedure while the patient is hospitalized. The procedure can be modified after the patient is discharged, and a clean technique can be used.

4. The patient's learning level should be assessed prior to teaching to determine the method of teaching that will be most appropriate. Refer to the procedure "Patient Education" for alternative methods of teaching for individual patients.
5. Since the learning levels of patients vary, this procedure must be adapted to the individual's learning needs. The procedure may need to be taught in short sessions over several days. Begin the instruction as early as possible so that the procedure can be mastered by the patient before discharge.
6. For optimal learning, written instructions and visual aids should be given to the patient along with the verbal instructions and demonstrations.
7. Since the patient will not need to use sterile technique after discharge, the nurse should coach and assist the patient through the sterile technique as necessary without emphasizing the sterile technique as a learning need.

NURSING ACTION/RATIONALE
1. Assemble all equipment.
2. Verify the physician's order.
3. Identify the patient.
4. Reinforce the nature and purpose of the procedure to the patient.
5. Provide privacy.
6. Provide adequate lighting.
7. Instruct the patient to attempt to urinate, if appropriate.
8. Provide soap and water and instruct the patient to wash and dry the perineal area.
9. Instruct the patient to wash his/her hands.
10. Assist the patient to a comfortable and convenient position for self-catheterization. The female is usually in a semi-Fowler's position with the knees drawn up and the legs separated. The male patient is usually in a semi-Fowler's position with legs flat. Once the patient has learned the procedure well, both males and females can do the clean procedure at home while sitting on the toilet.

11. Place all equipment within the patient's reach.
12. Open the catheterization tray.
13. Instruct the patient on applying the sterile gloves. Refer to the procedure "Sterile Gloving Technique," if necessary.
14. Place the sterile bed protector under the patient's buttocks.
15. Open the lubricant and empty the package onto the sterile bed protector.
16. Open the antiseptic solution and pour it over the cotton balls.
17. Place the mirror within the patient's line of vision if necessary.
18. Instruct the patient to:

Female
a. Place the collection container between the legs.
b. Separate the labia.
c. Cleanse the labia and meatus with antiseptic cotton balls, wiping from front to back and using one cotton ball for each stroke (Figure 6-5a).
d. Locate the meatus.
e. Grasp the catheter 3 inches from the tip and lubricate it.
f. Insert the catheter into the meatus (Figure 6-5b).

Male
a. Place the collection container between the legs.
b. Retract the foreskin if necessary.
c. Cleanse the head of the penis with antiseptic cotton balls, using a circular motion (Figure 6-6a).
d. Hold the penis at a right angle to the body with the non-dominant hand.
e. Grasp the catheter approximately 6 inches from the tip and lubricate it.
f. Insert the catheter while gradually lowering the angle of the penis to 60 degrees (Figure 6-6b).
19. Allow urine to drain completely.
20. Instruct the patient to pinch the catheter and withdraw it smoothly.
21. Instruct the patient to wipe the perineum dry. The male should reposition the foreskin if necessary.

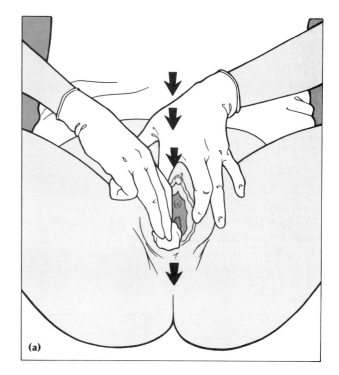

(a)

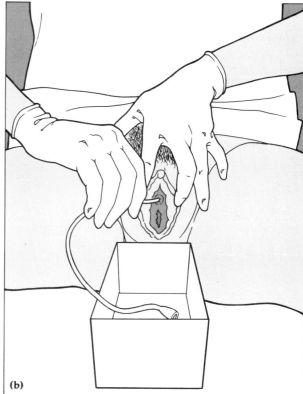

(b)

Figure 6-5. Self-catheterization technique for females. (a) Cleansing the female perineum and meatus. (b) Inserting the catheter into the female meatus.

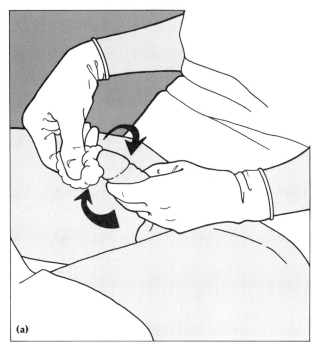

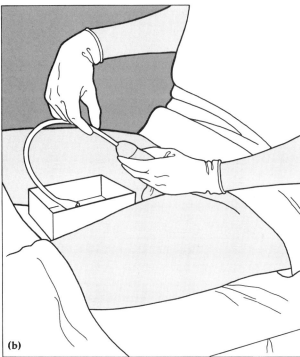

Figure 6-6. Self-catheterization technique for males.
(**a**) Cleansing the head of the penis. (**b**) Inserting the catheter into the penis.

22. Instruct the patient to remove the gloves and wash his/her hands.
23. Measure the urine if necessary, and discard.
24. Remove all equipment from the area and assist the patient to a comfortable position.
25. Wash the catheter in warm, soapy water and allow it to air dry. Store it in a plastic bag for the patient to take home and sterilize for reuse. This will eliminate the patient's need to purchase catheters following discharge.
26. Discard equipment or return it to the appropriate location.

PATIENT AND/OR FAMILY TEACHING

1. Explain self-catheterization and its purpose to the patient.
2. Explain the anatomy of the urinary tract if necessary.
3. Clarify the reason for sterile technique in the hospital.
4. Explain the variation to clean technique:
   a. There is no need to use antiseptic solution to clean the perineum or penis prior to inserting the catheter. Washing with soap and water is sufficient.
   b. Good handwashing is necessary; gloves are not necessary.
   c. Catheters can be resterilized and reused.
      (1) Catheters should be washed in soap and water and air-dried.
      (2) After several catheters have been used, they should be boiled for 20 minutes, air-dried, and stored in a clean towel or container for later use.
   d. A sufficient number of catheters should be available so that the boiling procedure would need to be done only once a day.
   e. The patient can do the clean procedure sitting on the toilet.
5. Instruct the patient on the schedule for catheterizations.
6. Instruct the patient on how to assess for a distended bladder.
7. Explain other therapeutic orders as appropriate.
8. Explain to the patient where necessary supplies can be obtained.

DOCUMENTATION

1. All patient teaching done and the methods used.
2. The patient's ability to demonstrate the procedure.
3. All written instructions and visual aids given to the patient.
4. The patient's reaction to performing the procedure.
5. Further learning needs of the patient.
6. Amount, color, clarity, and odor of urine.

Insertion and Removal of an Indwelling Foley Catheter

PURPOSE

1. Facilitate continuous drainage of urine from the bladder.
2. Obtain an accurate measurement of urinary output in severely ill patients.
3. Prevent urine from contacting an incision in the perianal area.

REQUISITES

Insertion

1. Sterile indwelling catheterization kit consisting of:
   a. Foley catheter with a 5 cc balloon (usually #16 Fr.) connected to a urinary drainage bag
   b. Urine specimen container
   c. Lubricant
   d. Antiseptic solution
   e. Fenestrated drape
   f. Gloves
   g. Forceps
   h. Cotton balls
   i. Prefilled syringe with sterile water
   j. Plastic-coated protector
2. Anchoring tape or catheter strap
3. Washcloth and towel
4. Bath blanket
5. Adequate lighting

Removal

1. Syringe (large enough to hold the contents of the balloon)
2. Disposable paper towel
3. Washcloth and towel
4. Exam gloves
5. Soap and water
6. Bed protector

GUIDELINES

1. Because of the risk of catheter-associated urinary tract infections, indwelling catheters should be used only when absolutely necessary and not soley to facilitate nursing care for the incontinent patient. Catheters should remain in place only as long as is medically indicated.
2. A physician's order is required for this procedure. The physician should order the size of the catheter and balloon to be inserted.
3. All indwelling catheters must be routinely connected to a closed drainage system.
4. Three-way Foley catheters are available for irrigation purposes. The method for insertion is the same.
5. Before the indwelling catheter is inserted, the balloon should be inflated with the sterile water to check for any defects and then deflated completely.
6. Refer to the procedure "Care and Maintenance of an Indwelling Catheter" for further information.

7. A sterile urine specimen may be obtained from the spigot of the drainage bag immediately after catheterization, since all equipment is considered sterile at that time.

NURSING ACTION/RATIONALE

Insertion

1. Follow the steps in the procedure "Urinary Catheterization" for the proper aseptic insertion of a catheter.
2. Attach the syringe to the balloon port of the catheter, after you have advanced the catheter 1½ inches beyond the point of urine flow.
3. Inject the water slowly into the balloon. Do not force the water. If the water will not inject easily or if the patient complains of pain, deflate the balloon completely and advance the catheter further, then reinflate.
4. Remove the syringe from the balloon port.
5. Pull on the catheter gently until you feel resistance. This will position the balloon correctly (Figure 6-7).

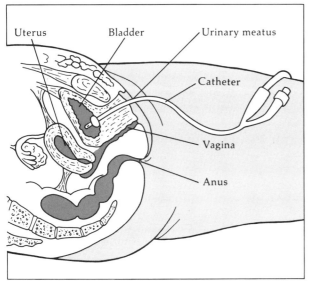

Figure 6-7. Indwelling Foley catheter in the correct position in a female patient.

6. Connect the drainage bag to the catheter, if not preconnected.
7. Tape the catheter to the patient or utilize a catheter strap. (See "Care and Maintenance of an Indwelling Catheter" for the taping procedure.)
8. Secure the urinary drainage bag below the level of the bladder and off the floor. Coil any extra tubing on the bed.
9. Wash the perineum or penis with soap and water to remove any lubricant or antiseptic on the skin.
10. Remove your gloves.
11. Remove drapes and protectors from the patient and position the patient comfortably.
12. Discard equipment or return it to the appropriate area.

Removal

1. Assemble all equipment.
2. Identify the patient.
3. Explain the procedure to the patient. Warn the patient that a slight burning sensation may be felt during removal.
4. Provide privacy and assist the female patient to a dorsal recumbent position or the male patient to a supine position.
5. Place bed protector under the patient's buttocks.
6. Wash your hands and put on exam gloves.
7. Remove the securing tape or the catheter strap.
8. Attach the syringe to the balloon port and aspirate the entire amount of water from the balloon.
9. Pinch the catheter off and remove with a steady gentle pull.
10. Wrap the catheter tip in a paper towel.
11. Wash the perineum or penis with soap and water and dry well.
12. Empty the drainage bag and measure the urine.
13. Remove the gloves and wash your hands.
14. Position the patient comfortably.
15. Discard equipment or return it to the appropriate area.

PATIENT AND/OR FAMILY TEACHING
Insertion
1. Explain proper care of an indwelling catheter as explained in "Care and Maintenance of an Indwelling Catheter."

Removal
1. Inform the patient that burning may occur on urination.
2. Instruct the patient to save all urine for measuring for at least 24 hours or as ordered by the physician.
3. Instruct the patient to notify the nurse:
   a. After urinating.
   b. If unable to urinate.
   c. If there is any burning on urination.
   d. If there is any blood in the urine.
   e. If any sensations of discomfort or pressure in the bladder area are experienced.
4. Instruct the patient to increase fluid intake to flush the bladder, if not medically contraindicated.

DOCUMENTATION
Insertion
1. Time of procedure and name of person who performed the procedure.
2. The patient's reaction to the procedure.
3. Specific parameters of assessment including:
   a. Amount, color, and clarity of the urine.
   b. Difficulties with the procedure.
   c. Presence of hematuria.
4. All patient teaching done and the patient's level of understanding.

Removal
1. Time of procedure and name of person who performed the procedure.
2. Amount, color, and clarity of urine in drainage bag.
3. All patient teaching done and the patient's level of understanding.

Care and Maintenance of an Indwelling Catheter

PURPOSE

1. Minimize the risk of catheter-associated urinary tract infection and its related problems.
2. Minimize trauma to the urethra.
3. Maintain cleanliness of the catheter and perineum.

REQUISITES

1. Soap and water
2. Washcloth and towel
3. Anchoring tape and safety pins, or catheter strap
4. Exam gloves
5. Alcohol sponges
6. Drape
7. Graduated collection container

GUIDELINES

1. All patients with indwelling catheters should have their urinary output assessed at regular intervals to ensure that adequate drainage is occurring.
2. Several protective nursing measures can be taken to reduce the risk of infection in patients who require indwelling catheters. They are:
   a. Staff should perform proper handwashing before and after every contact with the catheter, the drainage system, or the urine.
   b. Exam gloves should be worn as a protective measure during catheter care if a patient has a urinary tract infection.
   c. Infected and uninfected patients with indwelling catheters should be kept separated.
   d. Drainage bags should be secured to the bed or the wheelchair in such a manner that neither the bag nor the spigot touches the floor.
   e. Drainage bags should remain below the level of the patient's bladder.
   f. An unobstructed urine flow and a closed sterile drainage system should be maintained.
   g. Catheter tubing should be secured to the patient to prevent unnecessary movement or traction that may cause injury to the bladder or the urethra. Manipulation and movement of the catheter may also cause bacteria form the external meatus to travel up the catheter and enter the bladder.
   h. The patient should be taught the precautions to be taken with a catheter, as described in the Patient/Family Teaching section of this procedure.
   i. Avoid routine changing of the catheter or the drainage bag. The catheter and drainage bag should be changed if an obstruction of the system is suspected, if sediment is accumulating in the lumen of the tubing, or if the system has been contaminated.

NURSING ACTION/RATIONALE

1. Cleanse the perineal area daily with soap and water to promote good personal hygiene. This may have to be done more frequently if the patient is involuntary of stool or there is excessive drainage or blood. Cleanse the proximal third of the catheter with soap and water, washing away from the insertion site and manipulating the catheter as little as possible. Catheters that are heavily encrusted with drainage or blood should be changed.

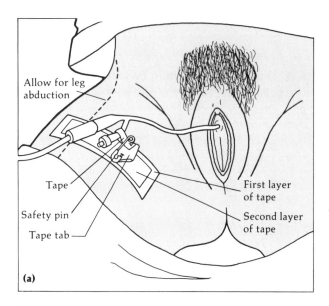

Allow for leg abduction

Tape

Safety pin

Tape tab

First layer of tape

Second layer of tape

(a)

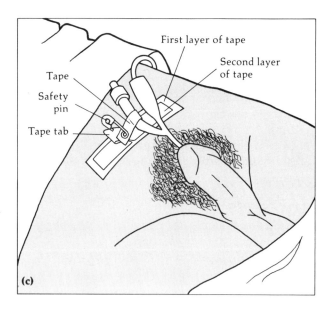

First layer of tape

Second layer of tape

Tape

Safety pin

Tape tab

(c)

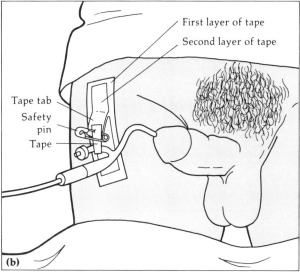

First layer of tape

Second layer of tape

Tape tab

Safety pin

Tape

(b)

Figure 6-8. Securing the catheter. (**a**) In female, catheter tubing secured to inner aspect of thigh. (**b**) In male, catheter secured horizontally. (**c**) In male, catheter secured to the lateral abdomen.

2. Secure the catheter tubing with tape or a catheter strap to the inner aspect of the female patient's thigh (Figure 6-8a). Tape the male catheter tubing horizontally to the thigh (Figure 6-8b) or to the lateral abdomen (Figure 6-8c). This will prevent pressure at the penoscrotal juncture.

3. Secure the catheter with tape and a safety pin in order to allow the catheter tubing to be freed for manipulation when necessary (Figure 6-9).
   a. Place a piece of flagged tape on the patient's skin in the appropriate location.
   b. Place a piece of flagged tape on the balloon port of the catheter.
   c. Pin the two flags of tape together.

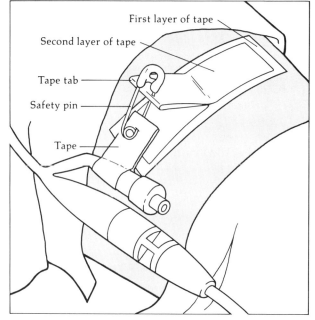

First layer of tape

Second layer of tape

Tape tab

Safety pin

Tape

Figure 6-9. Flagged tape on catheter and thigh secured with a pin.

4. Empty the catheter drainage bag at least every 8 hours, or as necessary. The level of urine should never reach the anti-reflux valve at the top of the drainage bag.
5. Cleanse the spigot on the drainage bag with a disinfectant sponge before and after emptying.

PATIENT AND/OR FAMILY TEACHING

1. Teach the patient the following infection prevention measures:
   a. Keep the drainage bag below the level of the bladder.
   b. Do not disconnect the catheter from the drainage tubing. If the catheter inadvertently becomes disconnected, notify the nurse.
   c. Do not place the drainage bag on the floor.
   d. Do not empty the drainage bag. Notify the nurse if it is full. If the patient will be emptying his/her own drainage bag, teach him/her how to cleanse the spigot before and after emptying.
   e. Notify the nurse if any pain or discomfort with the catheter is experienced.

2. Discuss with the patient the importance of maintaining a good fluid intake. Make specific plans for the number of glasses of fluid the patient should have, which will depend on the medical diagnosis.

DOCUMENTATION

1. The daily perineal cleansing and assessment of the perineal area.
2. Amount, color, and clarity of urine output.
3. Patient teaching done and the patient's level of understanding.

Aspirating a Small-Volume Fresh Urine Specimen from an Indwelling Catheter _____

PURPOSE
1. Obtain a fresh random urine specimen from a patient with an indwelling catheter without contaminating the closed drainage system.

REQUISITES
1. Rubber band or screw clamp
2. Sterile 2 cc or 10 cc syringe
3. Sterile 20 gauge needle
4. Alcohol sponge
5. Sterile specimen collection container
6. Identification label
7. Sign: "Urine Tubing Temporarily Clamped"

GUIDELINES
1. A closed drainage system should be maintained at all times to decrease the possibility that bacteria will enter the system and cause a urinary tract infection.
2. A laboratory requisition for a urine specimen should indicate the method used to obtain the urine.
3. The volume of the specimen needed will vary, depending on the laboratory testing methods. Refer questions to your laboratory technician.
4. Fresh urine specimens should be obtained for all laboratory tests. Urine specimens should be obtained with sterile equipment and placed in appropriate collection containers. Collection container lids should be secured to avoid spillage and/or contamination during transport.
5. A urine specimen collected from an indwelling catheter bag is not acceptable for laboratory testing unless it is the first urine drained into a new sterile bag.
6. Urine specimens should be refrigerated as soon as possible. Bacteria in the urine multiply at room temperature, causing inaccurate test results.

NURSING ACTION/RATIONALE
1. Assemble the equipment.
2. Identify the patient.
3. Explain the procedure.
4. Provide privacy.
5. Wash your hands.
6. Clamp the drainage tubing directly below the aspiration port with a rubber band or clamp to ensure a sufficient amount of pooled urine for a specimen (Figure 6-10).

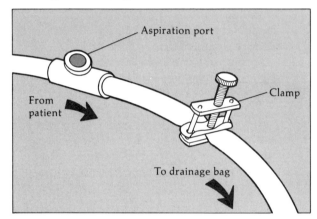

Figure 6-10. Drainage tube clamped below the aspiration port to pool urine.

7. Place a sign above the patient's bed, "Urine Tubing Temporarily Clamped."
8. Cleanse the aspirating port with an alcohol swab.
9. Expel air from the syringe.
10. Insert the needle into the aspirating port (Figure 6-11).

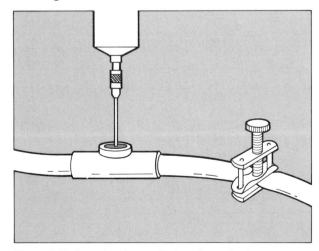

Figure 6-11. Inserting the needle into the aspirating port.

11. Withdraw the desired volume of urine.
12. Withdraw the needle.
13. Remove the rubber band or screw clamp so urine can drain freely into the drainage bag.
14. Remove the sign placed above the patient's bed.
15. Transfer the urine specimen from the syringe into the appropriate collection container.
16. Label the urine specimen and send it to the laboratory as ordered.
17. Dispose of the needle and syringe in the appropriate location.

PATIENT AND/OR FAMILY TEACHING

1. Explain the purpose for collecting the urine specimen.
2. Reinforce prior instruction on the maintenance of the catheter system. See procedure "Care and Maintenance of an Indwelling Catheter."

DOCUMENTATION

1. Amount, color, and clarity of urine specimen.
2. Time specimen was collected.
3. Time specimen was taken to the laboratory.
4. Any patient teaching done and the patient's level of understanding.

 # Manual Irrigation of an Indwelling Catheter

PURPOSE

1. Evacuation of blood clots, mucus, or sediment obstructing the flow of urine.

REQUISITES

1. Sterile disposable irrigation set consisting of:
   a. Asepto or piston syringe
   b. Graduated solution container
   c. Antiseptic wipes
   d. Graduated collection container
2. Bed protector
3. Sterile catheter plug and cap
4. Sterile gloves
5. Solution as prescribed by the physician (usually normal saline)
6. Drape or bath blanket

GUIDELINES

1. The risk that a urinary tract infection will develop in a patient with an indwelling catheter increases every time the closed system is opened. Breaking the system to irrigate a catheter should only be done as a last resort.
2. Catheters that become plugged by concentrated urine and sediment accumulations should be changed under sterile conditions, rather than irrigated.
3. The lumen of an obstructed catheter may sometimes be opened by gently milking the tube in the direction of the drainage bag to move small obstructions through the tubing.
4. Three-way catheters are available. They provide a separate lumen for irrigation, and the drainage system does not need to be interrupted. Three-way catheters should be used if frequent irrigations are anticipated.
5. A physician's order should be obtained before performing an open irrigation. The physician should designate the type and amount of irrigant to be used.

6. Strict aseptic technique must be used to perform this procedure. New sterile equipment must be used for each subsequent irrigation.
7. The procedure for instillation of medications varies slightly from this procedure. Refer to the procedure "Bladder Instillation."

NURSING ACTION/RATIONALE

1. Assemble all equipment.
2. Identify the patient.
3. Explain the procedure to the patient. Instruct the patient to report any discomfort during the procedure.
4. Provide privacy.
5. Assist the patient (male or female) to the dorsal recumbent position. Place a bed protector under the patient.
6. Drape the patient with a bath blanket, leaving only the catheter tubing exposed. The bath blanket can be wrapped and secured around the patient's legs.
7. Wash your hands.
8. Open sterile supplies, using aseptic technique.
9. Pour the irrigation solution into the solution container.
10. Cleanse the connection site between the drainage tubing and the catheter with antiseptic swabs.
11. Pinch the catheter and disconnect it from the tubing.
12. Insert a sterile catheter plug into the lumen of the catheter and cover the tip of the drainage tubing with the sterile cap. Secure the capped tubing to prevent it from falling to the floor.
13. Put on sterile gloves to prevent nosocomial infection.
14. Move the sterile collection container to the bed between the patient's legs.
15. Draw 50 cc of irrigating solution into the syringe, maintaining sterility of the barrel and tip.
16. Pinch the catheter while removing the catheter plug and insert the tip of the syringe into the lumen.
17. Inject the solution gently into the catheter. Do not force the solution. If the solution will not inject easily, reposition the patient and try injecting again. If unable to inject the solution, notify the physician.

18. Remove the syringe and allow the irrigating solution to drain into the collection container. If the solution does not drain, reattach the syringe and exert a small amount of pressure to withdraw the solution. If the catheter does not clear, inject approximately 20 cc of irrigant. Notify the physician if unable to drain the catheter. Do not inject more than 70 cc of solution without the catheter draining.
19. Repeat the above steps two to three times for complete irrigation or as the physician orders. Be sure all solution has drained before injecting more solution.
20. Reconnect the tubing to the catheter, using aseptic technique.
21. Remove the sterile gloves.
22. Reposition the patient comfortably.
23. Measure the amount of drainage in the collection container.
24. Discard equipment or return it to the appropriate area.

PATIENT AND/OR FAMILY TEACHING

1. Explain the procedure to the patient before you start.
2. Instruct the patient to notify the nurse if any of the following symptoms occur:
   a. Pain or discomfort in the bladder area.
   b. A sensation of needing to urinate.
   c. A feeling of fullness in the bladder.
3. Instruct the patient on increasing fluid intake if allowed and appropriate.
4. See "Care and Maintenance of an Indwelling Catheter" for further patient instruction.

DOCUMENTATION

1. Amount and type of irrigant used.
2. Amount, color, and clarity of return.
3. Any difficulties encountered in irrigating or draining the catheter.
4. The patient's reaction to the procedure.
5. All patient teaching done and the patient's level of understanding.

Bladder Irrigation
Through a Triple Lumen Foley Catheter _____

PURPOSE

1. Irrigate the bladder without interrupting the closed drainage system.
2. Dilute postoperative bleeding into the bladder to decrease the chance of clot formation.

REQUISITES

1. Sterile triple lumen Foley catheter, size as ordered by the physician (Figure 6-12)
2. Sterile 4000 cc drainage bag
3. Sterile bladder irrigation tubing
4. IV standard
5. Sterile irrigation solution as ordered by the physician (usually 3000 cc bag)
6. Sterile gloves
7. Antiseptic swabs
8. Sterile catheter plug

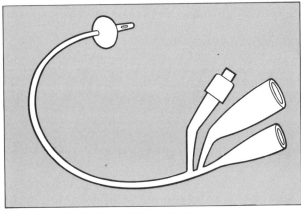

Figure 6-12. Triple lumen Foley catheter.

GUIDELINES

1. This procedure can be used for intermittent or continuous bladder irrigation.
2. All guidelines for "Care and Maintenance of an Indwelling Catheter" apply to a triple lumen catheter.
3. A physician's order is required to perform this procedure. The order should include the type of solution to be used, the rate of the irrigation, and whether the irrigation should be continuous or intermittent.
4. The physician may order a postoperative bladder irrigation to be infused at a rate that maintains a free flow of urine. In this case, the irrigation rate should be adjusted according to the color of returning drainage. If the drainage is bright red, the rate of the irrigation should be increased until the drainage becomes pink to clear in color. The rate can then be decreased to maintain that color of drainage. Vital signs should be monitored closely if the patient is being irrigated because of bleeding.
5. Close observation of intake and output is imperative to prevent complications from an obstructed catheter. Depending on the flow rate, the intake and output should be calculated hourly, or oftener if the rate is fast, to ensure that adequate drainage is occurring.
6. To determine an accurate output during a bladder irrigation, subtract the amount of irrigant used from the amount of drainage obtained. The difference is the patient's output of urine and blood.

7. If an obstruction occurs in the catheter, the irrigation should be shut off, and manual irrigation should be performed to remove the obstruction. When manual irrigant flows freely, the irrigation can be resumed.

8. Bleeding into the bladder is expected after urologic surgery. The bleeding usually decreases over 24 to 48 hours. Any bright-red drainage with numerous clots unresolved by irrigation should be reported to the physician immediately, since the patient may be bleeding arterially.

9. Strict sterile technique must be used throughout this procedure.

NURSING ACTION/RATIONALE

1. Assemble all equipment.
2. Identify the patient.
3. Explain the procedure to the patient. Warn the patient that bladder spasms may be experienced during the procedure.
4. Provide privacy.
5. Wash your hands.
6. Follow the procedure for "Insertion and Removal of an Indwelling Catheter" if the catheter is not already in place. Use a triple lumen catheter and a 4000 cc drainage bag.
7. Attach the irrigation tubing to the irrigation solution on the IV standard.
8. Fill the drip chamber with fluid and open the roll clamp to expel all air from the tubing.
9. Reclamp the tubing.
10. Put on sterile gloves.
11. Cleanse the connection between the Foley drainage bag and the catheter with antiseptic swabs.
12. Disconnect the drainage bag tubing from the large lumen of the catheter and cover with a sterile cap.
13. Connect the tubing of the 4000 cc drainage bag to the catheter.
14. Cleanse the connection between the small lumen and the catheter plug. If the catheter was just inserted this lumen will not be plugged.
15. Attach the irrigation tubing to the small lumen.
16. Open the clamp on the irrigation tubing and adjust the flow rate (Figure 6-13).

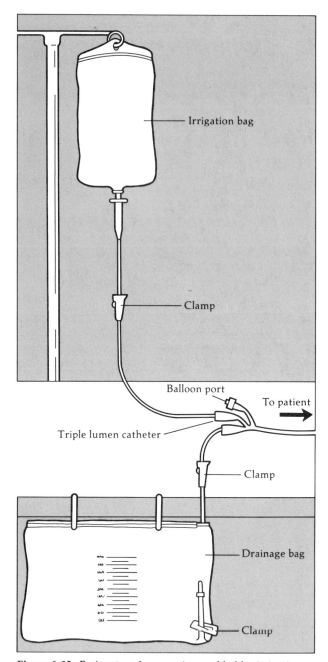

Figure 6-13. Basic set-up for a continuous bladder irrigation.

17. Add a new bag of irrigation solution by removing the drained bag and spiking the new bag with the irrigation tubing, using aseptic technique.
18. Empty the drainage bag when half full. Follow the procedure "Care and Maintenance of an Indwelling Catheter."

19. Discontinue the irrigation as ordered by the physician:
  a. Cleanse the connection on the small lumen of the catheter.
  b. Remove the irrigation tubing.
  c. Insert a sterile catheter plug.
  d. Change the large drainage bag to a conventional bag, following the steps described above.

PATIENT AND/OR FAMILY TEACHING

1. Instruct the patient before the procedure as previously described.
2. Instruct the patient to call for assistance to ambulate, if allowed.
3. Instruct the patient to report to the nurse any:
  a. Pain or discomfort.
  b. Feeling of fullness in the bladder.
  c. Sensation of a need to void.
4. Refer to the procedure "Care and Maintenance of an Indwelling Catheter" for other important areas of teaching for a patient with an indwelling catheter.

DOCUMENTATION

1. Catheter insertion, including the size, if not previously in place.
2. Type and amount of irrigation solution infused.
3. Amount, color, and clarity of drainage.
4. Presence or absence of clots or sediment.
5. Any problems encountered, such as an obstruction, and resolution of the problem.
6. An assessment of the patient's reaction to the procedure, including pain or discomfort, and vital signs.
7. Any patient teaching done and the patient's level of understanding.

Application of an External Catheter on an Adult Male _____

PURPOSE
1. Provide a dry environment for incontinent male patients.

REQUISITES
1. Urinary sheath kit containing the following items:
   a. Sheath or condom catheter
   b. Skin prep swabs
   c. Double-sided elastic adhesive
2. Soap and water
3. Washcloth and towel
4. Urinary drainage bag
5. Scissors (optional)
6. Bath blankets—2

GUIDELINES
1. The use of an external catheter on incontinent male patients decreases the risk of catheter-associated urinary tract infections that often accompany the use of indwelling catheters.
2. The main problems with external catheter devices are usually skin irritation or leakage from around the catheter. If the adhesive is applied too tightly, circulatory impairment of the penis may occur, causing tissue damage.
3. The catheter sheath should be changed at least daily; the drainage bag should be changed as necessary.
4. This is a clean procedure.

NURSING ACTION/RATIONALE
1. Assemble all equipment.
2. Explain the procedure to the patient.
3. Provide privacy and adequate lighting.
4. Assist the patient to a supine position.
5. Cover the upper torso and the legs with bath blankets. Cover the genitals with a towel until ready to begin.
6. Wash your hands.
7. Wash the penis and perineal area with soap and water and dry thoroughly. Retract the foreskin on an uncircumcised male to cleanse the glans, and ease the foreskin back into place after drying thoroughly.
8. Trim pubic hair with a scissors as necessary.
9. Coat the entire shaft of the penis using the skin prep swabs. Allow the skin to dry.

10. Apply the adhesive strip to the penis, starting at the base of the penis and wrapping in a spiral fashion (Figure 6-14a). The ends should not overlap. Do not wrap the tape tightly, since this may decrease the circulation in the penis.

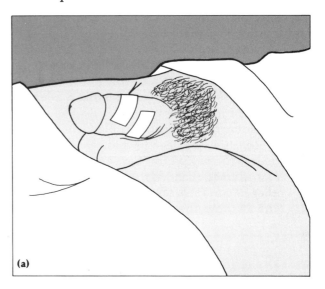

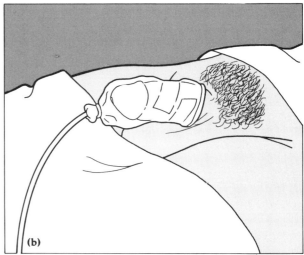

Figure 6-14. Applying external catheter to an adult male. (a) Wrap the double-sided adhesive strip in a spiral fashion starting at the base. (b) External catheter correctly applied.

11. Apply the external catheter by rolling the sheath over the end of the penis to the base. Allow ½ inch of space at the tip of the sheath to avoid pressure to the glans (Figure 6-14b).
12. Press gently to secure the sheath.
13. Connect the tubing to the catheter drainage bag.
14. Secure the drainage bag below the level of the patient's bladder.
15. Assist the patient to a comfortable position.
16. Discard equipment or return it to the appropriate area.
17. Assess the condition of the penis and the drainage system within 15 minutes after applying the catheter, then every hour for 3 hours, then every 4 hours. Assess for:
    a. Retracted foreskin.
    b. Skin irritation.
    c. Discoloration and/or edema.
    d. Leakage or pooling of urine in the sheath.

PATIENT AND/OR FAMILY TEACHING

1. Explain the procedure to the patient before you start.
2. Instruct the patient to keep the drainage bag below the bladder level to maintain adequate gravity flow.

3. Instruct the patient to notify the nurse of the following problems:
   a. Pain or swelling in the penis.
   b. Pooling of urine in the sheath.
   c. Leakage of urine around the sheath.
   d. Disconnection of the catheter and tubing.
4. Teach self-application when appropriate.

DOCUMENTATION

1. Application and effectiveness.
2. Regular assessments of the condition of penis and drainage system.
3. Patient's reaction to the procedure.
4. Daily change and cleansing.
5. Any teaching done and the patient's level of understanding.

Collection of a Midstream Urine Specimen

PURPOSE
1. Obtain a urine specimen uncontaminated by skin flora.

REQUISITES
1. Sterile midstream urine specimen kit containing the following:
   a. Specimen container
   b. Funnel
   c. Specimen container lid
   d. Specimen container label
   e. Antiseptic towelettes—3
2. Exam gloves (optional)

GUIDELINES
1. When the patient is expected to collect the specimen unassisted, specific verbal and written instructions should be given to the patient. The patient should be given an opportunity to ask questions. Patients should be assessed regarding their ability to understand and follow directions before being allowed to collect the specimen unsupervised.
2. In most cases the clean midstream urine specimen method of collection is satisfactory for laboratory testing provided the patient is cleansed correctly and the specimen is collected according to procedure.
3. If any part of the funnel, the inside of the cover, or the inside of the container is touched, the kit is considered contaminated and a new one should be obtained.
4. Alert patients on bedrest will need assistance with this procedure.

NURSING ACTION/RATIONALE
Ambulatory Patient
1. Assemble all equipment.
2. Identify the patient.

3. Instruct the ambulatory patient on the steps of urine collection. They are as follows:
   a. Wash your hands.
   b. Place the specimen container with the funnel attached on a counter or chair near the toilet, touching only the outside of the container.
   c. Place the specimen container lid on the counter, rim side up, taking care to touch only the outside surface.
   d. Remove all clothing from the waist down.
   e. Assume appropriate position:
      (1) *Female*—Sit on the toilet with legs spread far apart.
      (2) *Male*—Stand facing the toilet, or sit on the toilet with legs spread far apart.
   f. Open towelettes.
   g. Cleanse the perineal area:
      (1) *Female*
         (a) Separate the labia with the thumb and forefinger of the non-dominant hand.
         (b) Using downward strokes, cleanse one labium with a towelette and discard.
         (c) Cleanse the other labium and the meatus in the same fashion, using a separate towelette for each stroke, and discard.
         (d) Keep the labia separated.
      (2) *Male*
         (a) If uncircumcised, retract the foreskin before proceeding with the following steps.
         (b) Cleanse the head of the penis with a towelette, using a circular motion from the urethral opening to the outer diameter of the penis.
         (c) Discard towelette.
         (d) Repeat the procedure, using all the towelettes.
   h. Hold the specimen container by the outside surface and begin urinating into the toilet.

i. Place the specimen container under the stream of urine after a good flow has started. Remaining skin bacteria will be washed off with the first portion of the urine voided.

j. Fill the specimen container half full and remove from the stream. Void remainder of the urine into the toilet.

k. Place specimen container on a firm surface.

l. Dry the perineal area:
   (1) *Female*—Dry perineum from front to back with toilet tissue.
   (2) *Male*—Dry the head of the penis with toilet tissue. Ease foreskin back over glans in uncircumcised males.

m. Wash your hands.

n. Remove the funnel from the specimen container.

o. Screw on the sterile cover, touching only the outer surface.

p. Notify the nurse when the specimen has been collected.

4. Label the specimen and send it to the lab.

5. Discard all equipment or return it to the appropriate location.

Bedridden Patient

1. Assemble all equipment.
2. Identify the patient.
3. Assist the bedridden patient to obtain a urine specimen by the following steps:
   a. Place the patient on a bedpan in a semi-recumbent or semi-Fowler's position with legs spread.

b. Put on exam gloves.

c. Wash the perineum with soap and water.

d. Follow the cleansing and collection procedure described above.

e. Remove the bedpan after drying the patient.

f. Remove gloves.

g. Position the patient comfortably.

4. Label the specimen and send it to the laboratory.

5. Discard all equipment or return it to the appropriate area.

PATIENT AND/OR FAMILY TEACHING

1. Instruct the patient thoroughly prior to the procedure as stated in Nursing Action/ Rationale.

2. Emphasize the purpose of the procedure and the importance of following the procedure exactly.

DOCUMENTATION

1. Amount, color, odor, and clarity of urine.
2. Disposition of specimen.
3. Any patient teaching done and the patient's level of understanding.

Straining Urine for Renal Calculi

PURPOSE
1. Detect and recover renal calculi.

REQUISITES
1. Large-mouth bottle
2. Calculi strainer
3. Urine collector—bedpan or wide-mouth container
4. Sign: "Strain All Urine"
5. Labeled specimen container

GUIDELINES
1. Contributing factors to the development of kidney stones in a patient may be urinary tract infections, dehydration, concentrated urine, and inactivity.
2. The medical treatment for a patient who develops renal calculi varies, depending upon the chemical composition of the calculi; therefore it is important to have calculi analyzed to determine their composition.
3. Surgical intervention to remove calculi from the urinary tract may be indicated if the patient is unable to pass it when voiding. Most stones under 1 cm can be passed when voiding.
4. Passing renal calculi is usually painful, and the patient may require frequent analgesics.
5. Calculi may stick to the sides of the urinal. The male should void in a wide-mouth container to promote ease in visualizing the sides of the container for adhering calculi.
6. Most stones are easily crushed and need to be handled carefully when they are retrieved for testing.

NURSING ACTION/RATIONALE
1. Assemble all equipment.
2. Identify the patient.
3. Explain the purpose of the procedure to the patient.
4. Instruct the male patient to void in a wide-mouth container provided for that purpose. Instruct the female patient to void in a bedpan or a collection container placed in the toilet. Instruct the patient to save all urine and report all voidings to the nurse.
5. Label a large-mouth bottle with the patient's name and room number and place it with a strainer in the patient's bathroom or other designated area.
6. Place a "Strain All Urine" sign with the patient's name in an appropriate prominent location.
7. Pour all urine, after each voiding, through the strainer and into the large-mouth bottle.
8. Check the strainer for calculi or sediment after each straining.
9. Save all calculi retrieved, and inform the physician. Place calculi in a labeled specimen container and send it to the lab for analysis.
10. Rinse the strainer with running water after each use.
11. Measure the urine if indicated.
12. Discard the urine after each straining.
13. Change the calculi strainer as necessary.

PATIENT AND/OR FAMILY TEACHING
1. Instruct the patient prior to initiating the procedure as described in Nursing Action/Rationale.
2. Teach the patient health habits to minimize recurrence, such as increasing fluid intake if allowed and restricting dietary intake as ordered.
3. Teach the patient the urine straining procedure if it is to be continued following discharge.
4. Teach and reinforce the signs and symptoms of recurrence to be reported to the physician.

DOCUMENTATION
1. Amount, color, and clarity of urine.
2. Size and color of any calculi retrieved.
3. Disposition of calculi.
4. Notification of the physician, if appropriate.
5. Patient teaching and the patient's level of understanding.

Testing Urine
for Glucose and Acetone

PURPOSE
1. Determine the amount of glucose and/or ketone bodies in the urine.

REQUISITES
1. Specimen container
2. Test kit, as ordered by the physician

GUIDELINES
1. Glucose is normally found in the urine in trace amounts. In certain disease processes such as diabetes mellitus, the blood sugar concentration is high, and abnormal amounts of glucose are excreted in the urine. This is called glucosuria.
2. Acetone or ketone bodies are not normally found in the urine. Ketonuria (acetone in the urine) indicates incomplete fat metabolism. This can occur in diabetes mellitus, but is also found in cases of dehydration and starvation.
3. A variety of chemically treated strips or tablets are available to test for glucose and/or acetone in the urine. The type used will usually depend on hospital policy or physician preference.
4. Regardless of the product used for testing, several principles apply:
   a. The directions for completing the test accompany the product and must be followed exactly.
   b. Products must be stored in a tightly closed container to prevent moisture from accumulating on the tablet or strip and adversely affecting test results.
   c. Products should be stored at temperatures between 10 to 30°C (50 to 86°F). Storage at abnormally high or low temperatures will adversely affect the test results.
   d. Tablets or strips should not be used after the expiration date or if they are discolored.

e. Certain medications will account for false positive readings on some of the tests. The literature accompanying the product will identify these substances.
   f. The same product should be used consistently for any patient to ensure that any trends are accurately noted.
   g. Always use a fresh urine specimen.
5. Products are presently available to test a small drop of capillary blood to determine blood glucose concentration. These products can usually be used with a color chart, or they can be used in conjunction with a machine that gives a quantitative test result.
6. Urine testing of patients with diabetes mellitus is usually performed before meals and at bedtime.

NURSING ACTION/RATIONALE
1. Obtain a fresh urine specimen:
   a. If the patient has an indwelling catheter, following the procedure "Aspirating a Small-Volume Fresh Urine Specimen from an Indwelling Catheter."
   b. If the patient does not have a catheter, obtain a second voided urine specimen. Instruct the patient as follows:
      (1) Empty the bladder completely and discard the urine.
      (2) Drink a full glass of water, if allowed.
      (3) Void again in about 30 minutes and save the urine. This is the specimen to be tested.
2. Perform urine testing following directions on package insert accompanying the test product.

PATIENT AND/OR FAMILY TEACHING
1. Instruct the patient on the proper method of urine collection and the times the test will be done.
2. Demonstrate the test procedure to the patient if the patient will be expected to do the test after discharge. A correct return demonstration is evidence that the patient has learned.

3. Reinforce and clarify the physician's explanation of the disease process. Patients with diabetes mellitus will need comprehensive teaching in the following areas:
   a. The physiology of the disease process.
   b. Diet modifications.
   c. Medications—possibly insulin injections.
   d. Signs and symptoms of hypoglycemia.
   e. Skin care.
   f. Prevention of complications.

DOCUMENTATION
1. Time and results of test.
2. All patient teaching done and the patient's level of understanding.

Urostomy Disposable Appliance Change

PURPOSE
1. Permit visualization of the stoma and skin.
2. Prevent leakage and skin breakdown.
3. Control odor.
4. Prevent urinary tract infection.

REQUISITES
1. Correct size urinary ostomy appliance
2. Skin barrier (wafer)
3. Skin protector
4. Urostomy night drain tube and Foley drainage bag
5. Washcloth and towel
6. Washbasin
7. 4 × 4 gauze sponges
8. Clean scissors
9. Graduated container
10. Waste receptacle
11. Exam gloves

GUIDELINES
1. Urostomy is a general term used to describe a variety of surgical interventions for urinary diversion. When the urine is diverted to drain through an opening in the abdomen, a urinary drainage appliance must be worn at all times.
2. Patients having urinary diversion surgery must have comprehensive explanations and instructions pre- and postoperatively. Care should be taken to offer both psychological and emotional support.
3. There are many products available on the market to be used for a urostomy patient. The products selected will depend on patient need, cost, availability, and physician and hospital preference.
4. All urinary appliances have a valve on the bottom to drain urine and can be connected to night drainage.
5. Gravity flow aids in keeping urine away from the stoma, as does frequent emptying of the appliance. Appliances should be emptied when one-third full.
6. Early morning, before the patient drinks fluids, is the best time to change the urostomy appliance.
7. Bacteria thrive in concentrated alkaline urine. A urostomy patient should maintain a high fluid intake (8 to 10 glasses of water per day, unless contraindicated). Apple juice, prune juice, cranberry juice, and vitamin C tablets will help keep the urine more acid and decrease the chance of infection.
8. This is a clean non-sterile procedure. Because of the danger of nosocomial infection while the patient is hospitalized, it is best to maintain a closed drainage system. This avoids connecting and disconnecting tubes. However, the patient will need to be instructed on how to set up the night drainage system before going home.

9. Directions for application of the specific ostomy product being used always accompany the product. Refer to this insert, as the application technique may vary slightly from the procedure given here.
10. Immediately after surgery, urostomy appliances should be changed every 24 to 48 hours so that the condition of the stoma can be assessed. When the stoma is well healed, appliances can be changed every 48 to 72 hours.

NURSING ACTION/RATIONALE

1. Explain the procedure to the patient. Encourage participation.
2. Assemble all equipment.
3. Provide privacy and assist the patient to either a semi-Fowler's or a sitting position.
4. Wash your hands.
5. Put on exam gloves.
6. Remove the old appliance by gently pulling the adhesive on the pouch away from the skin while holding the skin securely. Place a 4 × 4 rolled gauze over the stoma to absorb any drainage.
7. Empty and measure the urine from the old drainage pouch and discard the pouch. If the pouch was connected to a night drainage bag, cleanse the connection with alcohol, disconnect the tubing from the pouch, and drain the drainage bag. Cover the end of the drainage tubing until ready to reconnect.
8. Use a washcloth to cleanse the skin around the stoma with soap and water. Rinse thoroughly, since residue on the skin will interfere with appliance adhesion. Pat the skin dry with a dry towel.
9. Assess the stoma and surrounding tissue for color, signs of irritation, and drainage.
10. Use a measure guide (which comes with ostomy pouches) to determine the correct size of the appliance needed (Figure 6-15). The smallest size that fits without touching the stoma is the right size. There should be no more than $\frac{1}{16}$ to $\frac{1}{8}$ inch of skin showing around the stoma.

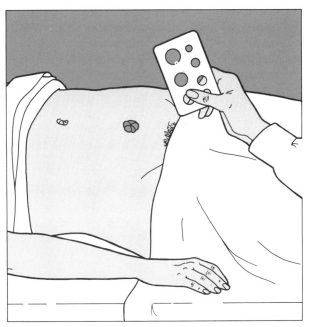

Figure 6-15. Use a measuring guide to determine the correct size of the appliance.

11. Use the measuring guide and draw a circle on the skin barrier (wafer), the same size as selected above.
12. Cut out the hole on the skin barrier.
13. Apply skin protectant 3 inches around the stoma in a thin layer. If using a spray product, cover the urostomy opening before spraying. If using skin gel, spread a thin layer on the skin with your finger. Allow to dry. This product will protect the skin from being irritated from the adhesives, and it also protects the first layer of skin when adhesives are removed.
14. Peel off the white backing from the skin barrier, center the hole over the stoma, and press firmly. Be sure the skin barrier adheres tightly, with no wrinkles.

15. Remove the white paper backing from the adhesive on the pouch, exposing the adhesive. Center the pouch hole over the skin barrier with the valve on the pouch pointing down and in a closed position (Figure 6-16).

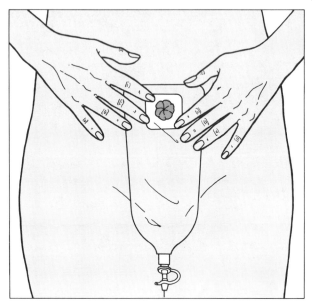

Figure 6-16. Center the appliance over the stoma and press down firmly.

16. Connect the night drain tube to the valve at the bottom of the pouch, then connect the other end of the drain tube to the Foley drainage bag attached to the side of the bed. If the patient will be out of bed most of the day, the night drain tube does not need to be connected.
17. Coil excess tubing on the bed to promote gravity flow drainage. Avoid kinks in the system.
18. Remove the exam gloves.
19. Position the patient comfortably.
20. Discard all equipment or return it to the appropriate area.
21. Wash your hands.

PATIENT AND/OR FAMILY TEACHING

1. Instruct the patient on how to measure the stoma, change the appliance, empty the appliance, and convert the appliance to a night drain system. A satisfactory return demonstration is evidence that the patient has learned.

2. Provide information and/or instruction to the ostomy patient both pre- and post-operatively in the following areas:
   a. The nature of the disease process and the surgical intervention.
   b. Prevention of urinary tract infection by good personal hygiene, maintaining a closed drainage system, proper cleansing of the stoma and skin, increasing the fluid intake, and diet modifications.
   c. Coping with skin problems and when to seek help.
   d. The importance of post-operative visits to the physician.
   e. Information about where additional supplies can be purchased.
   f. Resources, if appropriate, such as social service for financial counseling and insurance information.
   g. Availability of local ostomy groups and clinics including literature from these groups. Literature is also available from the American Cancer Society.

DOCUMENTATION

1. Time of appliance change and person performing the change.
2. Type and size of appliance used and method of application, along with preparation of skin.
3. Assessment of stoma and surrounding skin.
4. Amount, color, and clarity of urine.
5. The patient's reaction to the procedure.
6. All patient teaching done and the patient's level of understanding.

Peritoneal Dialysis: Temporary Catheter

PURPOSE
1. Assist the physician to insert the dialysis catheter.
2. Aseptically perform a fluid exchange.
3. Assist the physician to remove the dialysis catheter.

REQUISITES
Insertion
1. Sterile peritoneal dialysis procedure tray containing the following items:
   a. Local anesthetic
   b. 25 gauge, ⅝ inch skin wheal needle
   c. 5 cc disposable syringe
   d. 22 gauge, 1½ inch infiltration needle
   e. Scissors
   f. Peritoneal catheter as provided on tray
   g. 15 gauge, 3½ inch instillation needle
   h. Scalpel blade and rubber band
   i. Safety pin
   j. 8 inch extension set with L connection, Y injection site, and slide clamp
   k. Fenestrated drape
   l. Gauze sponges
   m. Prep sponges
   n. Antiseptic solution receptacle
2. Sterile gloves to fit physician and nurse
3. Antiseptic solution
4. Sterile precut 4 × 4 gauze sponges—2
5. Adhesive tape
6. Antiseptic ointment
7. Sterile suture thread (as ordered by the physician)
8. Sterile catheter cap

Exchange Procedure
1. Sterile peritoneal dialysis solution (amount and type as ordered by the physician) warmed to 37°C (98.6°F)
2. Sterile peritoneal dialysis administration tubing (Figure 6-17)
3. Sterile dialysis drainage bag
4. Sterile gloves
5. IV standard

Removal
1. Sterile suture removal kit
2. Antiseptic swabs
3. Sterile 4 × 4 sponges
4. Sterile gloves
5. Antiseptic ointment (optional)
6. Waste receptacle
7. Tape

GUIDELINES
1. Peritoneal dialysis is used as a substitute for kidney function during renal failure to remove toxic substances from the body, correct electrolyte imbalance, correct fluid imbalance, and control elevated blood pressure. It is also used as a therapeutic treatment for peritonitis.
2. Peritoneal dialysis works on the principle of molecules moving through a semipermeable membrane (the peritoneum) from an area of greater concentration to an area of lesser concentration.
3. Hypovolemic shock may occur if there is too rapid loss of fluid during dialysis. The patient's vital signs should be taken every 15 minutes during the first exchange and then every hour during subsequent exchanges.
4. Peritoneal infection is a major problem with peritoneal dialysis. Sterile technique must be maintained during the exchange procedure. The patient's temperature should be monitored closely for elevations. (Peritoneal drainage cultures are usually ordered at regular intervals during therapy.)
5. Peritoneal dialysis may be ordered as continuous or intermittent therapy.

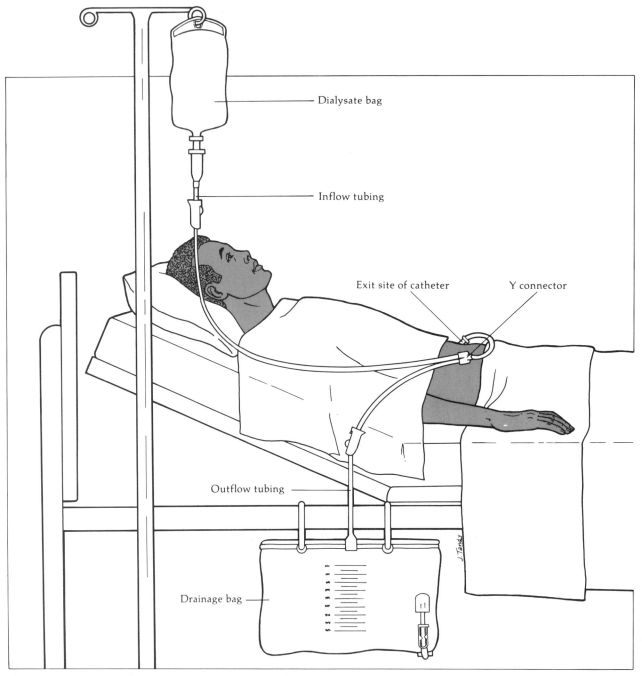

Figure 6-17. Basic set-up for a patient receiving a peritoneal dialysis exchange.

6. The requirement for a signed consent form for invasive procedures varies among hospitals. Refer to your hospital's policy manual.

7. Precautions should be taken when handling peritoneal outflow drainage, as with any body secretions that may contain contaminants.

8. The physician's order for peritoneal dialysis should specify the number of exchanges to be performed, the type of solution to be used, the amount of solution to be used for each exchange, the amount of time the fluid should remain in the peritoneum, and the maximum amount of fluid to be drained from the peritoneum during each exchange.

9. Peritoneal dialysis solution should be warmed to 37°C (98.6°F) to prevent abdominal discomfort from cramping.
10. The fluid balance is the difference between the amount of fluid infused into the peritoneum and the amount drained from the peritoneum. The patient's fluid balance is positive ($+$) if more fluid was infused than drained, and negative ($-$) if more fluid was drained from the peritoneum than was infused into the peritoneum.

NURSING ACTION/RATIONALE

1. Assemble all equipment.
2. Identify the patient.
3. Reinforce and clarify the physician's explanation of the procedure.
4. Obtain a permit if required.
5. Instruct the patient to void to empty the bladder. This will help to prevent perforation of the bladder when the trocar is introduced into the peritoneum.
6. Dress the patient in a hospital gown.
7. Obtain a baseline weight and baseline vital signs.
8. Assist the patient to a supine position.
9. Wash your hands.
10. Prepare the infusion by spiking the bag of dialysate with the peritoneal dialysis tubing. Prime the tubing with solution from the bag to the tip of the inflow tubing. The outflow tubing should be clamped.
11. Open the sterile supplies, using aseptic technique.
12. Assist the physician as required with insertion of the peritoneal catheter.
13. Connect the inflow end of the tubing to the peritoneal catheter, using strict aseptic technique.
14. Connect the drainage bag to the outflow tubing.
15. Unclamp the inflow tubing, allowing the warmed dialysate to run into the peritoneal catheter rapidly. The usual flow is 2 liters of solution infusing in 10 minutes.
16. Clamp the tubing from the solution bag just before the solution has drained completely into the peritoneum. This will prevent air from entering the tubing.

17. Allow the solution to remain in the peritoneum for the prescribed time, usually 30 to 60 minutes. Prepare the solution for the next exchange during this time, if another exchange is to be given.
18. Unclamp the outflow drainage tube and allow the solution to drain by gravity into the drainage bag. It will take approximately 10 to 20 minutes for the solution to drain completely. If the solution is not draining properly, rolling the patient from side to side, raising the head of the bed, or standing the patient, if allowed, will usually facilitate drainage. The physician may order only a limited amount of solution to be drained beyond what was infused during one exchange.
19. Clamp the drainage tube when the drainage ceases or when the prescribed amount of fluid has been drained.
20. Measure the outflow drainage and record.
21. Calculate the patient's fluid balance.
22. Repeat the above procedure for each subsequent exchange.
23. Assess the patient's vital signs regularly during therapy as described in the guidelines. Weigh the patient daily on the same scale.
24. Change the sterile dressing around the catheter daily, using aseptic technique. Inspect the site for signs of drainage, inflammation, or infection. Cleanse the area with antiseptic swabs and re-dress with sterile dressings.
25. Change the infusion tubing and drainage bag every 24 hours, using strict aseptic technique.
26. Assist the physician as required to remove the peritoneal catheter after the dialysis therapy is discontinued. Use aseptic technique.
27. Change the dressings following the removal of the catheter, as necessary, using aseptic technique. Scant drainage of fluid will continue for several hours after the catheter is removed.

PATIENT AND/OR FAMILY TEACHING

1. Instruct the patient prior to the procedure concerning:
   a. Insertion of the catheter.
   b. Procedure for dialysis.
   c. Frequency of vital sign checks during the procedure.
2. Instruct the patient to notify the nurse of:
   a. Feelings of pain or discomfort in the abdomen.
   b. Shortness of breath.
   c. Feelings of lightheadedness or dizziness.
   d. Feelings of being flushed or extremely warm or cold.
3. Instruct the patient to call for assistance in moving.
4. Instruct the patient to avoid touching the catheter tubing, connection, or insertion site.

DOCUMENTATION

1. Time of insertion of catheter, by whom, and any problems encountered.
2. Type and amount of solution infused for each exchange.
3. Amount, color, and clarity of drainage for each exchange.
4. Calculation of the patient's fluid balance following each exchange.
5. Assessment of the patient's vital signs, weight, and tolerance of the procedure.
6. Any dressing changes done and assessment of catheter site.
7. Tubing and drainage bag changes.
8. Time of removal of catheter, by whom, and any problems encountered.
9. All patient teaching done and the patient's level of understanding.

Arteriovenous Shunt Dressing Change

PURPOSE

1. Maintain the patency of the arteriovenous shunt.
2. Prevent complications with the shunt.
3. Assess the shunt exit sites.

REQUISITES

1. Exam gloves
2. Sterile gloves
3. Hydrogen peroxide solution
4. Sterile basin
5. Sterile 4 × 4 gauze sponges—4
6. Sterile scissors
7. Sterile 3 × 4 Telfa pad
8. Gauze roll—2 inch
9. Sterile cotton-tipped applicators
10. Antiseptic ointment
11. Waste receptacle
12. Washcloth and towel
13. Basin of warm, soapy water

GUIDELINES

1. An arteriovenous shunt is established for selected hemodialysis patients to provide an access to the arterial and venous system for hemodialysis treatment.
2. Patients in renal failure are more susceptible to infection. Any manipulation of the shunt or dressing should be performed using aseptic technique.
3. The most comon complications of a shunt are:
   a. *Infection.* This is manifested by an elevated white blood count, an elevated temperature, and drainage and/or redness at the exit side.

b. *Disconnection.* This complication is manifested by separation at the connection. Cannula clamps should be attached to the shunt dressings at all times. The two plastic shunt tubings should be clamped, the ends of the connection cleaned with antiseptic, the ends reconnected, and the clamps removed.

c. *Clotting.* This complication is manifested by dark blood in the tubing or a separation of blood and plasma. Notify the physician for orders for declotting the shunt. The shunt should be assessed for signs of clotting at least every 8 hours.

4. Blood pressures should not be taken, or venipunctures performed, on the affected extremity. The patient should be cautioned to refrain from wearing constricting clothing on the affected extremity.

5. Shunt dressings should be changed and the exit sites inspected every 24 hours or if dressings become soiled, loose, or wet.

NURSING ACTION/RATIONALE

1. Assemble all equipment.
2. Identify the patient.
3. Explain the procedure to the patient.
4. Provide privacy.
5. Provide adequate lighting.
6. Position the patient comfortably with the arteriovenous shunt extremity exposed.
7. Wash your hands.
8. Put on the exam gloves.
9. Remove the shunt clamps from the dressing. Place them in a clean area, within reach.
10. Remove the old dressings carefully and discard in the waste receptacle.
11. Assess the exit sites for redness and drainage. Assess the shunt for patency.
12. Remove the exam gloves.
13. Wash the patient's arm with soap and water and dry thoroughly. Do not wash around the shunt exit sites.
14. Pour the hydrogen peroxide solution into the sterile basin.
15. Dip a sterile cotton-tipped applicator into the hydrogen peroxide solution.

16. Cleanse one exit site with the applicator, starting from the site and moving out. Remove all exudate. Do not touch the exit site with a used applicator. Dry with a sterile 4 × 4 gauze sponge.
17. Cleanse the other side in the same manner with new sterile applicators. Dry with a sterile 4 × 4 gauze sponge.
18. Apply antiseptic ointment to each site, using sterile applicators.
19. Open sterile supplies, using aseptic technique.
20. Put on the sterile gloves.
21. Cut two slits into the sterile Telfa pad, using sterile scissors, and place it around the shunt as illustrated (Figure 6-18).

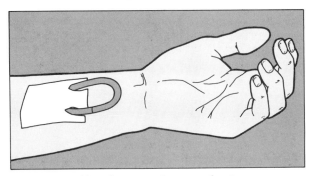

Figure 6-18. Telfa pad over arteriovenous shunt.

22. Apply one 4 × 4 sterile gauze under the shunt tubing and one over the shunt tubing, leaving a small portion of the shunt visible. Tape (Figure 6-19).

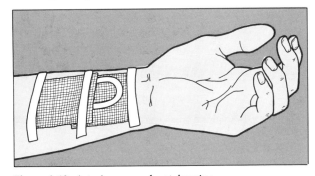

Figure 6-19. Arteriovenous shunt dressing.

23. Wrap the patient's arm with soft, flexible gauze around the shunt dressing area, leaving only one layer of gauze over the top of the loop so it may be pulled back for visualization of the shunt. Tape the end of the gauze.

24. Remove the sterile gloves.
25. Replace the shunt clamps on the proximal edge of the gauze.
26. Reposition the patient comfortably.
27. Discard equipment or return it to the appropriate location.

PATIENT AND/OR FAMILY TEACHING

1. Explain the procedure to the patient before starting.
2. Instruct the patient to avoid bumping the site of the shunt.
3. Instruct the patient to notify the nurse if the dressings become loose, soiled, or wet.
4. Instruct the patient and/or family to inspect the shunt for signs of clotting if the patient will be discharged with the shunt in place.
5. Teach the patient and/or family sterile dressing changes if the patient will be discharged.

DOCUMENTATION

1. Time of procedure and type of procedure performed.
2. Assessment of the cannula exit sites.
3. Assessment of patency of shunt.
4. All patient teaching done and the patient's level of understanding.

Unit 7

Musculoskeletal Procedures

PROCEDURES

Assisting the Physician with Bone Marrow Aspiration/Biopsy on the Adult Patient _____

PURPOSE

1. Assist the physician to collect bone marrow aspirant or bone biopsy specimens for laboratory analysis.

REQUISITES

1. Disposable sterile bone marrow biopsy tray, including:
   a. Single use sternal/iliac aspiration needle (1⅞ inch × 16 gauge)
   b. Single use bone marrow biopsy/aspiration needle (4 inch × 11 gauge)
   c. 10 cc syringe
   d. 5 cc syringe
   e. Needles (21 gauge, 25 gauge, and 20 gauge)
   f. Antiseptic
   g. Local anesthetic
   h. Scalpel blade with handle
   i. Specimen tubes containing 10% formalin for bone biopsy
   j. Slides and slide containers
   k. Sterile barriers
   l. Gauze sponges
   m. Adhesive strip or tape
2. Sterile gloves
3. Laboratory requisitions
4. Individual physicians vary in their preferences for the following items:
   a. Biopsy needle (disposable or non-disposable)
   b. Local anesthetic (amount and type)
   c. Sizes of syringes and needles

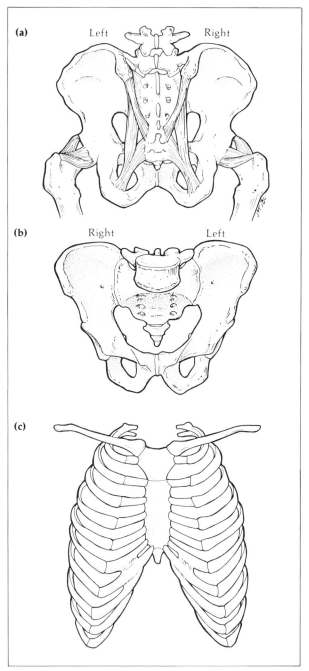

Figure 7-1. Alternative sites for bone marrow biopsy. **(a)** Posterior iliac crest. **(b)** Anterior iliac crest. **(c)** Sternum.

GUIDELINES

1. Bone marrow aspirations or biopsies are usually performed to:
   a. Diagnose cancer or hematologic disease processes.
   b. Isolate bacteria and other pathogens.
   c. Assess the patient's response to medical treatment.
2. The preferred sites for this procedure are:
   a. *Posterior iliac crest* (Figure 7-1a). The advantages for the selection of this site include: the procedure is performed where the patient cannot see it, no vital organs or major blood supply is nearby, and the iliac crests provide a large marrow cavity.
   b. *Anterior iliac crest* (Figure 7-1b). This site is within the patient's sight; otherwise it has the same advantages as the posterior iliac crest.
   c. *Sternum* (Figure 7-1c). Bone marrow aspirations can be done in this area, but the bone is too thin for biopsies to be done at this site. Precaution must be taken with this site since it is in close proximity to vital organs. An x-ray should be performed prior to the procedure to rule out an aortic aneurysm or an enlarged heart.
3. Following a bone marrow aspiration, the patient may experience pain or an aching sensation over the site for several days.
4. After the aspiration, it is important to apply pressure to the site to prevent bleeding or a hematoma formation.
5. The requirement for a signed consent form for invasive procedures varies among health care facilities. Refer to your hospital's policy manual.
6. Patient allergies should be determined prior to implementing the procedure.

NURSING ACTION/RATIONALE

1. Assemble all equipment.
2. Identify the patient.
3. Reinforce the physician's explanation of the procedure including:
   a. The reason for the procedure.
   b. Position required and the importance of remaining immobile.
   c. Any anticipated sensations of pressure or pain.
4. Obtain an informed consent, if required.
5. Provide adequate lighting.
6. Provide privacy.
7. Dress the patient in a clean hospital gown.
8. Assess baseline vital signs.
9. Assist the patient to a comfortable position desired by the physician. Expose the biopsy site.
10. Wash your hands.
11. Open the supplies, using aseptic technique.
12. Assist the physician as required.
13. Reassure the patient frequently.
14. Coach the patient to breathe deeply when experiencing pain during the procedure.
15. Have slides available for smearing the bone marrow aspirant and provide the specimen container with formalin for the bone specimen.
16. Cover the site with a sterile gauze sponge after the needle is removed and apply steady pressure to the site for 5 minutes.
17. Tape a sterile pressure dressing to the site and position the patient to add pressure to the biopsy site.
18. Send all labeled specimens to the laboratory with appropriate requisitions.
19. Discard equipment or return it to the appropriate area.
20. Keep a dressing over the site for 24 hours or as ordered by the physician.
21. Assess the patient's vital signs and the aspiration site for bleeding or inflammation every hour for 4 hours, then every 4 hours for 24 hours. Report any untoward signs to the physician.

PATIENT AND/OR FAMILY TEACHING

1. Instruct the patient regarding the procedure and the anticipated sensations that will be experienced during the procedure.
2. Instruct the patient to notify the nurse if any new symptoms occur, such as increased discomfort or bleeding.
3. Reinforce the physician's explanation regarding the patient's disease process.
4. Explain to the patient when the site will be inspected, and the frequency that the vital signs will be checked.

DOCUMENTATION

1. Type and time of procedure.
2. Name of physician performing procedure.
3. Any medication given, including dosage.
4. Site of biopsy or aspiration.
5. Disposition of specimen.
6. The patient's reaction to the procedure.
7. Specific parameters of assessment, including vital signs.
8. All patient teaching done and the patient's level of understanding.

Assisting the Physician with the Application of Skull Tongs

PURPOSE

1. Assist the physician with stabilizing cervical or thoracic fractures, dislocations, and/or subluxations.
2. Assist the physician in preventing any further sensory or motor impairment.

REQUISITES

1. Sterile skull tongs tray
2. Sterile pins (smooth or threaded)
3. Sterile wrenches
4. Sterile scalpel and blade
5. Antiseptic gauze
6. Razor or clipper
7. Antiseptic swabs
8. Antiseptic ointment
9. Local anesthetic
10. Sterile syringes (5 or 10 cc)
11. Sterile needles (25 and 22 gauge)

GUIDELINES

1. Patient support and instruction is of paramount importance, since this is an emotionally and physically traumatic experience.
2. Strict aseptic technique must be maintained, since this is an invasive procedure.
3. Tongs are usually used in conjunction with a specially designed bed or frame. Have the bed readily available for patient placement.
4. Insertion sites are in both temporal areas, usually 2 inches above the ears. The physician will indicate sites to be prepared.
5. The requirement for a signed consent form for invasive procedures varies among health care facilities. Refer to your hospital's policy manual.
6. Patient allergies should be determined prior to implementing the procedure.

NURSING ACTION/RATIONALE

1. Assemble all equipment.
2. Explain the procedure to the patient:
   a. Reinforce and clarify the physician's explanation of the procedure.
   b. Explain the effects of the local anesthetic.
   c. Explain the need for transfer to a specially designed bed or frame.
3. Obtain an informed consent, if required.
4. Provide privacy.
5. Provide adequate lighting.
6. Dress the patient in a hospital gown.
7. Obtain a baseline neurological assessment and baseline vital signs. Refer to the procedure "Neurological Assessment."
8. Wash your hands.
9. Prepare the insertion sites by cutting any hair and scrubbing with an antiseptic solution.
10. Open sterile supplies, using aseptic technique.
11. Assist the physician as required with insertion of the pins (Figure 7-2).

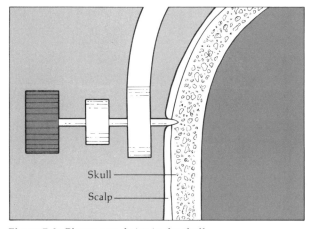

Figure 7-2. Placement of pins in the skull.

12. Assist the physician with pin care. The care and maintenance of the pins will be ordered by the physician. See the procedure "Skeletal Traction Pin Care."
13. Assist the physician and others with transfer of the patient to the special bed as indicated.
14. Assist the physician with traction rope placement.
15. Assess the weights and the patient's body position, making sure weights are hanging freely and the patient is in good body alignment.

16. Reassure the patient frequently.
17. Discard equipment or return it to the appropriate area. The wrenches should be displayed in an appropriate prominent location in the patient's room.
18. Assess vital signs, neurological signs, and other assessment parameters as indicated.

PATIENT AND/OR FAMILY TEACHING

1. Reinforce and clarify the physician's explanation of skeletal traction.
2. Inform and support the patient and family with factual information concerning:
   a. Purpose of skull tongs.
   b. Need for stabilization of the fracture.
   c. Correct body alignment.
   d. Need for continued assessment of the nervous system.
   e. Need for a special bed or frame.
3. Explain activity restrictions.
4. Reinforce the need to call the nurse when psychological support is needed or physical needs must be met.
5. Explain additional therapeutic orders as appropriate.

DOCUMENTATION

1. Time of procedure, local anesthetic used, duration of procedure, site of procedure, and name of physician performing procedure.
2. Use of any special bed or frame, traction used, and amount of weights.
3. The patient's tolerance of the procedure.
4. Assessment parameters of vital and neurological signs and any changes from the established baseline.
5. All patient teaching done and the patient's level of understanding.

Care of Skeletal Traction Pins _____

PURPOSE
1. Prevent complications by maintaining cleanliness of the skin at the pin site.

REQUISITES
1. Sterile suture kit containing:
   a. Forceps
   b. Scissors
2. Antiseptic swabs
3. Antiseptic gauze strips (optional)
4. Precut drain sponge—2
5. Sterile gloves
6. Sterile normal saline
7. Sterile 10 cc syringe
8. Needle (21 gauge)
9. Tape
10. Exam gloves
11. Waste receptacle

GUIDELINES
1. Skeletal traction pin care is done according to physician order or hospital policy. Verify prior to initiating the procedure.
2. Assess pin sites for edema, inflammation, and/or drainage, reporting any adverse findings to the physician.

NURSING ACTION/RATIONALE
1. Assemble all equipment.
2. Identify the patient.
3. Explain the procedure to the patient.
4. Wash your hands. Put on exam gloves.
5. Moisten old dressings with sterile saline, if necessary, before removal.
6. Remove old dressings and discard. Remove exam gloves.
7. Assess pin sites for drainage or inflammation.
8. Rewash your hands.
9. Prepare your supplies, using aseptic technique.
10. Cleanse around the sites with antiseptic swabs in a circular motion, moving from the pin site outward. Use one swab for each site. Discard swabs into the waste receptacle.
11. Apply sterile gloves.
12. If antiseptic gauze is ordered, apply a gauze strip (cut a 6- to 8-inch piece, using a sterile scissors) by winding it around the pin close to the skin (Figure 7-3).

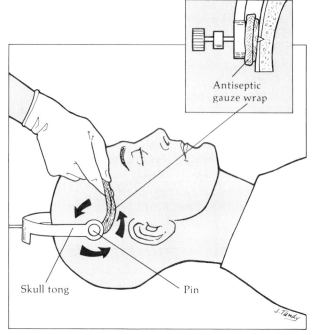

Figure 7-3. Application of antiseptic gauze strip.

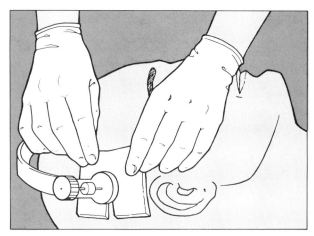

Figure 7-4. Application of precut drain sponge.

13. Slide precut drain sponge slit over the pin (Figure 7-4). Tape precut sponge to secure dressings.
14. Discard equipment and supplies or return them to the appropriate area. Reusable equipment must be labeled and used for the same patient.

PATIENT AND/OR FAMILY TEACHING

1. Explain the dressing change procedure and its purpose to the patient.
2. Reinforce the need to avoid touching the pin site and/or dressings.
3. Instruct the patient to notify the nurse if experiencing any unusual sensations at the pin sites.

DOCUMENTATION

1. Time and type of procedure done.
2. Condition of pin sites.
3. All patient teaching done and the patient's level of understanding.

Mechanical Turning Beds or Frames

PURPOSE

1. Minimize pressure on bony prominences.
2. Maintain immobility when necessary.
3. Decrease complications from immobility.

REQUISITES

1. Stryker CircOlectric bed with accessories (Figure 7-5) or
2. Roto-Rest Kinetic bed with accessories (Figure 7-6) or
3. Stryker Wedge frame with accessories (Figure 7-7)
4. Special bed linen for the bed used

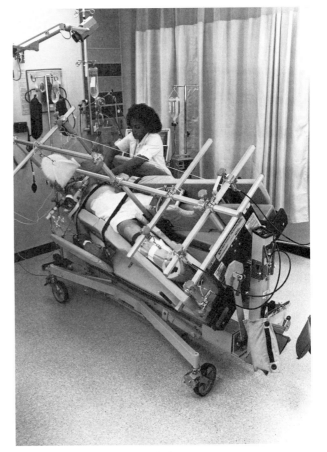

Figure 7-6. Roto-Rest Kinetic bed.

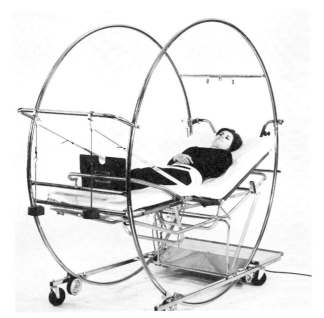

Figure 7-5. Stryker CircOlectric bed.

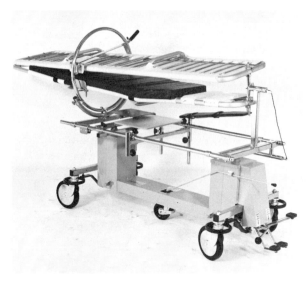

Figure 7-7. Stryker Wedge frame.

GUIDELINES

1. These special beds are used to provide immobile patients with the physiologic mobility needed to maintain functioning of all body systems.
2. The beds have application for a variety of patient problems including multiple fractures, extensive burns, paralysis, cardiovascular disease, spinal injuries, genitourinary problems, and most types of trauma.
3. The type of bed used will depend upon the needs of the patient, the physician's choice, the availability of the equipment, and the health care facility's policy. Besides the beds mentioned in Requisites, a number of other types of beds are available on the market.
4. Each bed operates differently. Any nurse caring for a patient on a special bed should thoroughly understand the operation, safety features, and capabilities of each bed.
5. Manufacturers supply operating manuals and inservice instruction to health care facilities who purchase or rent this equipment.
6. The operator's manual for the special bed should be kept with the bed at all times.
7. Because patients who need these beds usually have severe problems and because of the special turning features of these beds, the patient's anxiety level will be high. A competent, self-assured nurse who knows and understands the operation of the bed and recognizes the patient's anxiety can do much to lower the anxiety level.

8. Most of the beds are equipped so that one nurse can turn the patient and provide care unassisted. When possible, however, an assistant should be available to reassess safety bolts and straps before moving the patient. This will also help to decrease the patient's anxiety.
9. In addition to the mechanical bed, other supportive nursing measures should be provided for the patient, such as active or passive exercises. Consult with the physician before proceeding.
10. A physician's order is required to place a patient on any special bed.

NURSING ACTION/RATIONALE
Placing the Patient on the Special Bed

1. Verify the physician's order for the special bed.
2. Assemble all equipment.
3. Identify the patient.
4. Reinforce or clarify the physician's explanation for the use of the bed to the patient and/or family. Show the patient and/or family pictures of the bed and explain the major capabilities and safety features prior to transferring the patient to the bed.
5. Prepare the bed:
   a. Place the appropriate bed linen on the bed, securing the linen so it is wrinkle free.
   b. Assess all safety features and test the bed to ensure that it operates correctly.
6. Transfer the patient to the bed, using as many members of the health care team as is necessary to ensure patient safety. Position the patient in proper body alignment.
7. Assist the physician with the application of traction, if necessary.
8. Adjust any supports and safety straps, as necessary.
9. Assess all lines and tubes to ensure that they are free of kinks and are maintaining gravity flow, as appropriate.
10. Remain with the patient initially, provide reassurance, and answer all questions.
11. Place necessary equipment, including the call signal, within reach before leaving the patient's room.

Turning the Patient in the Special Bed

1. Verify the physician's order for turning.
2. Assemble all equipment.
3. Identify the patient.
4. Explain the procedure to the patient and reassure the patient as necessary.
5. Attach the frames and safety devices necessary for turning. Secure the assistance of a coworker to verify that all safety devices are secured.
6. Assess all drain tubes and intravenous lines to ensure correct positioning to prevent tension and kinking as the bed turns.
7. Inform the patient that you are going to start turning the bed. If patient cooperation is necessary, instruct the patient appropriately.
8. Turn the patient slowly and smoothly.
9. Readjust all safety features of the bed after turning.
10. Assess all tubes and lines as well as the position of the patient.
11. Assess the patient's skin condition and provide skin care as necessary.
12. Assess the patient's tolerance of the new position.
13. Place all necessary equipment, including the call signal, within the patient's reach, before leaving the patient's room.

PATIENT AND/OR FAMILY TEACHING

1. Reinforce and clarify the physician's explanation for the use of the bed.
2. Explain the bed capabilities and safety features prior to placing the patient on the bed.
3. Instruct the patient regarding any cooperation needed when turning.
4. Explain all procedures associated with the special bed prior to proceeding.
5. Explain activity restrictions.
6. Reinforce the need for the patient to call the nurse for assistance as necessary.
7. Explain other therapeutic or diagnostic orders as appropriate.

DOCUMENTATION

1. Time of patient transfer to bed and type of bed used.
2. Any accessory equipment attached, such as traction.
3. The patient's reaction and adjustment to the bed.
4. Time and position when turned and the patient's tolerance.
5. Safety features used, such as restraining straps.
6. An assessment of the patient's skin condition when turned, and any other appropriate assessment parameters.
7. All patient teaching done and the patient's level of understanding.

Assisting the Physician with a Cast Application

PURPOSE

1. Assist the physician with applying a cast and holding and positioning the body area.
2. Provide nursing support for the patient during the application of a cast.

REQUISITES

1. Plaster bandage
2. Stockinette
3. Casting tape
4. Exam gloves
5. Sheet wadding
6. Heavy felt or foam rubber
7. Moleskin adhesive
8. Plastic apron
9. Protective drapes
10. Walking heel (optional)
11. Cast knife
12. Cast bender
13. Large bandage scissors
14. Bucket
15. Plastic bag liners
16. Water and soap
17. Washcloth and towel

GUIDELINES

1. The purposes of cast applications are to:
   a. Keep fracture fragments aligned.
   b. Immobilize body parts that have been surgically reconstructed.
   c. Provide rest and support to injured or weakened extremities.
   d. Aid in nonsurgical correction of deformities.
   e. Provide rest and promote healing to a diseased bone or joint.
2. Nursing personnel should become familiar with the various casting materials the physician will be using and should assemble equipment as requested.
3. To add strength to the cast, plaster-impregnated gauze splints are sometimes used during application.
4. Thoroughly inspect the affected area before the cast application and if necessary cleanse the skin and dry thoroughly.
5. The affected body area may have to be positioned and held during the cast application. An assistant will be required if this is necessary.
6. An analgesic for the patient may be ordered by the physician prior to the cast application. Safety precautions should be considered.
7. A walking heel may be added to a leg cast if the patient will be allowed weight bearing on the cast at a later time.
8. Traditional plaster casts require up to 48 hours to dry. Care must be taken not to dent or bend the cast during the drying period. Plaster casts should be exposed to the air during the drying period.
9. New lightweight fiberglass casts require only 5 to 10 minutes to dry and facilitate increased activity levels more quickly.
10. Following cast applications to extremities, the extremity should be kept elevated, and ice bags should be applied to the affected site to control or prevent edema.

NURSING ACTION/RATIONALE

1. Assemble all equipment.
2. Identify the patient.
3. Reinforce and clarify the physician's explanation of the cast application including the reason for the cast, the position required, any medication available for pain, and any sensations of heat that may be experienced.
4. Obtain an informed consent for the procedure, if necessary.
5. Provide privacy.
6. Provide adequate lighting.
7. Protect the patient's clothing with a protective drape, or dress the patient in a hospital gown.
8. Wash the involved skin area and dry thoroughly if necessary.
9. Cleanse any open wounds and apply sterile dressings, using aseptic technique.
10. Inspect the patient's skin for irritation or redness.

11. Assess the need for an analgesic prior to the cast application.
12. Arrange the cast application materials in a convenient location for the physician.
13. Assist the physician with positioning the body area and the cast application as requested.
14. Elevate the wet extremity cast on a protected covered pillow. Keep the heel of the lower extremity cast off of the mattress until the cast has dried.
15. Remove any plaster from the patient's skin with a damp washcloth.
16. Apply ice bags to the affected site if swelling is anticipated at the trauma site.
17. Refer to the procedure "General Care of a Patient with an Extremity Cast."
18. Assist the patient to a comfortable position.
19. Place the call signal within reach.
20. Discard equipment or return it to the appropriate area.

PATIENT AND/OR FAMILY TEACHING

1. Reinforce and clarify the physician's explanation of the purpose for the cast, the position required, analgesics available, and any sensations that may be experienced.
2. Explain that the cast will feel warm following application because of the chemical reaction of the plaster and water.
3. Instruct the patient to inform the physician or nurse if severe pain is experienced during or following the cast application.

4. Instruct the patient to report any numbness or tingling in the affected body area.
5. Instruct the patient to keep the extremity elevated, if appropriate.
6. Explain that the cast must dry thoroughly before any pressure can be exerted on it.
7. Warn the patient to avoid:
   a. Getting the cast wet.
   b. Scratching inside the cast with sharp objects.
   c. Trimming or removing the cast.
8. Provide crutch-walking instructions, if appropriate.
9. Demonstrate any prescribed exercises and provide the opportunity for a return demonstration.

DOCUMENTATION

1. Type of cast applied and location.
2. Name of physician applying cast.
3. The patient's reaction to the procedure, any untoward reactions, and action taken.
4. Assessment of body area before and after cast application.
5. Any medications given.
6. Position of affected body area.
7. Condition of cast.
8. All patient teaching done and the patient's level of understanding.

General Care
of a Patient with an Extremity Cast

PURPOSE
1. Maintain the integrity of the cast.
2. Maintain proper circulation, sensation, and motion of the affected body part.
3. Maintain immobilization of the affected body part.

REQUISITES
1. Pillows protected by plastic covers or cast elevator aids
2. Moleskin tape

GUIDELINES
1. When a cast is initially applied, it will dry more quickly when exposed to the air.
2. Plaster casts dry from the inside to the outside and radiate heat until dry.
3. A moist cast needs to be handled with the palms of the hands to prevent indentations from fingers.
4. Plaster casts are somewhat porous and allow some air circulation to the skin underneath. Patients should be discouraged from decorating their casts with materials that would decrease the porosity of the cast.
5. To encourage venous return and reduce swelling, a casted extremity should be elevated above heart level.
6. Range-of-motion exercises are necessary for a patient limited to bedrest or whose activity is greatly reduced. See "Therapeutic Exercise and Positioning" procedure.
7. Any complaints of pain or irritation on the casted extremity should be investigated thoroughly for early identification of complications.
8. In cases of circulatory impairment, the physician may cut or remove the cast to increase the blood supply and to prevent irreversible damage to the extremity.
9. Depending on the type and location of the fracture, weight bearing may be restricted. Consult with the physician.

NURSING ACTION/RATIONALE
1. Explain to the patient the general care and precautions necessary for a cast.
2. Support and position the wet casted extremity in proper body alignment (Figure 7-8). Avoid uneven pressure on the wet cast. Reposition the patient every 30 minutes to promote even drying of the cast. Keep the casted extremity elevated.

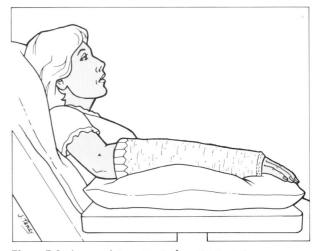

Figure 7-8. Appropriate support of a wet arm cast.

3. Assess the fingers or toes of the casted extremity every hour for the first 24 hours or until stable, then continue assessing every 4 hours. Assess and report any signs of decreased circulation or movement. They are:
   a. Change in the rate of capillary refill (Figure 7-9).
   b. Change in the color of the extremity to pale or cyanotic.
   c. Change in the skin temperature, either cooler or warmer.
   d. Increase in swelling.
   e. Numbness and tingling.
   f. Increase in pain or pressure.
   g. Decrease in movement (Figure 7-10).

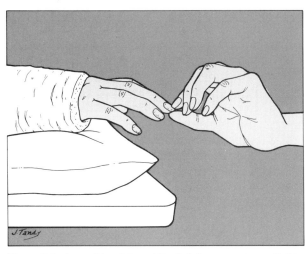

Figure 7-9. Assess blanching. After brief pressure is applied to the nailbed, the normal color should return rapidly.

4. Assess the casted extremity for signs of infection and report the following symptoms:
   a. Foul-smelling cast with or without drainage.
   b. Elevation in skin temperature.
   c. Increase in pain or pressure.
5. Assess any increase in drainage on the cast. Drainage is usually expected on a cast that covers an open wound. Outline drainage areas at least every 8 hours and mark with the date and time. Report any excessive increase in drainage or change in color or odor of the drainage.
6. Observe the cast for indentations, cracks, or weakened areas that may cause areas of pressure on the underlying extremity. Keep the cast clean and dry.

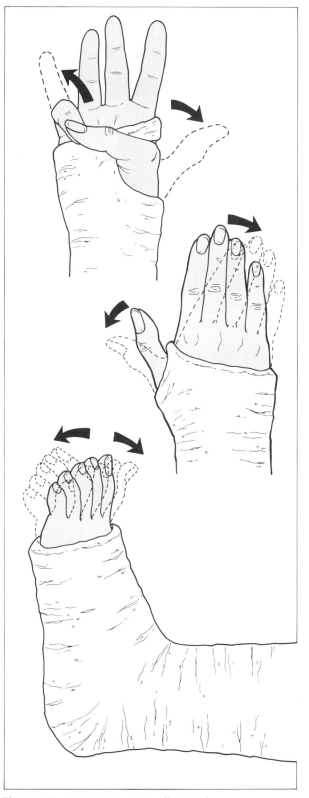

Figure 7-10. Assess movement as illustrated.

7. Inspect the skin integrity around the edges of the cast. Keep the skin clean and dry. If the cast has rough edges, apply moleskin tape in a "petaling" fashion (Figure 7-11).

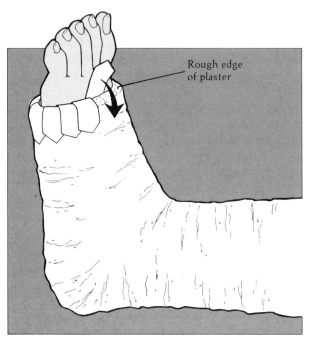

Rough edge of plaster

Figure 7-11. Applying moleskin tape to cast edges, slightly overlapping each piece.

8. Assist the patient with a heavy cast as necessary in moving and repositioning.
9. Encourage the patient to move the fingers or toes of the affected extremity frequently. This will increase the circulation to the extremity.
10. Assist the patient as necessary with activities of daily living.

PATIENT AND/OR FAMILY TEACHING

1. Reinforce and clarify the physician's explanation of the reason for the cast.
2. Instruct the patient concerning general cast care. Include:
   a. Precautions with a wet cast.
   b. Importance of keeping the cast clean and dry.
   c. Importance of not putting objects under the cast for scratching purposes.
   d. Any activity restrictions necessary.
   e. Keeping the extremity elevated.
   f. Importance of not damaging or removing the cast.
   g. Signs and symptoms of circulatory impairment.
3. Instruct the patient to notify the nurse for assistance with repositioning or ambulating, if allowed.
4. Instruct the patient to notify the nurse of any of the following symptoms:
   a. Increase in pain in the extremity.
   b. Pressure areas under the cast.
   c. Tingling or numbness.
   d. Swelling in the extremity.
   e. Decrease in movement of the extremity.
5. Teach the patient active exercises of the extremity as appropriate.
6. Assist with planning of home care as necessary.

DOCUMENTATION

1. All assessment parameters monitored.
2. Any complications, action taken, and results.
3. Any patient teaching done and the patient's level of understanding.

Assisting the Physician with a Cast Removal

PURPOSE
1. Assist the physician with removing a cast.
2. Provide nursing support for the patient during the removal of a cast.

REQUISITES
1. Cast cutter or saw
2. Cast spreader
3. Large bandage scissors
4. Lubricating skin oil
5. Warm water
6. Washcloth
7. Towel
8. Soap

GUIDELINES
1. Casts are most often removed by the physician following x-ray confirmation that the affected area has healed or before reapplication of another cast.
2. During cast removal the patient must be reassured that the cast cutter will not damage the skin.
3. Following cast removal, the affected area will not have normal function and mobility. Patients must be made aware of this and the rehabilitation process that is necessary to regain normal function.
4. Removal of dead skin that has accumulated under the cast may require softening with oil and/or soaking in warm water. This should be a gradual process to avoid skin irritation.

NURSING ACTION/RATIONALE
1. Assemble all equipment.
2. Identify the patient.
3. Reinforce and clarify the physician's explanation of the cast removal.
4. Reassure the patient that the cast cutter will not cut the skin. Demonstrate how it sounds and what it looks like.
5. Obtain an informed consent for the procedure, if necessary.
6. Provide privacy.
7. Provide adequate lighting.
8. Position the patient as required.
9. Protect the patient's clothing with a protective drape.
10. Wash your hands.
11. Arrange the cast removal equipment in a convenient location for the physician.
12. Assist the physician with the cast removal as required.
13. Assess the skin integrity and circulation of the affected area.
14. Wash the skin gently with soap and water, removing as much dead skin as possible. Pat dry.
15. Apply lubricating oil, if appropriate.
16. Assist the patient to a comfortable position.
17. Discard equipment or return it to the appropriate location.

PATIENT AND/OR FAMILY TEACHING
1. Explain what the patient is to expect when the physician removes the cast.
2. Explain and instruct the patient how to:
   a. Support the extremity.
   b. Maneuver the extremity.
   c. Care for the skin properly.
   d. Perform therapeutic exercises.
   e. Prevent dependent edema.
   f. Adjust to weakness.
   g. Relieve discomfort.
3. Caution the patient against scratching or vigorously rubbing the affected area.
4. Instruct the patient to notify the physician if any problems are experienced following discharge.
5. Provide crutch-walking instructions, if appropriate.
6. Encourage the patient to follow the physician's plan of care, including physician's office appointments.

DOCUMENTATION
1. Procedure and name of physician performing procedure.
2. The patient's reaction to the procedure.
3. All assessments, including skin condition and circulation in the area.
4. Treatment given to skin.
5. All patient teaching done and the patient's level of understanding.

Wrapping an Amputation

PURPOSE
1. Promote shrinkage of the stump area by minimizing edema and supporting the tissue.
2. Prepare the stump for an artificial extremity.

REQUISITES
1. Elastic roller bandage with clips
2. Dressings, as required
3. Tape

GUIDELINES
1. Amputations are performed for a variety of clinical problems including vascular disease, trauma, infectious processes, and carcinomas.
2. Immediate postoperative care following an amputation must include careful monitoring. Refer to the procedure "Postoperative Care."
3. Initially the physician will perform the stump dressing changes and apply the elastic roller bandage.
4. Stump bandaging should be done with the patient in a recumbent position and the stump area hyperextended.
5. Firm tension should be maintained on the stump at all times. The elastic bandage should be reapplied if any loosening occurs.
6. Care must be taken to apply the elastic bandage firmly without compromising circulation to the stump area.
7. The stump should be assessed frequently for redness, edema, color, sensation, and skin irritation.
8. Shaping and shrinking the stump is essential for measuring and fitting a comfortable prosthesis.

9. A second elastic bandage should be available to allow for washing and drying of soiled bandages.
10. Physical therapy exercises may be prescribed for the patient to prevent contractures and to promote physical strength in preparation for a prosthesis.

NURSING ACTION/RATIONALE
1. Assemble all equipment.
2. Identify the patient.
3. Explain the procedure to the patient, including the necessary positioning of the stump.
4. Provide privacy.
5. Assist the patient to a recumbent position with the stump hyperextended.
6. Wash your hands.
7. Remove the elastic roller bandage and rewind.
8. Inspect the stump area and change the dressing, if appropriate. Refer to the procedure "Sterile Dressing Change."
9. Reapply the elastic bandage smoothly using firm, even pressure (Figure 7-12):
   a. Anchor the bandage using a vertical recurrent turn over the anterior and posterior stump areas.
   b. Anchor the recurrent turns with several oblique turns toward the distal end of the stump.
   c. Reverse the direction of the oblique turns and wrap the bandage proximally.
   d. Anchor the elastic bandage around the waist area and clip or tape the end to a portion of the elastic bandage.

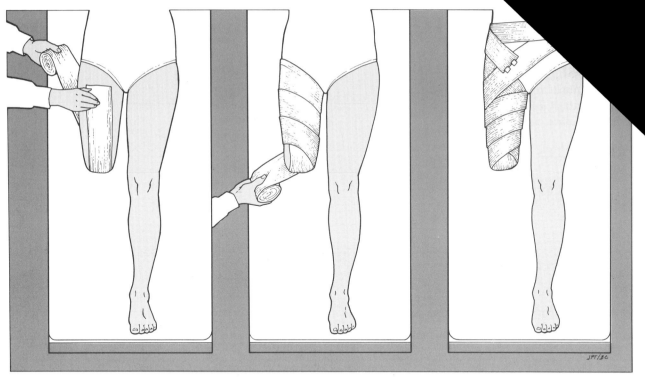

Figure 7-12. Applying an elastic bandage to an above-the-knee amputation.

10. Assess the bandage for smoothness and correct tension.
11. Assist the patient to a comfortable position.
12. Discard equipment or return it to the appropriate location.

PATIENT AND/OR FAMILY TEACHING

1. Explain the procedure and its purpose to the patient.
2. Instruct the patient to inform the nurse if the elastic bandage becomes loose or if pain is experienced in the stump area.
3. Teach the patient appropriate range-of-motion exercises for the extremity.
4. Teach the patient or family the procedure for applying the elastic bandage if wrapping will continue following hospital discharge.

DOCUMENTATION

1. Time of procedure and type of elastic bandage applied.
2. Assessment of stump area, including skin condition.
3. Any exercises performed with extremity.
4. The patient's reaction to the procedure.
5. All patient or family teaching done and the level of understanding.

apeutic

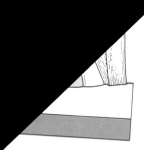

...le strength.

GUIDELINES

1. There are two basic types of range-of-motion exercises:
   a. *Passive exercise*—an exercise carried out for the patient by the nurse without participation of the patient.
   b. *Active exercise*—an exercise carried out by the patient with the assistance and supervision of the nurse.
2. Passive exercises are generally performed on:
   a. Semiconscious and unconscious patients.
   b. Elderly patients with limited mobility.
   c. Patients on complete bedrest.
   d. Patients with complete paralysis of extremities.
3. Active exercises are generally performed on:
   a. Patients with partially paralyzed extremities.
   b. Patients on bedrest unless contraindicated.
   c. Early postoperative patients unless contraindicated.
4. Definitions of range-of-motion terms are:
   a. *Flexion*—bending the various joints.
   b. *Extension*—straightening of the various joints.
   c. *Adduction*—movement of a limb toward the body's center.
   d. *Abduction*—movement of a limb away from the body's center.
   e. *Rotation*—turning or moving of a part around its axis.
   f. *Pronation*—turning downward.
   g. *Supination*—turning upward.
   h. *Inversion*—turning inward.
   i. *Eversion*—turning outward.
5. Range-of-motion exercises should be repeated approximately 7 to 10 times and done at least twice each day. Proceed slowly and carefully. Caution should be taken to not overtire the patient.

6. When planning an exercise program, consider the patient's age, diagnosis, vital signs, and duration of bedrest restriction. The physician should be consulted before a program of exercise is implemented.
7. Combinations of exercises are often prescribed by a physician and done by a physical therapist. Such exercises are:
   a. *Resistive-active:* an active exercise performed by the patient while working against a manual or a mechanical resistance for the purpose of increasing muscle strength.
   b. *Isometric–muscle setting:* the patient contracts and relaxes the muscle as much as possible without moving the joint for the purpose of maintaining strength.
8. Parts of the body on which range-of-motion exercises can be performed include the neck, fingers, wrist, forearm, elbow, shoulder, toes, foot, ankle, knee, hip, and trunk.
9. Therapeutic exercises may be performed on all body joints or only on those affected by a disease process.
10. Suggested appropriate times to perform exercises on the patient are during bath time and with evening cares.

NURSING ACTION/RATIONALE

1. Assess the patient and plan an exercise program suitable for the patient.
2. Explain the procedure to the patient, including the areas to be exercised and the role of the patient, if appropriate.
3. Provide privacy.
4. Provide suitable clothing to prevent restriction of movement.
5. Remove bed linen as appropriate.
6. Instruct the patient to lie in a comfortable supine position.
7. Perform the exercises or assist the patient to perform the exercises:

Flexion and Extension of the Wrist (Figure 7-13)
   a. Position the patient's arm out from the side of the body with the elbow bent and the hand pointed toward the ceiling.

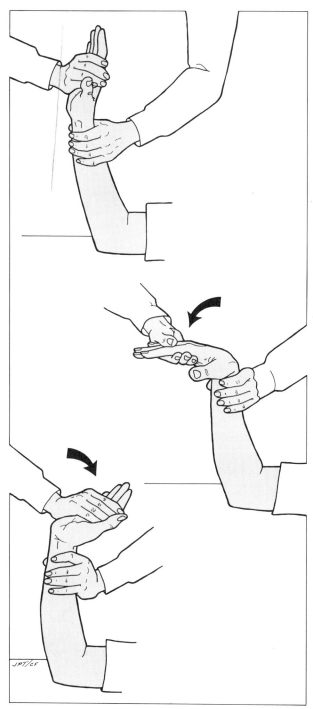

Figure 7-13. Flexion and extension of the wrist.

b. Hold the patient's hand with one hand and the wrist with your other hand.

c. Bend the patient's wrist forward as far as possible.

d. Bend the patient's wrist back as far as possible.

Flexion and Extension of the Elbow (Figure 7-14)

a. Position the patient's arm out from the side of the body with the palm of the patient's hand turned toward his or her body.

b. Place one hand above the patient's elbow and grasp the patient's hand with your other hand.

c. Bend the patient's elbow so that the hand is brought as close as possible to the shoulder.

d. Return to the starting position.

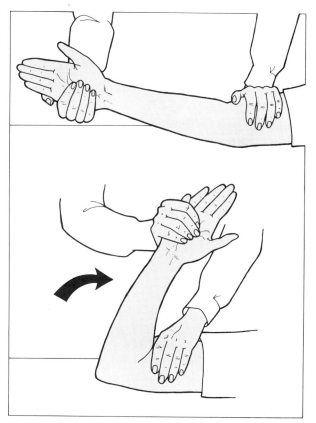

Figure 7-14. Flexion and extension of the elbow.

Pronation and Supination of the Forearm (Figure 7-15)

a. Position the patient's forearm away from the body with the elbow bent.

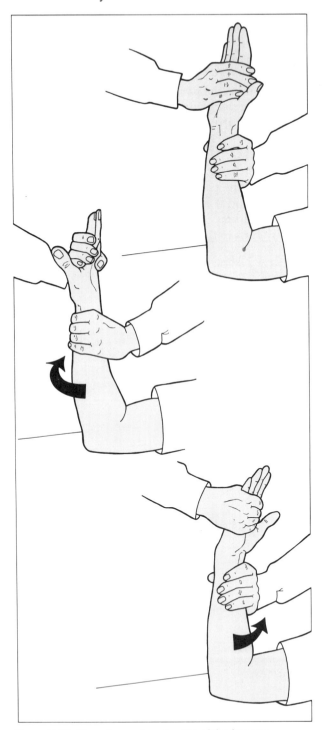

Figure 7-15. Pronation and supination of the forearm.

b. Place one hand on the patient's wrist and grasp the patient's hand with your other hand.

c. Turn the patient's forearm so that the palm faces away from the patient.

d. Return to the starting position.

e. Turn the patient's forearm so that the palm faces the patient.

f. Return to the starting position.

Flexion of the Shoulder (Figure 7-16)

a. Position the patient's arm next to the body.

b. Place one hand above the patient's elbow and hold the patient's hand with your other hand.

c. Lift the patient's arm straight into the air.

d. Return the arm to the starting position.

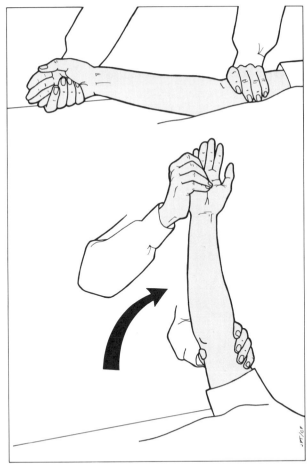

Figure 7-16. Flexion of the shoulder.

Abduction and Adduction of the Shoulder (Figure 7-17)

a. Position the patient's arm next to the body.
b. Place one hand above the patient's elbow and grasp the patient's hand with your other hand.
c. Move the patient's arm away from the body and toward you.
d. Return to the starting position.

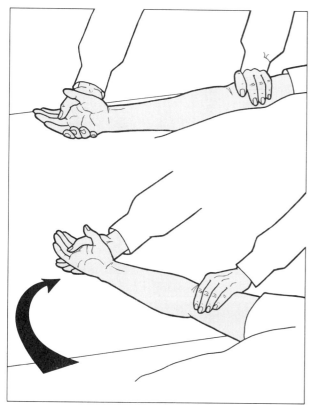

Figure 7-17. Abduction and adduction of the shoulder.

Rotation of the Shoulder (Figure 7-18)

a. Position the patient's arm out from the side of the body with the elbow bent.
b. Place one hand on the patient's upper arm near the elbow and grasp the patient's hand with your other hand.

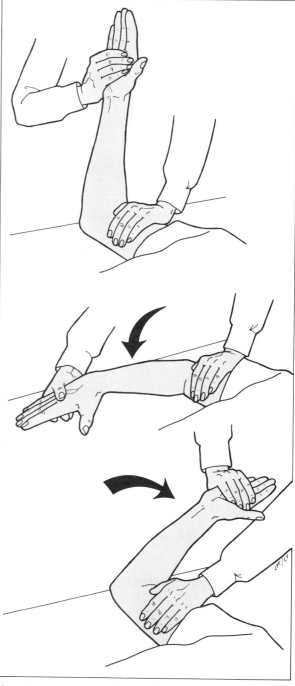

Figure 7-18. Rotation of the shoulder.

c. Move the forearm down until it rests on the bed, palm side down.

d. Return the arm to the starting position.

e. Move the forearm back until it rests on the bed, palm side up.

f. Return to the starting position.

Flexion and Extension of the Toes (Figure 7-19)

a. Grasp the patient's toes with one hand while holding the patient's foot firmly with your other hand.

b. Curl the toes down.

c. Straighten the toes and gently stretch them back.

d. Return to the starting position.

Inversion and Eversion of the Foot (Figure 7-20)

a. Grasp the top half of the patient's foot with one hand and grasp the ankle firmly with your other hand.

b. Turn the foot inward so that the sole faces toward the other foot.

c. Return to the starting position.

d. Turn the foot outward so the sole faces away from the other foot.

e. Return to the starting position.

Flexion and Extension of the Ankle (Figure 7-21)

a. Place one hand on the ball of patient's foot and one hand above the ankle. Keep the leg straight and the foot relaxed.

b. Bend the ankle, pointing the toes toward the patient's chest.

c. Return to the starting position.

d. Bend the ankle, pointing the toes away from the chest.

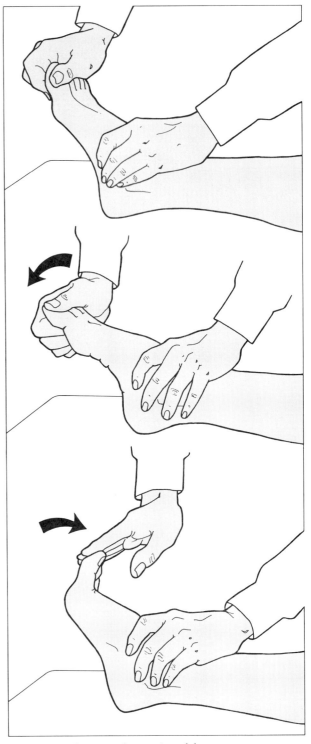

Figure 7-19. Flexion and extension of the toes.

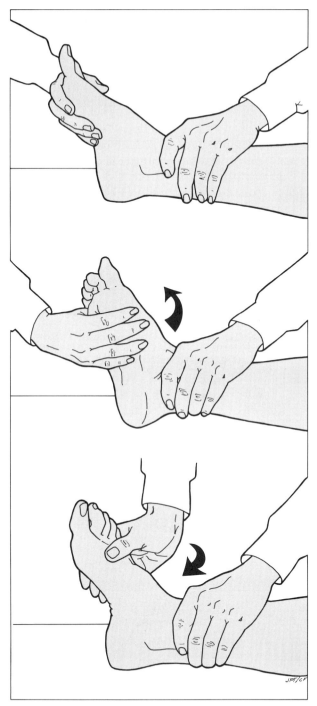

Figure 7-20. Inversion and eversion of the foot.

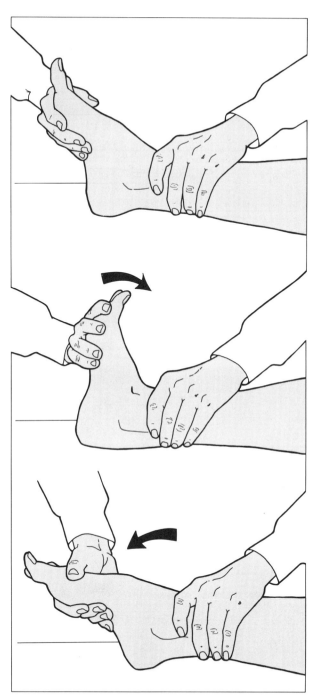

Figure 7-21. Flexion and extension of the ankle.

Flexion and Extension of the Knee (Figure 7-22)

a. Place one hand under the patient's knee and cup the heel in your other hand.

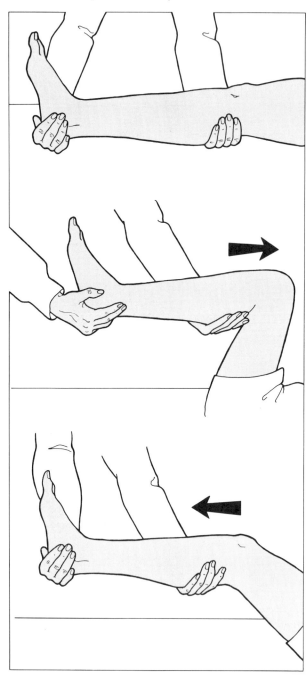

Figure 7-22. Flexion and extension of the knee.

b. Lift the leg, bending it at the knee and hip.
c. Continue to bend the knee toward the chest as far as it will go.
d. Lower the leg and straighten the knee by lifting the foot upward.
e. Return to the starting position.

Rotation of the Hip (Figure 7-23)

a. Place one hand above the patient's ankle and your other hand just above the knee.
b. Roll the leg away from you.
c. Roll the leg toward you.
d. Return to the starting position.

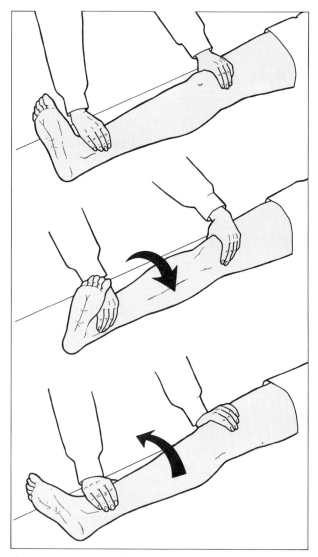

Figure 7-23. Rotation of the hip.

Abduction and Adduction of the Hip (Figure 7-24)

a. Place one hand under the patient's knee and cup the heel in your other hand.

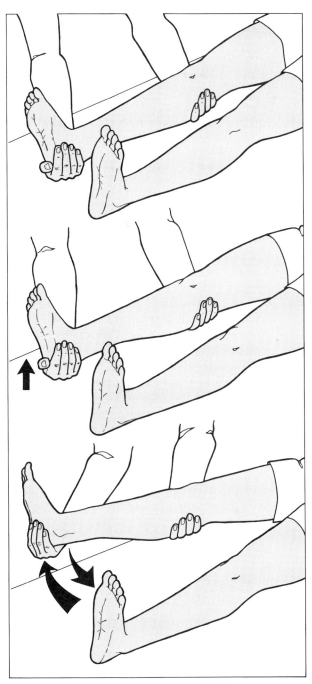

Figure 7-24. Abduction and adduction of the hip.

b. Keeping the patient's knee straight, lift the leg until the heel is about 4 inches from the bed.

c. Bring the leg toward you.

d. Move the leg away from you.

e. Return to the starting position.

8. Assess the patient for the effect of the exercise.

9. Place the patient in a comfortable position.

10. Replace the bed linens.

PATIENT AND/OR FAMILY TEACHING

1. Involve the patient and/or family in planning and implementing an exercise program.

2. Involve family members and teach them range-of-motion exercises by allowing them to observe and practice the exercises.

3. Assist the family in understanding their important role in the rehabilitation process.

4. Encourage the patient to practice the exercises as the disease process permits.

DOCUMENTATION

1. Degree of range of motion in each area exercised.

2. The patient's response to the exercises.

3. Any assessment parameters including pain, weakness, or change in vital signs.

4. Any patient and/or family teaching done, and the level of understanding and return demonstration techniques.

Positioning and Transferring the Patient

PURPOSE
1. Promote comfort.
2. Maintain good body alignment.
3. Decrease the complications related to immobility.
4. Decrease the possibility of injury to the patient and/or the nurse.

REQUISITES
1. Pillows (large and small)
2. Footboard
3. Drawsheet
4. Stretcher
5. Wheelchair
6. Bathrobe
7. Slippers
8. Blankets

GUIDELINES
1. One of the most successful nursing measures for preventing complications in the immobile patient is frequent changes in position.
2. Any patient confined to bed should be repositioned at least every 2 hours unless contraindicated.
3. The patient's body should always be in good alignment to prevent strain and contractures.
4. Additional supportive devices, such as splints or braces may be required to maintain correct body alignment in the comatose or paralyzed patient.
5. The linen on the patient's bed should always be clean, smooth, and dry.
6. The schedule for repositioning the patient should be planned with the patient whenever possible. Analgesics can be given in advance of the scheduled repositioning if moving is a painful experience for the patient.
7. Moving a patient with injuries or pain can cause anxiety. The procedure should be done carefully while providing support and reassurance to the patient.
8. When appropriate the patient should assist with the move. This will provide the patient with some control, independence, and exercise.
9. To prevent accidents or injuries, the wheels of the bed, stretcher, and/or wheelchair must always be locked when transferring a patient.
10. Good body mechanics should be used when moving or lifting a patient. The principles of good body mechanics are:
    a. Stand close to the patient.
    b. Keep your back straight.
    c. Tighten your abdominal and pelvic muscles.
    d. Utilize the muscles of your thighs when lifting.
11. Depending on the patient's condition, the patient can be placed in a variety of positions in bed. Some of the positions that can be utilized are:
    a. *Supine position* (Figure 7-25). The patient is positioned on his or her back. The spine and legs should be straight. The patient's arms are at his or her side with the hands prone. A pillow under the head and shoulders prevents hyperextension and flexion of the neck. A footboard can be used to maintain the feet at right angles to the legs to prevent plantar flexion.
    b. *Fowler's position* (Figure 7-26). The patient lies in the supine position with his or her head near the top of the bed. The head of the bed is elevated 45 degrees (90 degrees for high-Fowler's and 30 degrees for semi-Fowler's). The knee gatch is raised slightly unless contraindicated. A footboard can be used to maintain the feet at right angles to the legs. Pillows can be placed for support as needed:
       (1) Behind the shoulders and head to prevent flexion and hyperextension of the neck.
       (2) Behind the lower back to prevent posterior convexity of the lumbar spine region.
       (3) Under the thighs to prevent hyperextension of the knees.
    c. *Prone position* (Figure 7-27). The patient is placed on his or her abdomen with the head to one side and the arms flexed toward the shoulders. A pillow is placed under the patient's head to prevent hyperextension and flexion of the neck.

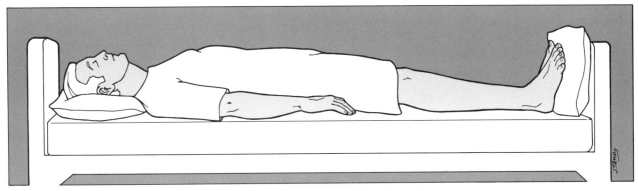

Figure 7-25. Supine position.

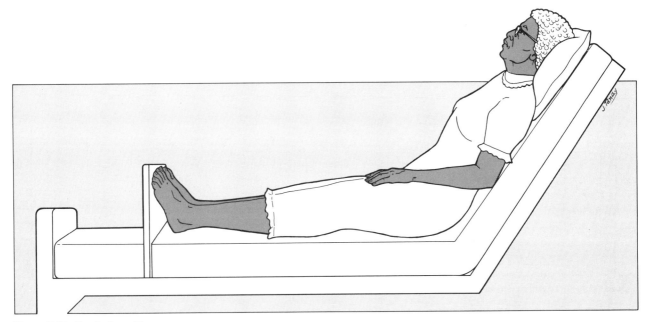

Figure 7-26. Fowler's position.

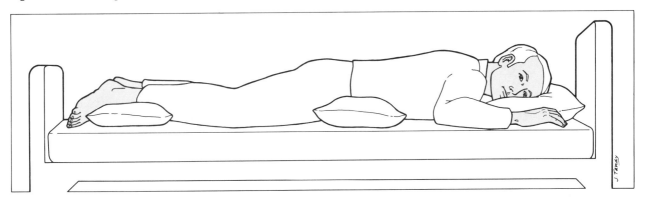

Figure 7-27. Prone position.

A small pillow under the ankles prevents plantar flexion and a pillow under the abdomen provides comfort and prevents hyperextension of the lower spine.

d. *Side-lying position* (Figure 7-28). The patient is placed on his or her right or left side with the arms to the front. The underlying arm is flexed toward the head alongside or on the pillow. A pillow under the head and shoulders supports the sternocleidomastoid muscles. A pillow under the upper arm prevents adduction of the arm and internal rotation of the shoulder. The upper leg is flexed slightly with a pillow under it for support. This prevents adduction and internal rotation of the thigh.

e. *Sim's position* (Figure 7-29). The patient is placed on the right or left side with the lower arm behind him or her and the upper arm flexed toward the shoulder. The upper leg is flexed slightly more than the lower leg and a pillow is placed under the upper leg. A pillow under the head prevents flexion and hyperextension of the neck.

NURSING ACTION/RATIONALE

1. Assemble all equipment.
2. Identify the patient.
3. Explain the repositioning or transferring procedure to the patient. Explain to the patient any active or passive participation that will be necessary.

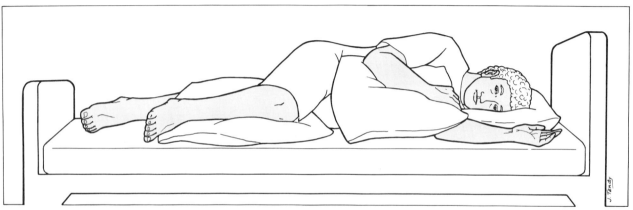

Figure 7-28. Side-lying position.

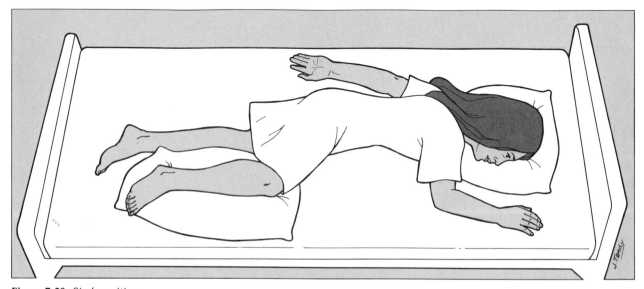

Figure 7-29. Sim's position.

4. Request assistance from other personnel if necessary.
5. Provide adequate lighting.
6. Provide privacy.
7. Wash your hands.
8. Remove any pillows or supports from the bed.
9. Raise the bed to a comfortable height.
10. Lower the siderail on the side of the bed on which you will be working.
11. Move the patient in bed as necessary, using one of the following methods or a combination of methods:
   a. *Moving the patient to the side of the bed.* This movement is used when changing bed linen, when positioning a patient for a procedure, or in preparation for dangling a patient (Figure 7-30).
      (1) Place the bed in a flat position.
      (2) Position yourself close to and facing the side of the bed.
      (3) Stand with your feet apart and your knees flexed to provide a solid base.
      (4) Place the patient's arm closest to you across the patient's chest.
      (5) Place one of your arms under the patient's shoulder, supporting the patient's head and neck.
      (6) Place your other arm under the patient's lower spine (Figure 7-30a).
      (7) Pull the upper part of the patient's body toward you by rocking backward onto your heels.
      (8) Place one arm under the patient's waist and the other arm under his or her thighs. Move the buttocks toward you in the same manner (Figure 7-30b).
      (9) Place one arm under the patient's thighs and the other arm under the patient's calves. Move the patient's legs and feet toward you in the same manner (Figure 7-30c).

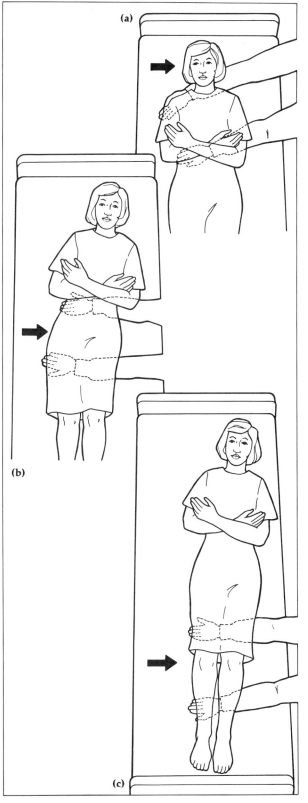

Figure 7-30. Repositioning the patient to the side of the bed.

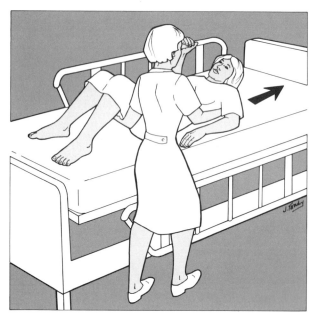

Figure 7-31. Repositioning the patient up in bed with the patient assisting.

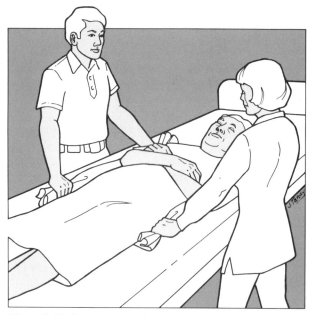

Figure 7-32. Repositioning the patient up in bed with the assistance of two nurses.

b. *Repositioning the patient up in bed with the patient assisting.* This movement is usually used to promote comfort and to place the body in good alignment (Figure 7-31).

   (1) Instruct or assist the patient to flex his or her knees, place the feet flat on the bed, and grasp the siderail closest to his or her shoulder on the far side of the bed.

   (2) Position yourself with your feet apart and your knees flexed close to the side of the bed.

   (3) Place one arm under the patient's shoulder and the other under the patient's thighs.

   (4) Instruct the patient that on the count of three you will both move simultaneously.

   (5) Pull the patient up in bed on the count of three by rocking forward on your front leg.

c. *Repositioning the patient up in bed using two nurses.* This movement is used for a patient who is obese or unable to assist (Figure 7-32).

   (1) Place a drawsheet under the patient, extending from the shoulders to the buttocks.

   (2) Stand on each side of the bed with both siderails down and the bed flat.

   (3) Fold the patient's arms across the patient's chest.

   (4) Position yourselves with your feet apart and your knees flexed close to the side of the bed.

   (5) Roll up the drawsheet close to the patient's side, grasping it near the patient's shoulders and the buttocks.

   (6) Move the patient up in bed by sliding the drawsheet toward the head of the bed while rocking forward onto the balls of your feet.

d. *Turning a patient from a supine to a side-lying position* (Figure 7-33).

   (1) Move the patient to the side of the bed so that the side of the body that he or she is to lie on is nearest the center of the bed.

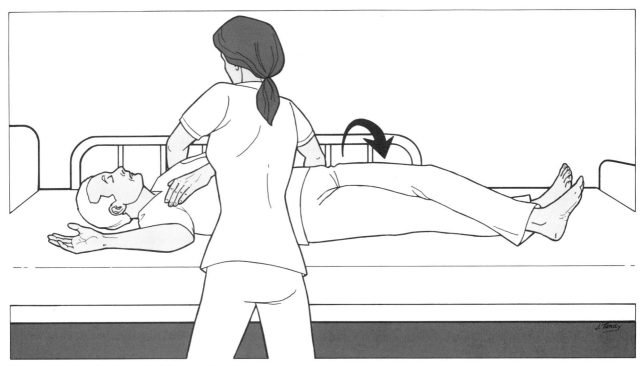

Figure 7-33. Turning the patient from back to side.

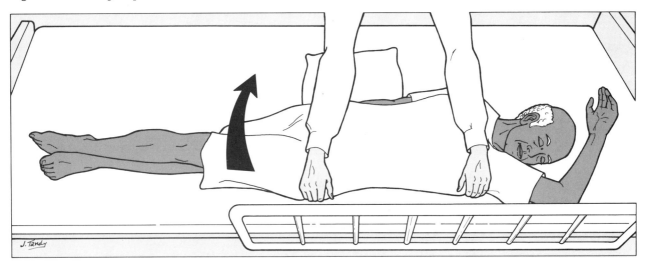

Figure 7-34. Turning the patient from back to abdomen.

(2) Raise the siderail on that side of the bed.

(3) Move to the other side of the bed and lower the siderail on that side.

(4) Position yourself with your feet apart and your knees flexed close to the side of the bed.

(5) Position the patient's near arm toward you.

(6) Place the patient's far arm across the patient's chest.

(7) Grasp the patient's far shoulder and hip.

(8) Roll the patient toward you and place the necessary pillows for support.

e. *Turning the patient from a supine to a prone position* (Figure 7-34).

(1) Follow the steps for moving a patient to the side of the bed.

(2) Raise the siderail on that side and move to the other side of the bed. Lower the siderail on that side.

(3) Position yourself with your feet apart and your knees flexed close to the side of the bed.

(4) Place the abdominal support pillow, if appropriate, on the bed so the patient can be rolled onto it (Figure 7-27).

(5) Place the patient's far arm over the patient's head and the near arm alongside his or her body. Turn the patient's face away from you.

(6) Grasp the patient's far shoulder and hip.

(7) Roll the patient on his or her side while rocking backward onto your heels.

(8) Roll the patient onto his or her abdomen by means of the same motion.

(9) Place the necessary pillows required for support and adjust the patient's position as necessary.

f. *Logrolling the patient.* This movement is used when straight body alignment must be maintained. Two nurses are required and three may be necessary for an obese patient (Figure 7-35).

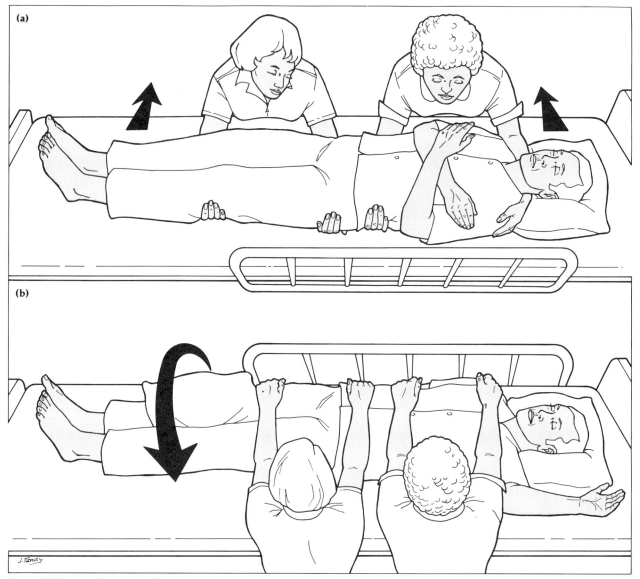

Figure 7-35. Logrolling the patient.

(1) Position yourselves with your feet apart and your knees flexed close to the side of the bed.

(2) Fold the patient's arms across the patient's chest.

(3) Place your arms under the patient so that a major portion of the patient's weight is centered between your arms. The arm of one nurse should support the patient's head and neck (Figure 7-35a).

(4) On the count of three, move the patient to the side of the bed, rocking backward onto your heels and keeping the patient's body in correct alignment.

(5) Raise the siderail on that side of the bed.

(6) Move to the other side of the bed.

(7) Place a pillow under the patient's head and between the patient's legs. Position the patient's near arm toward you.

(8) Grasp the far side of the patient's body with your hands evenly distributed from the shoulder to the thigh (Figure 7-35b).

(9) On the count of three, roll the patient to a side-lying position, rocking backward onto your heels.

12. Transfer the patient out of bed, using one of the following methods as appropriate:

a. *Transferring the patient onto a stretcher.* Two nurses are necessary for the procedure if the patient is obese or is unable to assist (Figure 7-36).

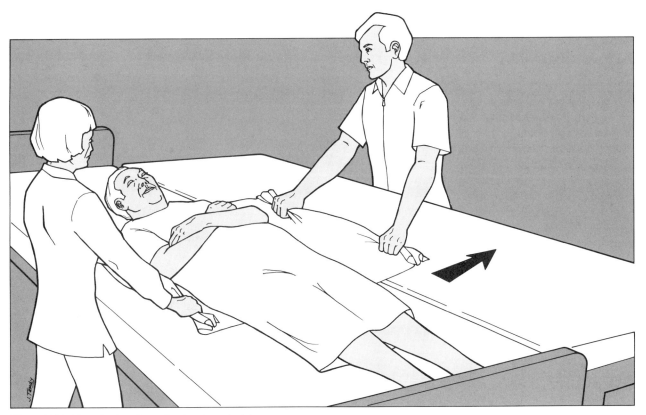

Figure 7-36. Transferring the patient on to a stretcher.

(1) Adjust the bed to a flat position with the height the same level as the stretcher.

(2) Place a drawsheet under the patient, extending from the shoulders to the buttocks, by rolling the patient from side to side.

(3) Assist the patient to the side of the bed or move the patient to the side of the bed by using the drawsheet. To do this, roll the drawsheet close to the patient on the side of the bed to which the patient will be moved. Grasp the sheet at the shoulder and buttock level of the patient and pull while rocking backward onto your heels.

(4) Place the stretcher close to and parallel with the side of the bed. Cushion any gap between the stretcher and the bed with pillows and blankets.

(5) Lock all wheels on the bed and the stretcher.

(6) Stand on the outside of the stretcher. If two nurses are participating, the other nurse should stand on the far side of the bed.

(7) Roll the drawsheet close to the patient and grasp the drawsheet at the shoulders and thighs. Move the patient onto the stretcher by pulling on the drawsheet while rocking backward onto your heels.

(8) Fasten the safety straps on the stretcher and raise the siderails.

b. *Transferring a patient into a wheelchair when the patient can assist:*

(1) Move the patient to the side of the bed.

(2) Raise the head of the bed to a 90 degree angle.

(3) Lower the level of the bed so that the patient's legs will be able to reach the floor.

(4) Place the wheelchair parallel to the head of the bed, facing the foot of the bed. Fold the footrests out of the way and lock the wheelchair in place.

(5) Position yourself with your feet apart and your knees flexed close to the side of the bed.

(6) Assist the patient onto his or her side facing you.

(7) Place one arm behind the patient's back, supporting his or her neck, and the other hand on his or her upper thigh. Pivot the patient into a sitting position on the edge of the bed, rocking backward onto your heels.

(8) Dress the patient in a bathrobe and slippers if desired. Allow the patient to sit for a few minutes to allow the circulatory system to adjust, to prevent orthostatic hypotension.

(9) Position yourself again with your legs apart and your knees flexed facing the patient.

(10) Grasp the patient around the waist. Instruct the patient to put his or her arms on your shoulders.

(11) Assist the patient to a standing position by straightening your knees and supporting the patient's knees inside your own knees (Figure 7-37).

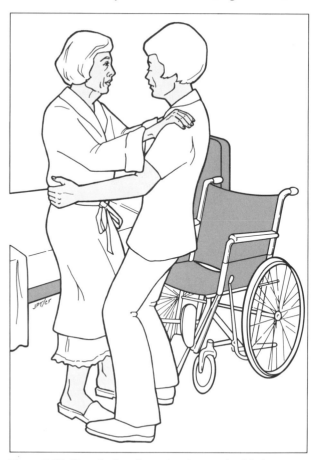

Figure 7-37. Transferring the patient into a wheelchair.

(12) Pivot toward the wheelchair, supporting the patient in the same manner until the patient is standing in front of the wheelchair.

(13) Flex your knees again to lower the patient into the wheelchair.

(14) Position the patient so that his or her back is straight against the back of the chair. Lower the footrests, placing the patient's feet on them. Cover the patient's lap with a blanket if desired.

13. Lower the height of the bed and adjust the siderails if the patient was only repositioned in bed.

14. Place the call signal within the patient's reach.

15. Discard equipment or return it to the appropriate area.

PATIENT AND/OR FAMILY TEACHING

1. Explain the method and reasons for moving the patient before beginning the procedure.

2. Answer any questions the patient has about the move.

3. Explain the reasons for the patient's activity limitations.

4. Teach the appropriate positioning and transfer techniques to the family, if the patient will be confined to bed at home.

5. Teach the patient exercises that can be done while confined to bed to improve muscle tone and prevent pressure sores.

DOCUMENTATION

1. Patient's position before the move as well as the new position.

2. Assessment of the patient's skin condition.

3. Any skin care and range-of-motion exercises performed.

4. The patient's reaction to the move.

5. All patient teaching done and the patient's level of understanding.

Assisting with Ambulation

PURPOSE
1. Increase the patient's mobility.
2. Decrease the possibility of patient accidents and injuries.
3. Assist the patient to use assistive devices correctly.

REQUISITES
1. Ambulation belt
2. Cane
3. Crutches
4. Walker
5. Bathrobe and slippers or shoes

GUIDELINES
1. Exercise is essential to normal functioning of the cardiovascular and musculoskeletal systems as well as being beneficial to the other systems of the body. Likewise, immobility is detrimental to psychophysiological homeostasis.
2. Any patient who has been confined to bed for more than a few days may be weak and unsteady when ambulating.
3. A physician's order for ambulating a patient should state the type and method of assistance and the length of practice time.
4. When ambulating a patient, walk on the patient's affected side unless the patient tends to lean toward the person assisting him or her. In such circumstances, walk on the patient's unaffected side so that his or her weight will be shifted in that direction.
5. Be aware of the immediate environment so that you know where the patient can sit down should he or she become weak or dizzy while ambulating.
6. Canes, walkers, and crutches must be the appropriate size for the patient in order to be effective. Refer questions to the physical therapist.
7. Make certain that the cane, walker, or crutches to be used have rubber caps on the tips of the legs to prevent slipping.

8. The patient may find it difficult to adjust to dependence on a cane, walker, or crutches. Offer the patient emotional support and frequent praise for his or her accomplishments.
9. The physical therapy department is a good resource to consult regarding ambulation, especially with canes, walkers, and crutches.

NURSING ACTION/RATIONALE
1. Assemble all equipment.
2. Check the physician's orders for the ambulation order as well as the type of assistance, the gait, and the length of practice time.
3. Identify the patient.
4. Explain to the patient why and how you will be helping him or her to walk. Explain how his or her assistance will be required.
5. Assess the patient's strength and ability to ambulate, as well as any previous experience with walking aids.
6. Assess baseline vital signs, if appropriate.
7. Request assistance from other personnel, if necessary.
8. Provide adequate lighting.
9. Provide privacy.
10. Wash your hands.
11. Apply an ambulation belt to the patient's waist, if desired.
12. Assist the patient to sit on the side of the bed. (Refer to the procedure "Positioning and Transferring the Patient.")
13. Dress the patient in a robe and sturdy non-skid slippers or shoes. The male patient may want to wear pajama pants to cover his legs.
14. Allow the patient to sit for a few minutes with his or her feet resting on the floor so that the circulatory system can adjust prior to standing, to prevent orthostatic hypotension.

15. Slowly assist the patient to stand. If a cane or a walker is being used, teach the patient to stand, using the cane or walker for support. The patient should place one hand on the cane or walker, while pushing off from the bed with the free hand and shifting the weight forward to the legs. If the patient is using crutches, have him or her grasp both crutches in one hand at the waist grip, then push off from the bed with the free hand, using the crutches vertically for support.

16. Assist the patient with ambulation by one of the following methods:

Ambulation with Support

This method is used when the patient has been in bed for more than a few days.

a. Bring your arm around the patient's waist or hold onto the back of the ambulation belt. Flex your outside arm at a 90 degree angle and have the patient rest his or her inside arm or hand on your hand for support (Figure 7-38).

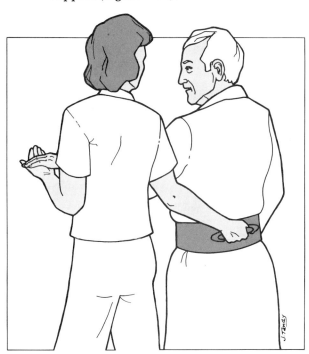

Figure 7-38. Ambulating with the assistance of one nurse using the ambulation belt.

b. If two nurses are needed to ambulate the patient, one should stand on either side of the patient. With your inside hands, hold the patient's upper arms. With your outside hands, hold the patient's hands (Figure 7-39).

c. Walk slowly and evenly alongside the patient, copying the speed and length of the patient's steps. When one nurse is assisting, step with the leg opposite to the one the patient is using. When two nurses are assisting, step with the same leg as the one the patient is using to help the patient feel balanced and secure.

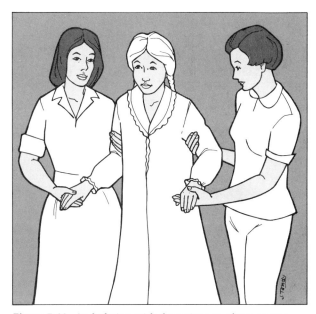

Figure 7-39. Ambulating with the assistance of two nurses.

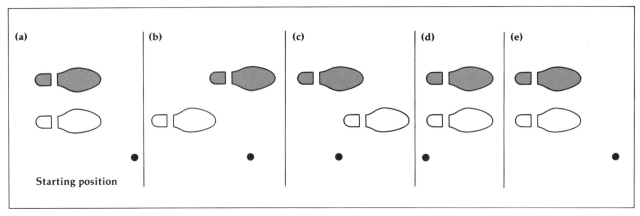

Figure 7-40. Walking with a cane.

Ambulation with a Cane

This method is used for added balance and when one leg is slightly weaker (Figure 7-40).

a. Instruct the patient to hold the cane on the unaffected side with the elbow slightly flexed and to place the tip of the cane about 6 inches in front of and 6 inches to the side of the foot.

b. Instruct the patient as follows:

   (1) Move the affected leg forward, parallel to the cane.

   (2) Move the unaffected leg forward so that the heel is just beyond the cane.

   (3) Move the affected leg forward so that it is even with the unaffected leg.

   (4) Move the cane forward 6 inches to the front and side of the patient.

   (5) Repeat the sequence. If less support is needed, the cane and the affected leg can be moved together.

c. Walk next to, but slightly behind, the patient on the affected side. Offer support as needed.

Ambulation with a Walker

This method is used when more support and balance are required.

a. Place the walker in front of the patient. Instruct the patient to grasp the hand grips.

b. Instruct the patient to use the muscles of the arms and upper body to help support his or her weight.

c. Instruct the patient to move the walker and the affected leg forward about 6 inches. Move the unaffected leg forward, parallel to the affected leg. Repeat the sequence.

d. Walk next to, and slightly behind, the patient on the affected side. Offer support as needed.

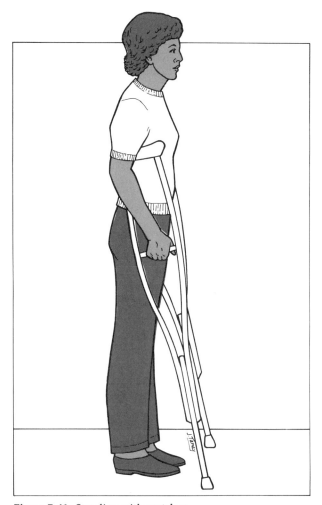

Figure 7-41. Standing with crutches.

Ambulation with Crutches

This method is used when the patient has limited use of one or both of the lower extremities.

a. Instruct the patient to stand in correct body alignment with the tip of the crutches 6 inches in front of and 6 inches to the side of the feet. The hands and arms, not the axillae, should bear the weight. The elbows should be flexed about 30 degrees (Figure 7-41).

b. *Four-point gait* (Figure 7-42). This is used when the patient can bear some weight on both extremities.
   (1) Move the right crutch forward.
   (2) Move the left foot forward.
   (3) Move the left crutch forward.
   (4) Move the right foot forward.

c. *Three-point gait* (Figure 7-43). This is used when the patient should not bear any weight on the affected leg.

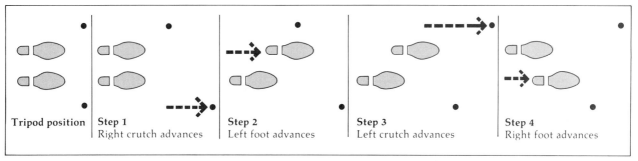

Tripod position | Step 1 Right crutch advances | Step 2 Left foot advances | Step 3 Left crutch advances | Step 4 Right foot advances

Figure 7-42. Four-point gait.

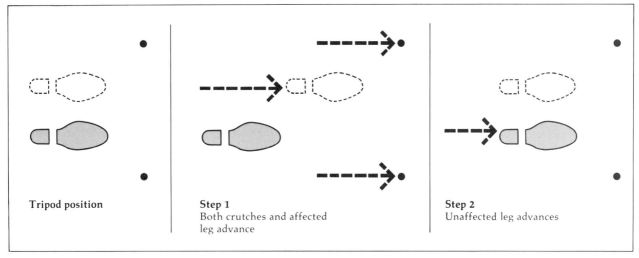

Tripod position | Step 1 Both crutches and affected leg advance | Step 2 Unaffected leg advances

Figure 7-43. Three-point gait.

(1) Move the affected leg and both crutches forward together.

(2) Move the unaffected leg forward.

d. *Two-point gait* (Figure 7-44). This is used when the patient can bear some weight on both extremities.

    (1) Move the right leg and the left crutch forward together.

    (2) Move the left leg and the right crutch forward together.

e. *Swing-through gait* (Figure 7-45). This is used for patients with paralyzed lower extremities. Walk next to but slightly behind the crutch-walking patient on the affected side. Offer support as needed.

    (1) Move both crutches forward together.

    (2) Move both legs forward together beyond the crutches.

    (3) Move about 6 inches for each move or step. Repeat the sequence in rhythm.

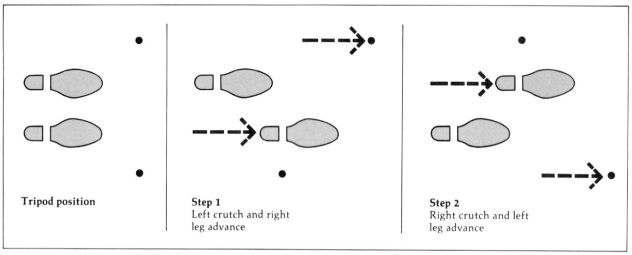

Tripod position

Step 1
Left crutch and right leg advance

Step 2
Right crutch and left leg advance

Figure 7-44. Two-point gait.

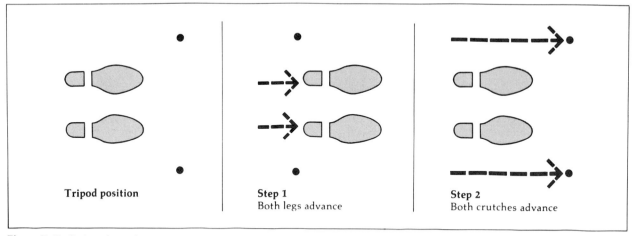

Tripod position

Step 1
Both legs advance

Step 2
Both crutches advance

Figure 7-45. Swing-through gait.

17. Assess the patient's balance and offer positive reinforcement appropriately.
18. Be alert for signs that the patient is falling. If the patient begins to fall, try to help the patient regain balance. If unsuccessful, assume a broad stance and ease the patient backward slowly to the floor. Request assistance of other health team members to return the patient to bed.
19. Ambulate the patient for the required length of time.
20. Assist the patient back to bed to a comfortable position by reversing the technique used to get the patient out of bed.
21. Evaluate the patient's response to the exercise. Assess vital signs if necessary.
22. Return all equipment to the appropriate area.

PATIENT AND/OR FAMILY TEACHING
1. Explain the technique and the reasons for ambulation to the patient.
2. Answer any questions the patient has about ambulating or use of the cane, walker, or crutches.
3. Teach the patient how to handle different situations with a cane, walker, or crutches (e.g., stairs, chairs).

4. Teach the patient the appropriate body alignment and body mechanics associated with ambulation.
5. If the patient will need assistance with ambulation after discharge, teach the family the appropriate techniques.
6. Teach the patient exercises to strengthen muscles for walking.

DOCUMENTATION
1. The patient's ability to ambulate or use one of the supportive devices.
2. The distance the patient was able to ambulate.
3. An assessment of the patient's condition before and after exercise.
4. All patient teaching done and the patient's level of understanding.
5. The patient's psychological response to the need for assistance with ambulation.

Unit
8
Sensorineural Procedures

PROCEDURES

Eye Irrigation

PURPOSE
1. Cleanse the eye and remove secretions.
2. Remove an irritating chemical or foreign body.
3. Treat an inflammatory process.
4. Relieve congestion and pain.
5. Lubricate the eye of the comatose patient.

REQUISITES
1. Sterile eye irrigation tray containing:
   a. Bulb syringe or eyedropper
   b. Solution container
   c. Cotton balls in a medicine glass
2. Sterile irrigation solution (type and amount as ordered by the physician)
3. Sterile normal saline (if not the solution ordered for irrigating)
4. Emesis basin
5. Bed protector
6. Waste receptacle
7. Towel

GUIDELINES
1. A physician's order is required to perform this procedure.
2. Extreme care must be taken during this procedure to avoid injuring the eye or surrounding tissue.
3. To avoid injury to the cornea when separating the eyelids, position your fingers above and below the eyelids so pressure is placed on the cheekbone and brow.
4. The patient should be positioned with the head tilted toward the affected eye to prevent contamination of the other eye.
5. Precautions should be taken to prevent the irrigation solution from flowing into the ear.
6. The tip of the syringe or eyedropper should not touch any part of the eye.
7. The irrigating solution should be at room temperature.
8. Before any medications are administered, patient allergies should be assessed.

NURSING ACTION/RATIONALE
1. Assemble all equipment.
2. Verify the physician's order.
3. Identify the patient.
4. Explain the procedure and its purpose to the patient. Caution the patient not to touch the eyes during any part of the procedure.
5. Provide privacy.
6. Assist the patient to a supine position with the neck slightly extended and the head tilted slightly toward the affected eye.
7. Cover the surrounding area with a bed protector.
8. Wash your hands.
9. Pour the sterile normal saline over the cotton balls to moisten them, using aseptic technique.
10. Pour the irrigation solution into the solution container, using aseptic technique.
11. Place the emesis basin along the contour of the patient's face, supporting the basin with a towel if necessary (Figure 8-1).

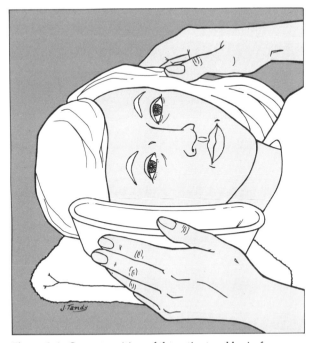

Figure 8-1. Correct position of the patient and basin for an eye irrigation.

12. Cleanse the eyelids with the moistened cotton balls, starting with the inner canthus and cleansing outward. Use a new cotton ball with each stroke.
13. Fill the irrigation syringe or dropper with the irrigating solution.
14. Separate the eyelids with your forefinger and thumb, resting your fingers on the cheekbone and brow (Figure 8-2).

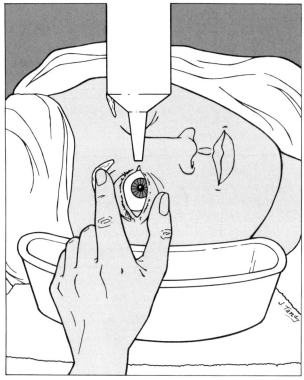

Figure 8-2. Position of the fingers and syringe for an eye irrigation.

15. Irrigate *gently* by directing the flow of solution from the inner canthus along the conjunctival sac (Figure 8-2).
16. Irrigate until the prescribed amount of solution has been used.
17. Wipe the eyelids with a moistened cotton ball after the irrigation has been completed.
18. Position the patient comfortably.
19. Discard equipment or return it to the appropriate location.
20. Wash your hands.

PATIENT AND/OR FAMILY TEACHING
1. Explain the procedure, its purpose, and the cooperation needed from the patient before starting.
2. Instruct the patient to notify you if any discomfort is felt during the procedure.
3. Instruct the patient regarding safety precautions if the irrigation was done because of a chemical irritant or foreign body in the eye.

DOCUMENTATION
1. Procedure and time performed.
2. Type and amount of solution used.
3. Color and characteristics of solution returned.
4. The patient's reaction to the procedure.
5. All patient teaching done and the patient's level of understanding.

Care of the Artificial Eye

PURPOSE

1. Cleanse the eye prosthesis and eye socket.
2. Prevent complications with the eye prosthesis or eye socket.

REQUISITES

1. 3 × 3 gauze sponges
2. Small basin
3. Cotton balls moistened with water
4. Bed protector
5. Mild soap
6. Eye irrigation syringe (optional)
7. Emesis basin
8. Tap water faucet, or a small basin filled with tap water
9. Small labeled storage container

GUIDELINES

1. The care of an artificial eye for a hospitalized patient should closely resemble the care routine that the patient has been using at home.
2. The patient or family should be consulted regarding the usual care regimen, and this information should be placed on the patient care plan.
3. The patient's record should clearly indicate that the patient has an artificial eye.
4. There are two kinds of artificial eyes, plastic and glass. The glass eye is heavy and can break if dropped. The plastic eye is much lighter and is unbreakable, but it can be scratched and chipped easily.
5. Excessive tearing, drainage, crusting, or irritation indicates a need to cleanse both the eye and the socket. Frequency of cleansing will vary.

6. Once a prosthesis has been removed, it should be cleansed immediately to prevent secretions from adhering to the surface of the prosthesis.
7. The eye prosthesis should be stored in water or contact lens solution in a labeled container when not in use.
8. Most eye prostheses are designed to be worn day and night.
9. If the patient is capable of performing any part of the eye care procedure, allow the patient to do as much of the care as possible. Assist the patient as necessary.

NURSING ACTION/RATIONALE

1. Assemble all equipment.
2. Identify the patient.
3. Explain the procedure to the patient. Encourage patient participation if appropriate.
4. Provide adequate lighting.
5. Assist the patient to a semi-Fowler's position.
6. Wash your hands.
7. Cover the bottom of the small basin with gauze and fill the basin half-full with mild soap and water.
8. Cleanse the eyelid with cotton balls soaked in warm tap water.
9. Remove the eye prosthesis:
   a. Raise the upper eyelid with the index finger of your dominant hand and depress the lower eyelid with your thumb. Cup your other hand below the eye to receive the prosthesis.

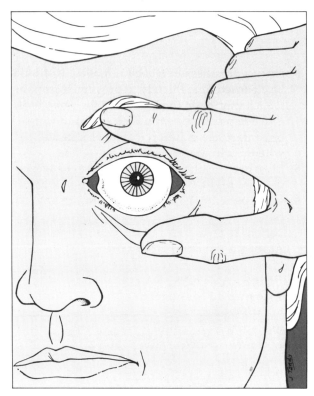

Figure 8-3. Removal of an eye prosthesis.

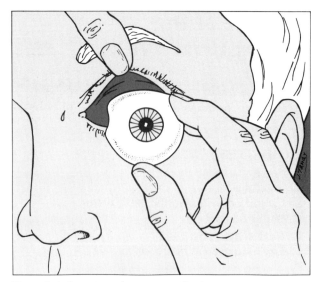

Figure 8-4. Insertion of an eye prosthesis.

    b. Apply slight pressure with your index finger between the brow and the prosthesis. The prosthesis will slip out (Figure 8-3).

10. Place the eye prosthesis in the soap and water solution.
11. Cleanse around the edge of the eye socket with moistened cotton balls.
12. Irrigate the eye socket, following the procedure "Eye Irrigation," if this is the patient's usual routine or if the physician has ordered the irrigation.
13. Cleanse the prosthesis by rubbing it between your index finger and thumb in the warm soapy water.
14. Rinse the prosthesis under warm running tap water after placing a towel liner in the sink prior to rinsing. Do not dry the prosthesis.
15. Reinsert the prosthesis (Figure 8-4).
    a. Raise the upper eyelid with your index finger or thumb.
    b. Slide the prosthesis, with the marked edge toward the nose, under the upper eyelid as far as possible.

    c. Depress the lower lid, allowing the prosthesis to slide into place.
    d. Pull the lower lid forward to cover the edge of the eye prosthesis.
16. Wipe the eyelid with a cotton ball to remove moisture. Wipe toward the nose to prevent disloding the prosthesis.
17. Discard equipment or return it to the appropriate location.

PATIENT AND/OR FAMILY TEACHING
1. Explain the procedure to the patient, if necessary. Encourage patient participation.
2. Teach the patient to perform the procedure, if appropriate.

DOCUMENTATION
1. Date, time, and procedure performed.
2. An assessment of the condition of the eye prosthesis and the eye socket.
3. Patient participation in the procedure.
4. Patient's reaction to the procedure.
5. All patient teaching done and the patient's level of understanding.

Removal of a Contact Lens

PURPOSE

1. Remove a contact lens for a patient unable to do so independently.

REQUISITES

1. Contact lens storage case or two small plastic labeled containers with lids
2. Soaking solution (type normally used by the patient)
3. Towel
4. Suction cup (optional)
5. Scotch tape (optional)

GUIDELINES

1. On admission, the nursing history should include the type of contact lens the patient wears, the wearing schedule, and the routine for care. The family should be advised to bring the necessary equipment to the hospital for the care of the lenses.
2. Most contact lens wearers also have corrective eyeglasses. If the patient will be unable to insert and remove the lenses while in the hospital, he/she should be advised not to wear them while hospitalized, unless absolutely necessary.
3. There are two general types of contact lenses, hard and soft. These two types of contacts require different cleaning and care and slightly different methods of insertion and removal.
4. The following general principles apply to the safe handling of both types of contact lenses:
   a. Hands must be washed immediately before handling lenses.
   b. Lenses should not be worn in the presence of noxious fumes or vapors such as hairspray.
   c. Hard lenses can be scratched or broken easily. Soft lenses tear easily.
   d. Lenses should not be worn when the eyes are reddened or irritated or if an eye infection is present.
   e. Medications should not be placed in the eye with lenses in place unless specifically ordered by the physician.
   f. Lenses should be handled over a smooth flat surface. Close the drain when handling the lenses over the sink.
   g. Lenses that have dropped should not be picked up with fingernails or sharp objects but should be lifted by wetting the fingertip to allow the lens to adhere.
   h. Hard lenses are generally stored dry or in special soaking solution. Soft lenses are stored in sterile normal saline without a preservative.
5. The patient's routine care of the contact lenses should be recorded in detail on the nursing care plan if the nursing staff will need to assist the patient.
6. The patient's medical record should be clearly marked that the patient is a contact lens wearer.
7. Patients who can insert, remove, and manage the care of the contact lenses may need only minimal assistance from the nurse. The nurse should assist the patient as the patient directs.
8. In an emergency, contact lenses can be removed and placed in the appropriate solution and cleaned at a later time.
9. The following procedure describes the removal of the contact lenses for a patient who has become dependent and is unable to remove the lenses.
10. If the nurse is unable to locate the lens in the eye, or is unable to remove the lens successfully, the physician should be notified.

NURSING ACTION/RATIONALE

1. Assemble all equipment.
2. Identify the patient.
3. Explain the procedure to the patient.
4. Provide adequate lighting.
5. Provide privacy.
6. Assist the patient to a semi- or high-Fowler's position, if allowed.

7. Place a clean towel over the patient's chest.
8. Wash your hands and dry thoroughly.
9. Assess the location of the contact lens. The lens should be lying directly over the cornea. If the lens has been displaced to the sclera, instruct the patient to close the eye and carefully slide the lens toward the cornea by *gently* rubbing the lid directly over the lens toward the cornea.
10. Remove the lens.

Hard Lens
a. Place your index finger on the outside corner of the eye.
b. Cup your other hand under the eye.
c. Pull gently on the outside corner of the eye toward the temple. The contact lens will pop out.

Soft Lens
a. Separate the eyelids with your thumb and middle finger of one hand.
b. Place your index finger gently on the lower edge of the contact lens and slide the lens down onto the sclera.
c. Compress the lens gently, allowing air to enter under the lens, breaking the suction with the eye.
d. Release the top eyelid and remove the lens with your index finger and thumb while still holding the lower lid down with your middle finger.
e. A suction cup for contact lens removal or a piece of rolled tape with the adhesive to the outside, touched gently against the lens, will also work to remove the lens.

10. Place the lens in the storage case with the designated solution or in a container of lens solution specifically labeled with the patient's name and the words "Right" and "Left."
11. Remove the other lens in the same manner.
12. Assess the eye for redness or irritation.
13. Reposition the patient comfortably.
14. Store the clearly labeled contact lens case or containers in a safe location.
15. Discard equipment or return it to the appropriate location.
16. Wash your hands.

PATIENT AND/OR FAMILY TEACHING
1. Explain the procedure to the patient before starting.
2. Advise the patient not to wear the contact lenses while in the hospital, if unable to care for them properly.

DOCUMENTATION
1. Time of removal and type of contact lens removed.
2. Solution used for storage of contact lenses.
3. Any problems encountered with the procedure.
4. An assessment of the eye.
5. Disposition of the lenses after removal.
6. All patient teaching done and the patient's level of understanding.

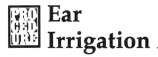 **Ear Irrigation**

PURPOSE

1. Remove an obstruction from the external auditory canal.
2. Cleanse the auditory canal of secretions.
3. Relieve congestion and pain.

REQUISITES

1. Sterile ear irrigation tray containing:
   a. Irrigating syringe
   b. Solution container
   c. Cotton balls
2. Sterile solution (amount and type as ordered by the physician)
3. Sterile solution thermometer
4. Bed protector
5. Emesis basin
6. Waste receptacle

GUIDELINES

1. A physician's order is required for this procedure.
2. Care must be taken when irrigating the ear so that the fragile components of the inner ear are not damaged.
3. The irrigating solution must be directed into the upper auditory canal. If the solution is directed toward the center of the canal, it will push the plugging substance back against the eardrum and may cause injury.
4. The temperature of the solution should be 37°C to 40.5°C (100°F to 105°F). Solutions above or below this temperature may cause dizziness.
5. The solution should not be administered with force. Use a gentle irrigating stream to remove secretions.
6. During the irrigation the nurse must allow for a return flow of irrigant to prevent pressure in the ear canal.
7. If the patient's ear is impacted with hard wax, the physician may prescribe eardrops for several days to soften the wax before the ear irrigation.
8. Before administering any new medications, assess for any patient allergies.

NURSING ACTION/RATIONALE

1. Assemble all equipment.
2. Verify the physician's order.
3. Identify the patient.
4. Explain the procedure to the patient.
5. Assist the patient to a sitting or high-Fowler's position with the head tilted slightly toward the affected ear.
6. Place a bed protector around the patient's shoulder.
7. Wash your hands.
8. Open the tray, using aseptic technique, and pour the irrigating soution into the solution container.
9. Cleanse the outer ear of any surface discharge with cotton balls and discard in the waste receptacle.
10. Fill the syringe with solution, and expel all the air from the syringe.
11. Direct the patient to hold the emesis basin directly under the ear (Figure 8-5).

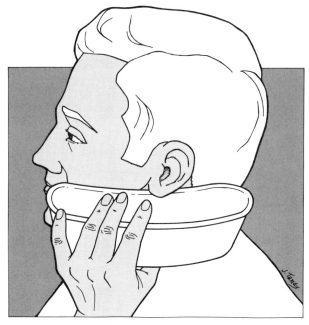

Figure 8-5. Placement of the emesis basin for an ear irrigation.

12. Grasp the auricle and pull upward and backward.
13. Introduce the tip of the syringe ¼ inch into the auditory canal.
14. Inject the stream of irrigating solution gently into the upper ear canal (Figure 8-6).
15. Observe for any pieces of wax or other materials as the irrigating solution returns.
16. Stop the procedure if the patient experiences pain, dizziness, or other adverse symptoms.
17. Irrigate the ear canal with 50 cc of solution or as ordered, then assess the ear canal with an otoscope to determine if the canal is clear. If not, repeat the procedure.

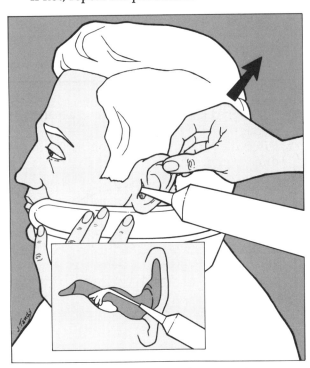

Figure 8-6. Directing the irrigating solution into the upper ear canal.

18. Assist the patient to lie on the affected side for several minutes to completely drain the canal of all irrigating solution.
19. Cleanse the ear and surrounding skin with cotton balls dipped in soapy water to remove any residual wax or irrigating solution. Dry this area with cotton balls.
20. Assess hearing.
21. Discard equipment or return it to the appropriate location.

PATIENT AND/OR FAMILY TEACHING
1. Explain the procedure and its purpose to the patient.
2. Instruct the patient to notify the nurse if any pain, discomfort, or dizziness is felt.
3. Instruct the patient, as appropriate, never to introduce foreign objects into the ear.
4. Instruct patients with a history of ear infections to avoid introducing contaminated water into the ear when swimming or bathing. Earplugs can be used.

DOCUMENTATION
1. Procedure and time performed.
2. Type and amount of irrigating solution used.
3. Amount, color, and consistency of returns along with a description of any solid particles.
4. An assessment of the ear canal and hearing ability.
5. The patient's tolerance of the procedure.
6. All patient teaching done and the patient's level of understanding.

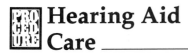 **Hearing Aid Care**

PURPOSE

1. Provide care of a hearing aid for a dependent patient.

REQUISITES

1. Hearing aid
2. Pipe cleaner or toothpicks
3. Disposable tissues
4. Moistened and dry cotton balls
5. Replacement batteries (size as specified by the patient)
6. Carrying case or plastic labeled container lined with gauze

GUIDELINES

1. There are four types of hearing aids (Figure 8-7). The insertion, removal, and care of these aids differ slightly.
   a. Body-worn hearing aid.
   b. Eyeglass hearing aid.
   c. Behind-the-ear hearing aid.
   d. In-the-ear hearing aid.
2. Hearing aids only amplify sound. If the patient hears distorted sounds without the hearing aid, the aid will not eliminate the distortion but will only amplify the sound heard.
3. When communicating with a hearing-aid user:
   a. Draw the person's attention by addressing him/her by name and wait for the person to face you before beginning the conversation.
   b. Speak clearly and naturally—don't shout. Speaking slowly and distinctly is helpful.
   c. Always face the person while talking. Do not exaggerate lip movements.
   d. Treat the hearing-aid wearer in all other aspects as you would any other patient.
4. Hearing aids should not be exposed to heat, dust and dirt, or humidity. They must be handled carefully to avoid bumps or falls that could damage the delicate mechanisms of the aid.
5. The admission history of a hearing-aid user should include the patient's wearing and cleaning schedule. This information should be placed on the nursing care plan.

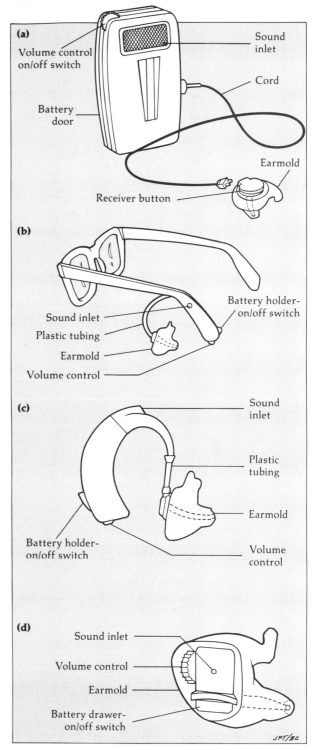

Figure 8-7. Types of hearing aids. (**a**) Body-worn hearing aid. (**b**) Eyeglass hearing aid. (**c**) Behind-the-ear hearing aid. (**d**) In-the-ear hearing aid.

6. The family should be requested to bring extra replacement batteries to the hospital to be used if necessary.
7. If the hearing aid does not function properly, certain checks can be done before contacting the family or the hearing-aid dealer for assistance. Signs of a problem with the aid may be volume weakness, sound distortion, feedback (whistling), or complete malfunction.
   a. Check that the aid is turned on and the volume control is adjusted.
   b. Check that the battery is positioned properly or change the battery.
   c. Check the plastic tubing for cracks, breaks, loose connections, twists, or kinks.
   d. Check the earmold channel for wax or debris.
   e. For an aid equipped with a telephone switch, be sure the aid is not set for use with a telephone.

NURSING ACTION/RATIONALE

1. Assemble all equipment.
2. Identify the patient.
3. Explain the procedure to the patient, if appropriate.
4. Provide privacy.
5. Provide adequate lighting.
6. Assist the patient to a semi- or high-Fowler's position, if allowed.
7. Wash your hands.
8. Remove the hearing aid:
   a. Turn the aid off. The on-off switch is on the battery holder.
   b. Grasp the receiver button in the ear between your index finger and thumb.
   c. Twist slightly to disengage the upper portion of the earmold, lifting up and outward simultaneously.
   d. Remove the amplifier from the clothing if removing a body-worn aid.
9. Inspect the earmold for dirt or wax clogging the earmold channel.

10. Carefully dislodge any wax or dirt in the earmold channel, using a pipe cleaner or a toothpick. Wipe the outside of the earmold with a soft dry tissue.
    a. Do not attempt to disconnect the plastic tube from the earmold or receiver.
    b. Do not use water, alcohol, or any other fluid on the earmold, since this can damage the intricate mechanism.
11. Change the battery, if necessary:
    a. Open the battery cover gently.
    b. Note carefully which way the battery is placed in the compartment.
    c. Turn the receiver over so the battery falls out into the palm of your hand.
    d. Replace the new battery in the same position as the old battery.
    e. Close the battery cover.
12. Store the hearing aid in the carrying case or a padded plastic container, clearly labeled, if the hearing aid will not be replaced at this time.
13. Cleanse the patient's outer ear with moistened cotton balls, and dry the ear with dry cotton balls.
14. Replace the hearing aid into the patient's outer ear.
    a. *Body-worn hearing aid:*
       (1) Clip the aid to the clothing.
       (2) Guide the cord and earmold assembly to the ear.
       (3) Hold the receiver between your thumb and forefinger and insert the long process of the earmold into the canal.
       (4) Use your free hand to pull down on the earlobe while pushing upward and inward at the bottom of the earmold to seat it correctly.
    b. *Eyeglass hearing aid:*
       (1) Slip the glasses on. Make sure the plastic tube is free of kinks.
       (2) Insert the long process of the earmold into the ear canal.
       (3) Twist the upper portion of the earmold into the contour of the outer ear.
       (4) Use your free hand to pull down on the earlobe while pushing upward and inward at the bottom of the earmold to seat it correctly.

   c. *Behind-the-ear hearing aid:*
     (1) Slip the aid over the ear. Make sure the plastic tube is free of kinks.
     (2) Insert the long process of the earmold into the ear canal.
     (3) Twist the upper portion of the earmold into the contour of the upper part of the ear.
     (4) Use your free hand to pull on the earlobe while pushing upward and inward at the bottom of the earmold to seat it correctly.
   d. *In-the-ear hearing aid:*
     (1) Hold the aid between your thumb and index finger and insert the long process of the earmold into the ear canal.
     (2) Twist the upper portion of the earmold into the contour of the upper ear.
     (3) Use your free hand to pull on the earlobe while pushing upward and inward at the bottom of the earmold to seat it correctly.

15. Turn the aid on and adjust the volume to the patient's specifications.
16. Reposition the patient comfortably.
17. Discard equipment or return it to the appropriate location.

PATIENT AND/OR FAMILY TEACHING

1. Explain each procedure to the patient before starting.
2. Instruct the patient on proper care of the hearing aid, if necessary.
3. Instruct the patient to notify the nurse if any problems with the hearing aid are experienced.

DOCUMENTATION

1. Type of hearing aid and ear the aid is used in (on the nursing care plan).
2. Cleaning and maintenance of the aid and battery changes, if appropriate.
3. Any problems with the aid, interventions, and results.
4. An assessment of the patient's hearing, if appropriate.
5. All patient teaching done and the patient's level of understanding.

Assisting the Physician with a Spinal Lumbar Puncture

PURPOSE

1. Assist the physician in obtaining cerebral spinal fluid for diagnostic examination.
2. Assist the physician to determine the pressure of the cerebral spinal fluid and to relieve intracranial pressure if necessary.
3. Assist the physician to administer medication into the spinal fluid.

REQUISITES

1. Sterile disposable lumbar tray, including:
   a. Spinal needle with stylet (size as ordered by physician)
   b. 5 cc syringe
   c. Sterile needles (25 gauge, 1½ inch, and 20 gauge, 1½ inch)
   d. Manometer with three-way stopcock
   e. Sterile barriers
   f. Local anesthetic
   g. Antiseptic
   h. Adhesive strip
   i. Test tubes with cap
2. Sterile gloves

GUIDELINES

1. Spinal lumbar puncture is usually performed to assist the physician in diagnosing neurological disease, to relieve intracranial pressure, or to administer medication.
2. The patient must be relaxed during the procedure, since straining produces a false increase in the pressure readings.
3. Spinal lumbar puncture is a relatively safe procedure, and serious side effects are rare. Headache is by far the most common side effect.
4. Closely monitor the patient for symptoms such as headache, vertigo, syncope, nausea, tinnitus, respiratory distress, or any change in vital signs during and after the procedure, and inform the physician immediately.
5. Assist the physician with the Queckenstedt's test. The physician will instruct you on how to proceed. The Queckenstedt's test is done to determine if there is an obstruction between the cranial cavity and the lumbar puncture needle.

6. To minimize and/or prevent postpuncture headache, the patient should be instructed to remain supine for several hours and to increase clear fluid intake if not contraindicated.
7. Closely monitor a patient who has increased intracranial pressure and who has had a spinal lumbar puncture. Watch for early signs of further increase in pressure and notify the physician immediately.
8. The requirement for a signed consent form for invasive procedures varies among health care facilities. Refer to your hospital's policy manual.
9. Patient allergies should be determined prior to implementing the procedure.

NURSING ACTION/RATIONALE

1. Assemble all equipment
2. Identify the patient.
3. Reinforce and clarify the physician's explanation of the procedure.
   a. Pre- and postspinal puncture care.
   b. The reason for the spinal puncture.
   c. The sensations associated with the local anesthetic.
   d. The anticipated sensation of pressure.
   e. The necessity of proper positioning.
4. Obtain an informed consent if required.
5. Instruct the patient to empty his or her bladder.
6. Provide adequate lighting.
7. Dress the patient in a clean hospital gown.
8. Assist the patient to the position desired by the physician. Positions usually are:
   a. Sitting on the edge of the bed with feet on a chair (Figure 8-8).
   b. Lying on either side near the edge of the bed with chin to chest and knees to forehead. This position attains maximal widening between intervertebral spaces (Figure 8-9).

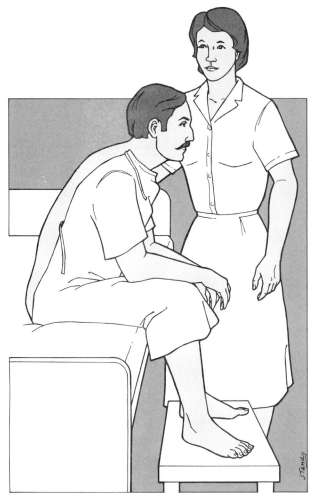

Figure 8-8. Sitting position for a lumbar puncture.

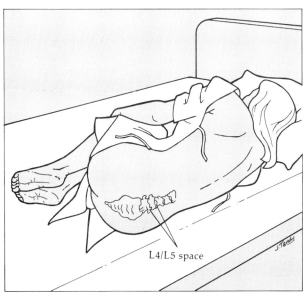

L4/L5 space

Figure 8-9. Lateral position for a lumbar puncture.

9. Wash your hands.
10. Assess baseline neurological and vital signs. Refer to the procedure "Neurological Assessment."
11. Open the supplies in a convenient location, using aseptic technique.
12. Assist the physician as required. Assist with the Queckenstedt's test as directed by compressing the patient's jugular vein first on one side, then on the other, and finally both sides simultaneously for 10 seconds.
13. Assist the patient to maintain the required position.
14. Give the patient constant support and reassurance.
15. Apply the adhesive strip to the puncture site after the physician removes the spinal needle.
16. Place the patient in a supine position.
17. Send all labeled spinal fluid specimens to the laboratory with appropriate requisitions.
18. Discard equipment or return it to the appropriate area.
19. Assess the patient's neurological and vital signs every 4 hours for 24 hours or as ordered. Assess the puncture site at the same time intervals.
20. Provide an increased fluid intake for the patient for at least 24 hours unless contraindicated.

PATIENT AND/OR FAMILY TEACHING
1. Reinforce and clarify the physician's explanation of the disease process.
2. Explain the positioning for the procedure and sensations that may be experienced.
3. Explain postprocedure care and rationale, including:
   a. Positioning and activity restrictions.
   b. Frequency of vital signs and neurological assessment.
   c. Importance of increasing fluid intake.
4. Instruct the patient to notify the nurse if any symptoms occur such as tinnitis, vertigo, or headache.
5. Instruct the patient to call the nurse for any assistance needed.

DOCUMENTATION

1. Type and time of procedure.
2. Name of physician performing procedure.
3. Any medication given, including dosage.
4. Amount and appearance of spinal fluid.
5. Disposition of specimen.
6. The patient's reaction to the procedure.
7. Specific parameters of assessment, including vital signs and neurological assessment.
8. All patient teaching done and the patient's level of understanding.

Neurological Assessment

PURPOSE

1. Establish a baseline neurological assessment.
2. Recognize neurological trends and changes in the patient's condition.
3. Provide an evaluation tool for reference when evaluating the patient's neurological status.

REQUISITES

1. Flashlight
2. Tongue blade
3. Clean safety pin
4. Neurological Record (Figure 8-10)

GUIDELINES

1. A neurological assessment is a simple, quick assessment tool used in combination with a complete neurological examination.
2. The physician's order will dictate the frequency of neurological assessments.
3. Dangerous trends that need to be reported to the physician are:
   a. Any pupillary reaction changes, especially with a decrease in the level of consciousness.
   b. Any decrease in the level of consciousness from a baseline assessment or from patient normalcy.
   c. Any sensory or motor loss or decline.
   d. Any marked changes in vital signs.

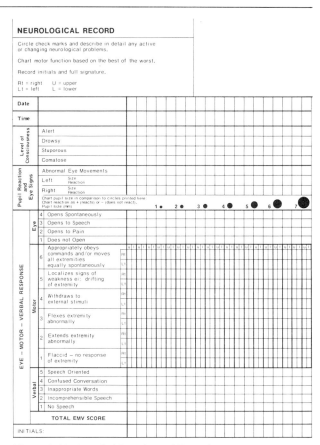

Figure 8-10. Sample Neurological Record.

4. Other significant neurological symptoms include:
   a. Nausea and vomiting.
   b. Seizure activity.
   c. Visual field disturbances.
   d. Headache.
5. Certain significant changes in the patient always require a more frequent neurological assessment, such as:
   a. Regression in the level of consciousness.
   b. Any procedure that may alter neurological vital signs.
   c. Any deterioration in condition.
6. Close monitoring of a patient who has signs of increased intracranial pressure is crucial. If the early signs of increasing intracranial pressure are not recognized, irreversible brain damage can occur.
7. Assess neurological signs prior to any procedure, when beginning a tour of duty, or before any surgical and/or emergency intervention.
8. Document the neurological assessment clearly and accurately in the nurses' notes. Use descriptive wording rather than generalizations. The neurological record should be a clear, concise, up-to-date record.
9. The neurological assessment record is a tool for evaluating and recording the patient's level of consciousness, pupil response, and motor-verbal response based on the Glasgow Coma Scale. The points given to the patient (according to patient response) are added after each neurological assessment to determine an overall EMV (eye, motor, verbal) score. A fully conscious patient would score 15 points. A comatose patient would score 3 points.
10. Definition of the Glasgow Coma Scale Points include:

Eye Response
4 points   Eyes open spontaneously.
3 points   Eyes open in response to speech.
2 points   Eyes open in response to pain.
1 point   Eyes do not open in response to painful stimuli.

Motor Response
6 points   The patient obeys commands appropriately and moves all extremities equally and spontaneously.
5 points   The patient is still able to obey commands, but exhibits weakness such as drifting of an upper extremity.
4 points   The patient will purposefully try to remove a painful stimulus.
3 points   The patient flexes an extremity abnormally.
2 points   The patient extends an extremity abnormally.
1 point   The patient has no motor response to painful stimuli in any extremity.

Verbal Response
5 points   The patient is oriented to person, place, and time.
4 points   The patient is not oriented but is able to communicate.
3 points   The patient speaks in a disorganized manner. The words and phrases make little or no sense.
2 points   The patient's response is moaning or groaning sounds.
1 point   The patient does not respond.

11. Definitions of the levels of consciousness listed on the neurological record to be used by the examiner for assessing changes in the patient are as follows:
    a. *Alert:* An alert patient is oriented to time, place, and person. The patient responds immediately and is able to recall remote and recent events.
    b. *Drowsy:* A drowsy patient is oriented to person and disoriented to time and place. The patient is usually lethargic and may alternate between cooperative and uncooperative behavior. The patient is easily aroused but falls back to sleep.

c. *Stuporous:* A stuporous patient is disoriented to time, place, and person but usually oriented to himself/herself. Repeated vigorous and continuous external stimulation is necessary to get the patient to respond. Behavior may be combative.

d. *Comatose:* A comatose patient is not arousable. There is little or no response to painful stimuli.

12. Early signs of clouding of consciousness such as the patient losing memory of recent events and insight into his/her physical condition are to be observed closely and reported. (Refer to the procedure "Assessment of Level of Consciousness.")

13. When assessing the level of consciousness, be aware of any medication that the patient is receiving and its effect on the patient. The effects of the medication may mask the neurological assessment of the patient.

14. The pupillary status must be evaluated along with the level of consciousness of the patient. Be aware that an alert patient with a dilated pupil may have had direct injury to the orbit. Eye protheses, cataracts, or eye lesions may also alter pupil responses. All pupillary changes should be reported to the physician. (Refer to the procedure "Pupillary Assessment.")

15. As intracranial pressure rises, tentorial herniation may occur, resulting in the compression of the brain stem. Symmetrical or asymmetrical pupil dilation reflects this possible occurrence, and it must be reported to the physician.

16. Each motor and verbal neurological assessment is the patient's best response to a maximal stimulus. The examiner determines the stimuli needed and the best motor and verbal response.

17. Accurate description and interpretation of postural positioning must be done. Examiners must be careful to interpret definitions consistently.

18. Frequent monitoring of vital signs is important. Changes in pulse and blood pressure are late neurological signs of increased intracranial pressure. Changes in vital signs should be reported immediately.

19. If the patient cannot follow commands, apply pressure to produce a patient response. Record the stimulus needed to produce the response. Observe and record all signs or types of responses and/or weaknesses produced. Record specific normal and abnormal flexion and extension produced. Report any regression from the established baseline. (Refer to the procedure "Motor and Sensory Assessment.")

20. All responses must be assessed bilaterally to detect lateralizing signs of neurological deterioration.

21. If the patient is not awake, the motor response best indicates the patient's level of consciousness.

NURSING ACTION/RATIONALE

1. Assemble all equipment.
2. Verify the physician's order for the frequency of the neurological assessment.
3. Identify the patient.
4. Explain the procedure to the patient, including the frequency of the neurological assessment and any patient participation.
5. Assist the patient to a supine position unless contraindicated.
6. Assess the patient's vital signs including:
   a. Blood pressure.
   b. Apical heart rate and rhythm.
   c. Radial and femoral pulses bilaterally.
   d. Respiratory rate and rhythm.
   e. Temperature.
7. Assess the patient's level of consciousness:
   a. Establish awareness by calling out the patient's name, touching the patient, shaking the patient for a response, and/or applying a painful stimulus.
   b. Establish orientation to time, place, person, and the patient's own self.
8. Darken the room slightly.
9. Assess the patient's pupillary reaction and eye signs:
   a. Evaluate pupils for size, equality, and reaction to light. Use the standard pupil gauge chart and the neurological record (see Figure 8-10).
   b. Assess consensual response.
   c. Assess eye signs and movement.
10. Relight the room.

11. Assess the patient's motor response.
    a. Test bilateral arm strength.
    b. Test bilateral leg strength.
12. Assess the patient's sensory response by testing bilateral body areas for the patient's ability to distinguish between dull and sharp.
13. Assess the patient's verbal response.
14. Reposition the patient as indicated.
15. Notify the physician of any changes.
16. Discard equipment or return it to the appropriate location.

PATIENT AND/OR FAMILY TEACHING

1. Explain the procedure and its purpose to the patient, including any patient participation.
2. Reinforce and clarify the physician's explanation of the disease process.
3. Encourage the family to reorient and stimulate the patient, if appropriate.
4. Instruct the family regarding neurological assessment, both orally and in writing, if the patient is to be discharged.

DOCUMENTATION

1. Date, time, and results of all neurological assessments including:
    a. Level of consciousness.
    b. Pupillary reaction.
    c. Motor and sensory function.
    d. Vital signs.
2. Total Glasgow Scale points, if appropriate.
3. Description of all behaviors and responses.
4. All patient teaching done and the patient's level of understanding.

Assessment of Level of Consciousness

PURPOSE

1. Determine the patient's level of consciousness.

REQUISITES

1. Neurological Record (see Figure 8-10)

GUIDELINES

1. The single most important assessment indicator of brain function is the level of consciousness. It varies from alertness to deeply comatose with many variable identifiable stages in between. Identification of these stages requires careful observation.
2. Specific criteria should be established for the following descriptive terms (refer to the procedure "Neurological Assessment" for definitions):
    a. Alert
    b. Drowsy
    c. Stuporous
    d. Comatose
3. The patient's condition will determine the amount and type of stimulus needed to evoke a response. Avoid pressure stimulus that will cause injury to the patient if pressure must be applied to obtain a full response from the patient.
4. Types of pressure to elicit a response are:
    a. Sternal pressure.
    b. Supraorbital pressure.
    c. Pinching the trapezius muscle between the patient's neck and shoulder.
    d. Pressure to nailbeds.
    e. Pressure to the Achilles tendon.
5. The following specific responses help to assess the level of consciousness:
    a. Patient's orientation to time, place, and person.
    b. Patient's ability to carry out commands.
    c. Patient's response to a painful stimuli, if necessary.

6. Orientation deteriorates in the following sequence:
   a. Time
   b. Place
   c. Others
   d. Self
7. Assess and evaluate factors, other than neurological concerns, that may cause disorientation; for example:
   a. New surroundings.
   b. Untoward side effects of medication.
   c. Darkness.
8. Establish normalcy for each patient. Consider such things as:
   a. Hearing deficit.
   b. Inability to understand speech.
   c. Previous physical weaknesses.
9. Indicate on the Neurological Record if the patient cannot respond verbally because of intubation, oral injuries, or dysphasia.
10. During assessment and evaluation of speech and language, it is important to know the patient's educational level, principal language, and his or her socioeconomic background.

NURSING ACTION/RATIONALE

1. Assemble all equipment.
2. Identify the patient.
3. Arouse the patient to the fullest and to his or her highest functioning level. Explain the procedure and its purpose, if appropriate.
4. Have the patient carry on a conversation. Ask questions such as:
   a. What year is it?
   b. What is your name?
   c. Where are you?
   d. What is your home address?
5. Evaluate the patient's level of orientation and behavior.
6. Evaluate the patient's best verbal response and his or her alertness and coherency.
7. Reorient the patient if he or she shows signs of confusion.
8. Ask the patient to carry out simple commands such as:
   a. Stick out your tongue.
   b. Smile.
   c. Raise your arms.
9. Evaluate the patient's best motor response.
10. Test patient response with physical stimuli if the patient is stuporous or lower in the level of consciousness, using an appropriate stimulus to evoke a response.
11. Apply pressure or pain to elicit a full response.
12. Check for corneal and gag reflexes.
13. Assess vital signs.
14. Position the patient comfortably, and if appropriate, position the patient to prevent aspiration.

PATIENT AND/OR FAMILY TEACHING

1. Explain to the family why it is important to know the patient's level of consciousness.
2. Explain the methods of eliciting the best response.
3. Explain the importance of clearing the patient's thinking.
4. Explain the importance of providing a clock, newspaper, or calendar to reorient the patient, if appropriate.

DOCUMENTATION

1. Level of consciousness, using established descriptive terms.
2. Amount and kind of pressure or pain applied to elicit a response.
3. Notification of the physician regarding any abnormal response or change.
4. All patient teaching done and the level of understanding.

Pupillary Assessment

PURPOSE

1. Determine cranial nerve damage through an assessment of pupillary response.

REQUISITES

1. Flashlight
2. Small object (pen)
3. Neurological Record (see Figure 8-10)

GUIDELINES

1. The oculomotor (III), trochlear (IV), and abducens (VI) nerves control the eye movements. The basic eye tests are done to test all three cranial nerves (III, IV, and VI).
2. The oculomotor nerve also controls the muscles that hold the upper eyelid open and the muscles that constrict the pupil. Therefore, additional specific testing must be done for that nerve.
3. The consensual light reflex reaction is the reaction of the opposite pupil when light is shown in one of the pupils. The opposite pupil should react to light because of the communication fibers between the two oculomotor cranial nerves.
4. Abnormalities of size, reactivity, and symmetry of the pupils may not always signify the presence of an intracranial space-occupying lesion. Direct orbital trauma may cause a pupil to be abnormally large or small, and certain medications may affect pupil size and reaction.
5. Refer to the Neurological Record (Figure 8-10) for the standard chart to judge pupil size. Each health care facility should have its own standard pupil size chart.
6. Assess pupils under the same lighting each time and be sure that the pupils are receiving the same amount of ambient light.
7. Report all unusual eye responses to the physician.

NURSING ACTION/RATIONALE

1. Assemble all equipment.
2. Identify the patient.
3. Explain the procedure to the patient, if appropriate.
4. Reduce room light to a minimum.
5. Observe the appearance of the pupils by holding the eyelids open if necessary, and assess size and shape of both pupils.
6. *Light reaction.* Direct a bright flashlight into one eye while keeping the patient's other eye closed. Angle the flashlight on the side of the patient's face and bring it to the front of the eye. Repeat the procedure on the other eye. Note the reaction (Figure 8-11).

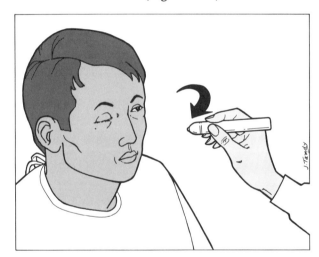

Figure 8-11. Assess individual pupillary light reaction.

7. *Equality of pupils.* Bring the flashlight to the front of the patient's face, about 6 inches from the nose, and check for equality of pupils.
8. *Consensual reaction.* Direct the flashlight into one eye, watching for constriction of the pupil of the other eye.
9. *Eye movement.* Observe whether the right and left eye move together and follow the object in all directions.
   a. *Conscious patient:*
      (1) Instruct the patient to keep the head still and follow the movement of the object with his or her eyes.

(2) Hold an object, such as a pen, about 18 to 20 inches in front of the nose of the patient (Figure 8-12**a**).

(3) Move the pen up, down, sideways, and diagonally, always returning to the central point after each movement (Figure 8-12**b**).

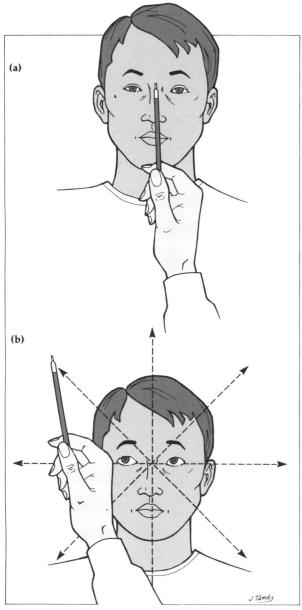

Figure 8-12. Assessing eye movement. (**a**) Initial step. (**b**) Move the pen up, down, sideways, and diagonally.

b. *Unconscious patient:* Open the patient's eyelids and observe random movement of the pupil.

10. Assist the patient to a comfortable position.

PATIENT AND/OR FAMILY TEACHING

1. Explain the procedure and its purpose to the patient and/or family member.

2. Explain the value of testing eye responses, especially in the unconscious patient.

DOCUMENTATION

1. Date, time of exam, and all pupillary responses.

2. Notification of the physician regarding all abnormal eye responses.

3. All patient teaching done and the patient's level of understanding.

Motor and Sensory Assessment

PURPOSE

1. Assess the patient's neurological status through motor and sensory responses.

REQUISITES

1. Cotton-tipped applicator
2. Clean safety pin
3. Cotton
4. Clean dull instrument
5. Neurological Record (see Figure 8-10)

GUIDELINES

1. An accurate description and interpretation of postural positioning must be done. Examiners must be careful to interpret definitions consistently.

   a. *Purposeful movement:* The patient carries out commands and attempts to remove a painful stimulus.

   b. *Non-purposeful movement:* The patient exhibits random purposeless movement in response to a very painful stimulus. The two types of non-purposeful movement are:

   (1) *Decerebrate posturing:* Rigid extension of the arms with adduction and pronation. The lower extremities are stiffly hyperextended with plantar flexion (Figure 8-13).

   (2) *Decorticate posturing:* Flexion of the arms, wrists, and fingers with hyperextension of the lower extremities, which are rotated internally (Figure 8-14).

   c. *Flaccid:* Absence of motor response.

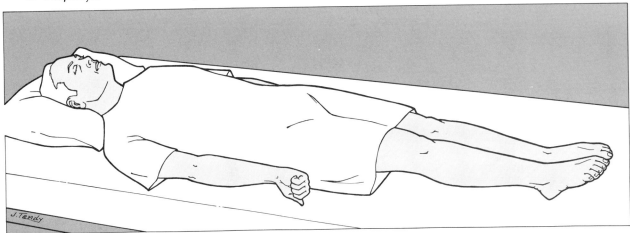

Figure 8-13. Decerebrate posturing.

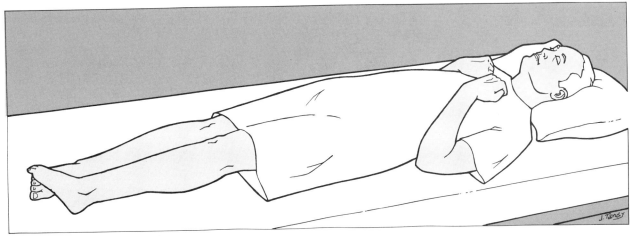

Figure 8-14. Decorticate posturing.

2. If the patient can follow commands, two tests for bilateral motor strength include:

    a. *Arm strength:* Ask the patient to extend the arms in front of him or her while keeping eyes closed and palms up. If there is a weakness, one arm may drift downward and away from midline (Figure 8-15).

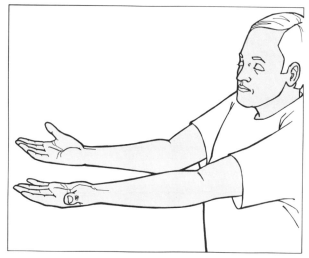

Figure 8-15. Testing arm strength.

    b. *Leg strength:* Assist the patient to a supine position. Ask the patient to raise one leg at a time with the knee straight. If there is weakness, the leg will lift with difficulty and fall easily (Figure 8-16).

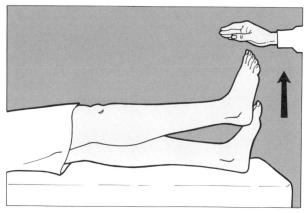

Figure 8-16. Testing leg strength.

3. Assess accuracy and ease of movement as you have the patient carry out commands. This will provide an assessment of the patient's condition.

4. Assess motor response by observing the patient's overall ability to move. You can detect slight weakness or paretic extremities by observing the patient's daily activities.

5. Sensory function can be tested to determine the patient's ability to distinguish between dull and sharp sensations. Test identical locations on each side of the patient's body simultaneously. The patient's sensory perception should be bilaterally equal.

6. During testing for sensory ability, confine your testing to areas of the body that have very little hair, such as the:

    a. Foot

    b. Lower leg

    c. Hand

    d. Back

    e. Abdomen

7. Report immediately to the physician if there is a change from the established baseline in the patient's status regarding pain, temperature, and/or touch sensation.

8. The examiner determines the best response that the patient can make with either arm or leg. Any change from the established baseline should be reported to the physician.

NURSING ACTION/RATIONALE

1. Assemble all equipment.

2. Identify the patient.

3. Explain the procedure and its purpose, if appropriate.

4. Test motor and sensory function.

Motor Function/Coordination

    a. Observe spontaneous movements during daily activities.

    b. If the patient can follow commands, test:

        (1) Arm strength.

        (2) Grip strength.

        (3) Leg strength.

        (4) Facial muscles.

    c. Instruct the patient to hold one arm straight out from the side of the body, then bring the arm around to the face to touch his or her nose with the index finger. Repeat this step with the opposite arm.

d. Instruct the patient to place his or her heel on the opposite knee and to slide the heel down the lower leg to the foot. Repeat this step with the opposite leg (Figure 8-17).

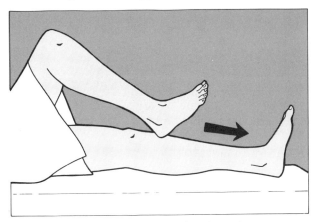

Figure 8-17. Sliding the heel of one foot down the opposite leg.

e. If the patient cannot follow commands, observe for:
   (1) Drooping of the mouth.
   (2) Inability to close the eyelids.
   (3) Asymmetry of facial muscles.
   (4) Clumsily moving extremities.
   (5) Externally rotated lower extremities.
   (6) Inability to use an extremity.
f. If necessary, use a stimulus to produce a response.

Sensory Function
a. Ask the patient to close his or her eyes.
b. Touch various parts of his or her body and ask if he or she feels the touch and can identify the location.

c. Grasp the right large toe and point the toe toward the face. Have the patient identify the position. Randomly move the toe up or down and ask the patient to identify the position after each move.
d. Grasp the left toe and repeat the procedure as above.
e. Ask the patient to identify the temperature (warm/cold) of any object.
f. Instruct the patient to open both eyes.
5. Assist the patient to a comfortable position.

PATIENT AND/OR FAMILY TEACHING
1. Explain the procedure and the purpose of the examination.
2. Give specific instructions for each testing method just prior to performing the test.

DOCUMENTATION
1. Date, time, and response for each assessment.
2. Stimulus needed to produce the response:
   a. Command
   b. Pain
   c. Spontaneous
3. Notification of the physician regarding any abnormal response.
4. All patient teaching done and the patient's level of understanding.

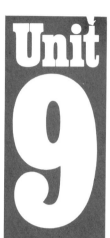

Unit 9

Integumentary/ Gynecological Procedures

PROCEDURES

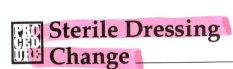

Sterile Dressing Change

PURPOSE

1. Promote wound healing.
2. Prevent wound infection.
3. Provide for assessment of the wound.

REQUISITES

1. Sterile dressings as appropriate
2. Sterile gloves
3. Exam gloves
4. Antiseptic swabs
5. Tape
6. Waste receptacle
7. Bath blanket, if appropriate

GUIDELINES

1. A physician's order is required for the dressing change procedure. In some cases, the physician may prefer to perform the first dressing change after surgery.
2. The dressing may be reinforced if unexpected excessive wound drainage occurs and the physician has not written an order for a dressing change. The physician should be notified.
3. Sterile dressing changes are performed to provide wound care, inspect the wound, and apply a clean sterile dressing.
4. Wounds should be inspected carefully for redness, edema, skin irritation, type of drainage, and progression of healing.
5. Wound infections are generally manifested by redness, edema, and pain at the incision line along with purulent drainage from the wound.
6. Infection control protocol should be implemented if a wound infection occurs.
7. Surgical or traumatic wounds should be observed closely for hemorrhage during the first 24 hours.
8. Remove old dressings slowly and carefully. If sticking occurs, sterile normal saline may be applied to loosen the dressing.
9. When removing tape, pull it straight away from the skin while holding the skin taut to reduce pain. If frequent dressing changes are required, Montgomery straps may be indicated to prevent skin irritation from the repeated tape removal (Figure 9-1).

10. A variety of dressings are available for dressing changes. The size of the wound, amount of drainage, and physician preference will dictate the type of dressings used.

NURSING ACTION/RATIONALE

1. Assemble all equipment.
2. Verify the physician's order.
3. Identify the patient.
4. Explain the procedure to the patient, including the importance of not touching the exposed wound.
5. Provide privacy.
6. Assist the patient to the most appropriate position for the dressing change.
7. Clear a clean work area for the dressing change supplies.
8. Provide adequate lighting.
9. Wash your hands.
10. Open all dressings and supplies, using aseptic technique.
11. Expose the dressing to be changed. Drape the patient, if appropriate.

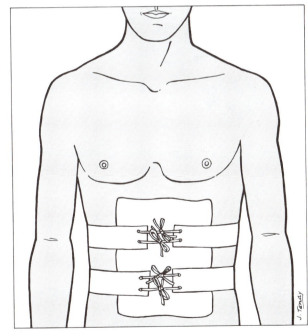

Figure 9-1. Montgomery straps.

12. Place the waste receptacle near your work area.
13. Loosen the tape on the dressing.
14. Put on the exam gloves.
15. Remove the dressing slowly, taking care not to dislodge any drains. Avoid contaminating the wound with the edges of the dressing, the tape, or your non-sterile gloves. Touch only the outer surface of the dressings.
16. Assess the dressing for the amount, color, consistency, and odor of drainage and discard in the waste receptacle.
17. Remove the exam gloves and discard in the waste receptacle.
18. Inspect the wound and surrounding skin for appearance, presence of drainage, and approximation of wound edges.
19. Cleanse the wound with antiseptic swabs, holding each swab with the tip down. Cleanse the wound in the following sequence:
    a. Cleanse the incision line from the proximal to distal end by rolling the swab gently over the center of the incision (Figure 9-2). Discard the swab.

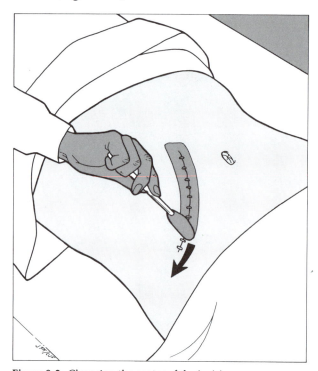

Figure 9-2. Cleansing the center of the incision.

b. Cleanse one side of the incision line from the proximal to the distal end by rolling the swab along the side of the incision covering approximately 1 inch of adjacent tissue (Figure 9-3). Discard the swab.

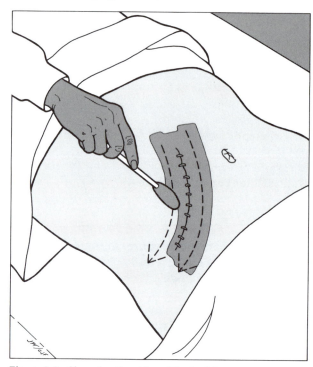

Figure 9-3. Cleansing the sides of the incision.

c. Cleanse the opposite side of the incision in the same manner.

d. Cleanse the area around the drain, if appropriate, by working around the drain in a circular pattern, moving the swab away from the drain (Figure 9-4). Discard the swab.

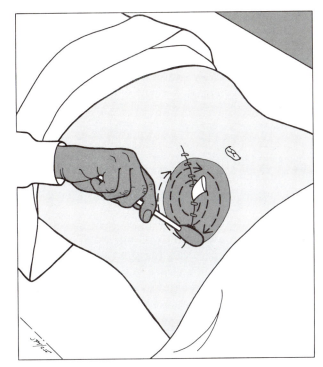

Figure 9-4. Cleansing around the drain.

20. Put on the sterile gloves.

21. Apply the sterile dressing, using aseptic technique and taking care not to contaminate your sterile gloves:

a. Apply a precut 4 × 4 gauze around the drain, if present, to protect the skin area.

b. Cover the entire incision, using heavier dressings over drain site areas.

22. Remove the gloves and discard.

23. Secure the dressings with tape.

24. Assist the patient to a comfortable position.

25. Discard equipment or return it to the appropriate area.

26. Wash your hands.

PATIENT AND/OR FAMILY TEACHING

1. Explain the procedure to the patient, including the frequency of dressing changes.

2. Instruct the patient to notify the nurse if the dressing becomes soiled or if incisional pain is experienced.

3. Instruct the patient that analgesics are available for incisional pain, if appropriate.

4. Explain to the patient the importance of not handling the dressing or the incision.

5. Teach the patient and/or family the dressing change procedure if dressings are to be changed at home. Provide a return demonstration opportunity.

DOCUMENTATION

1. Time of dressing change and type of dressing.

2. Amount, color, consistency, and odor of any drainage.

3. Specific assessment parameters including condition of skin, drain site, and incision line.

4. The patient's reaction to the procedure, including any pain experienced.

5. Any patient and/or family teaching done and the level of understanidng.

Intermittent Wound Irrigation

PURPOSE

1. Cleanse the wound of debris or drainage.
2. Stimulate the formulation of granulation tissue and promote wound healing.
3. Instill medication into a wound.

REQUISITES

1. Sterile irrigation set including:
   a. Asepto syringe
   b. Solution container
   c. Solution receptacle
   d. Sterile barrier
2. Sterile 3 × 3 gauze sponges
3. Sterile dressings as appropriate
4. Exam gloves
5. Sterile gloves
6. Irrigation solution as prescribed
7. Mask, if required
8. Sterile red rubber catheter (optional)
9. Bed protector
10. Waste receptacle

GUIDELINES

1. A physician's order is required for the wound irrigation procedure. Request that the physician demonstrate any specific technique desired for the irrigation.
2. Wound irrigation is a sterile procedure and requires careful aseptic technique.
3. Although wound irrigations may be performed with solutions at room temperature, warming the solution to body temperature will reduce the patient's discomfort.
4. Refer to the procedure "Isolation Precautions" for the specific care of a patient with a wound infection.
5. Refer to the procedure "Sterile Dressing Change" for the specific procedure for changing a sterile dressing.
6. Patient allergies should be assessed before administering any new medications.

NURSING ACTION/RATIONALE

1. Assemble all equipment.
2. Verify the physician's order.
3. Identify the patient.
4. Explain the procedure to the patient. Instruct the patient to inform you if any burning or pain occurs.
5. Provide adequate lighting.
6. Provide privacy.
7. Position the patient to facilitate solution flow through the wound and into the solution receptacle.
8. Place a bed protector under the area to be irrigated.
9. Wash your hands.
10. Expose the wound area. Drape the patient, if necessary.
11. Put on the exam gloves.
12. Remove the wound dressing and discard in the waste receptacle. Inspect the wound for appearance and amount of drainage.
13. Remove the exam gloves and discard.
14. Open the irrigating set and sterile dressings, using aseptic technique.
15. Pour the irrigating solution into the solution container.
16. Position the solution collection receptacle in the proper position for the return flow of solution.
17. Apply the sterile gloves.
18. Fill the Asepto syringe with irrigating solution and instill directly into the wound or through a catheter that has been placed gently in the wound.
19. Direct the solution over the entire wound. Use your non-dominant hand to manipulate the solution collection container.
20. Continue irrigating until the prescribed amount of solution has been used.
21. Dry the wound with sterile 3 × 3 gauze sponges held in your sterile dominant hand.
22. Reapply sterile dressings, using aseptic technique.
23. Remove the sterile gloves.
24. Assist the patient to a comfortable position.
25. Discard equipment or return it to the appropriate location.

PATIENT AND/OR FAMILY TEACHING

1. Explain the procedure to the patient before you start. Instruct the patient to avoid touching the wound area.
2. Instruct the patient to inform the nurse if burning or pain is experienced during the procedure.
3. Reinforce and clarify the physician's explanation of the disease process.
4. Explain any additional therapeutic orders.

DOCUMENTATION

1. Time of irrigation.
2. Type and amount of solution used.
3. Assessment of wound, including amount and type of drainage and appearance of wound and surrounding skin.
4. The patient's reaction to the procedure.
5. Color, consistency, and odor of solution returned.
6. All patient teaching done and the patient's level of understanding.

Wound Suction

PURPOSE

1. Provide continuous or intermittent drainage from a wound.
2. Maintain adequate suction on a wound for removal of debris and fluid.

REQUISITES

1. Suction unit
   a. Portable wound suction unit such as a Hemovac, electric or wall vacuum continuous unit, or intermittent suction unit
2. Graduated container
3. Antiseptic wipes
4. Irrigation set including:
   a. Irrigation syringe
   b. Solution container
   c. Solution receptacle
   d. Sterile barrier
5. Irrigation solution, as prescribed
6. Sterile gloves

GUIDELINES

1. Wound suction may be used postoperatively to collect wound drainage or may be used for infected wounds to control a large volume of drainage.
2. Placement of independent continuous suction units and drainage catheters is performed by the physician.
3. Wound drainage systems must be maintained using aseptic technique, since they are potential sources of infection.
4. Wound drainage systems should be assessed frequently for patency or loss of suction.
5. Independent wound suction units provide a constant, gentle suction for wounds with lesser amounts of drainage.
6. Electric or wall vacuum continuous or intermittent suction units are generally used for open, copiously draining wounds.
7. Irrigation of clogged drainage tubes requires a physician's order.
8. Refer to the procedure "Isolation Precautions" for the specific care of a patient with a wound infection.
9. Refer to the manufacturer's recommendations for activating and emptying independent suction units.

NURSING ACTION/RATIONALE

1. Assemble all equipment.
2. Identify the patient.
3. Explain the procedure to the patient.
4. Provide privacy.
5. Position the patient to facilitate access to the suction catheter area.
6. Provide adequate lighting.
7. Wash your hands.

Independent Suction Unit (Figure 9-5)

1. Activate the unit:
   a. Remove the plug cap aseptically and place the portable suction unit upright on a firm surface.
   b. Compress the suction unit as flat as possible.
   c. Replace the plug cap immediately.
   d. Position the suction unit to prevent kinking of the tubes or dropping of the unit.
   e. Assess the suction unit for proper compression and patency.

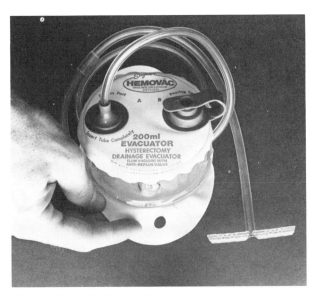

Figure 9-5. Synder Hemovac.

2. Empty the unit:
   a. Remove the plug cap, using aseptic technique.
   b. Invert the suction unit over the graduated container and empty the contents.
   c. Return the unit to an upright position and reactivate the unit as described previously.
   d. Measure the drainage and discard.
3. Discard equipment or return it to the appropriate location.
4. Wash your hands.

Electric or Wall Vacuum Continuous or Intermittent Wound Suction Unit

1. Activate the unit:
   a. Plug the unit into an electrical outlet or attach to a wall system vacuum.
   b. Connect the suction tube to the drainage tube, using aseptic technique.
   c. Tape the connection. Ensure that the tubing is not pulling on the drainage tube.
   d. Turn the suction unit on "Low" unless specifically ordered differently.
   e. Assess the suction system for proper functioning.
2. Empty the unit:
   a. Turn the suction unit off.
   b. Empty the drainage bottle.
   c. Measure the drainage and discard.
   d. Reattach the drainage bottle.
   e. Turn the suction unit on and assess for proper function.
3. Discard equipment or return it to the appropriate location.
4. Wash your hands.

Irrigation of Wound Drainage Tubes

1. Open the irrigation set, using aseptic technique.
2. Pour the irrigating solution into the solution container.
3. Place the sterile barrier under the connection site.
4. Cleanse the connection site with an antiseptic wipe. Allow it to dry.
5. Disconnect the drainage tubing from the suction tubing and place the ends of both carefully on the sterile barrier.
6. Put on the sterile gloves.
7. Draw the irrigating solution into the syringe, maintaining asepsis of the irrigating tip.
8. Instill the prescribed amount of irrigating solution gently into the drainage tube.
9. Allow the return solution to flow into the solution receptacle.
10. Repeat the irrigation if necessary, maintaining aseptic technique.
11. Reconnect the suction tubing to the drainage tube.
12. Remove your gloves.
13. Reactivate the suction unit.
14. Discard equipment or return it to the appropriate location.
15. Wash your hands.

PATIENT AND/OR FAMILY TEACHING

1. Explain the procedure and its purpose to the patient.
2. Instruct the patient to inform the nurse if experiencing any discomfort.
3. Reinforce and clarify the physician's explanation of the disease process.
4. Explain any additional therapeutic orders.

DOCUMENTATION

1. Type of wound catheter and suction.
2. Amount, color, characteristics, and odor of drainage.
3. Amount and type of irrigation solution used and color, consistency, and odor of solution returned.
4. The patient's reaction to the procedure.
5. Function of suction system.
6. Any assessment of the wound area or dressing.
7. All patient teaching done and the patient's level of understanding.

PROCEDURE Sterile Warm Moist Compresses

PURPOSE

1. Apply warm, moist heat to an open body area.

REQUISITES

1. Sterile premoistened (normal saline or water) gauze sponges in a foil pack
2. Electric foil pack heater
3. Sterile gloves
4. Sterile abdominal pad
5. Waterproof protector
6. Exam gloves
7. Circulating water pad (optional)
8. Medications and dressings appropriate for wound care
9. Waste receptacle

GUIDELINES

1. A physician's order is required for this procedure.
2. Sterile warm moist compresses are applied to enhance healing; relieve inflammation, burning, and itching; soften exudate; promote drainage; and relieve discomfort.
3. The therapeutic effect of warm, moist compresses results from vasodilatation of the local blood vessels, increasing circulation in the area.
4. Sterile compresses should always be used over unhealed incisions, open wounds, or orifices such as the eyes.
5. A corner of the compress should be applied first to determine if the compress is too hot.
6. Patients who are comatose or have decreased sensation must be assessed closely for their tolerance to the heat application.
7. If desired, an additional heat source such as a circulating water pad may be applied over the compress to maintain heat for a longer period of time.
8. "Wet to dry" dressings are applied in the same manner as sterile warm moist compresses. The purpose of a "wet to dry" dressing is to debride the wound. The moist dressing remains on the wound until completely dried and is then removed along with any dead tissue.

NURSING ACTION/RATIONALE

1. Assemble all equipment.
2. Plug in the electric foil pack heater and activate the heater according to the manufacturer's instructions.
3. Place up to six unopened dressings in the heater with the peel flaps facing out.
4. Heat the packs for at least 5 minutes. If more than two dressings are being heated, rotate them, heating an additional 3 minutes for each dressing.
5. Identify the patient.
6. Explain the procedure to the patient.
7. Provide adequate lighting.
8. Provide privacy.
9. Position the patient comfortably with the area for treatment accessible.
10. Wash your hands.
11. Expose the affected area. Drape the patient if required.
12. Put on the exam gloves.
13. Remove soiled dressings. Discard into the waste receptacle.
14. Assess the wound for appearance, amount of drainage, odor, and skin condition.
15. Remove the exam gloves. Discard in the waste receptacle.
16. Wash your hands.
17. Open the wet dressing package and the dry abdominal pad, creating a sterile field with the wrappers.
18. Put on the sterile gloves.

19. Apply the wet dressings to the affected site.
20. Verify with the patient that the dressings are not too hot. Lift the corner slightly to check for signs of hyperthermia.
21. Cover the wet dressings with a sterile abdominal pad.
22. Remove the sterile gloves and discard.
23. Tape the dressing securely in place.
24. Cover the abdominal pad with a waterproof protector to aid in retaining the heat and moisture. Do *not* cover a "wet to dry" dressing.
25. Instruct the patient to notify the nurse if any discomfort develops.
26. Assist the patient to a comfortable position.
27. Discard equipment or return it to the appropriate location.
28. Leave the dressings in place for the length of time ordered. Compresses cool after about 30 minutes.
29. Apply an additional external heat source, if appropriate.
30. Remove the dressings after the prescribed time, using exam gloves. Discard in the waste receptacle.
31. Reapply appropriate sterile dry dressings, following the procedure "Sterile Dressing Change."
32. Discard equipment or return it to the appropriate area.

PATIENT AND/OR FAMILY TEACHING

1. Explain the procedure and its purpose to the patient.
2. Reinforce and clarify the physician's explanation of the disease process and the reason for the treatment.
3. Explain any additional therapeutic orders.
4. Instruct the patient to notify the nurse regarding any discomfort during the procedure.
5. Explain any activity restrictions necessary to ensure that the compresses stay in place.
6. Teach the patient or a family member how to make and apply warm compresses at home, if required following discharge.

DOCUMENTATION

1. Time of procedure, type of moisture used, and length of application.
2. Assessment of affected area, including appearance, amount of drainage, odor, and general condition.
3. The patient's reaction to the procedure.
4. All patient teaching done and the patient's level of understanding.

Non-Sterile Warm Moist Compresses

PURPOSE

1. Apply warm, moist heat.

REQUISITES

1. Compress machine
2. Lifting forceps
3. Compress cloth
4. Waterproof protector
5. Distilled water
6. Funnel
7. Circulating water pad (optional)

GUIDELINES

1. Non-sterile warm moist compresses are used over areas of the body where the skin is intact to relieve pain and congestion, localize infections, increase circulation, and aid in muscle relaxation.
2. The non-sterile compress should not be used over an open wound.
3. There is danger of burning the patient if the compress is too hot. A corner of the compress should be applied lightly to the patient's skin to determine tolerance to the temperature.
4. Patients that are comatose or have decreased sensation must be assessed closely for tolerance to the heat application.
5. The following procedure describes compresses prepared with a compress machine. If a compress machine is not available, the procedure can be performed using a towel soaked in hot tap water and wrung out.
6. If desired, an additional external heat source such as a circulating water pad may be applied to maintain heat for a longer period of time.

NURSING ACTION/RATIONALE

1. Assemble all equipment.
2. Wash your hands.
3. Prepare the compress machine according to manufacturer's recommendations.
4. Identify the patient.
5. Explain the procedure to the patient.
6. Moisten the compresses, using tap water only. Wring the cloth nearly dry and place it in the compress tray. Close the cover.
7. Using a pumping motion, press the lever down slowly three times, then wait 6 seconds.
8. Remove the compresses from the machine with a lifting forceps and take them to the patient's room in the waterproof protector.
9. Provide privacy.
10. Position the patient so that the affected area is exposed. Drape the patient, if appropriate.
11. Wash your hands.
12. Remove any used compresses and discard appropriately.
13. Assess the affected area for appearance and general condition.
14. Test the temperature of the compress with your hand.
15. Apply the compress carefully, testing one corner of the compress against the patient's skin to determine tolerance to the temperature.
16. Verify with the patient that the dressing is not too hot. Lift the corner of the compress to check for signs of hyperthermia.
17. Apply the waterproof protector over the compresses to aid in retaining the heat and the moisture.
18. Apply an additional external heat source, if appropriate.
19. Instruct the patient to call the nurse if any discomfort develops.
20. Leave the compresses on for the length of time ordered. Compresses cool after 30 minutes.
21. Assist the patient to a comfortable position.
22. Discard equipment or return it to the appropriate area.

PATIENT AND/OR FAMILY TEACHING

1. Explain the procedure and its purpose to the patient.
2. Reinforce and clarify the physician's explanation of the disease process.
3. Explain any additional therapeutic orders.
4. Instruct the patient to notify the nurse regarding any discomfort during the procedure.
5. Explain any activity restrictions necessary to ensure that the compresses stay in place.
6. Teach the patient or a family member how to make and apply warm compresses at home, if required following discharge.

DOCUMENTATION

1. Time of procedure and length of application.
2. Assessment of affected area, including appearance and general condition.
3. The patient's reaction to the procedure.
4. All patient teaching done and the patient's level of understanding.

 # Light Therapy

PURPOSE

1. Provide dry heat to the skin surface or mucous membranes.

REQUISITES

1. Gooseneck lamp or heat cradle
2. Light bulb (25, 40, or 60 watt)
3. Bath blanket
4. Exam gloves
5. Waste receptacle
6. Supplies for a sterile dressing change, if appropriate

GUIDELINES

1. A physician's order should be obtained before performing this procedure.
2. Heat lamps and cradles supply dry heat that increases circulation to an area, promotes drying, and aids in healing.
3. Heat lamps are usually gooseneck lamps that may be used to treat decubitus ulcers or small surface areas. The distance between the lamp and the patient is determined by the strength of the light bulb, the pigmentation of the skin, and the sensitivity of the skin. In general, a safe guide is:
   a. 25 watt light bulb—distance of 14 inches.
   b. 40 watt light bulb—distance of 18 inches.
   c. 60 watt light bulb—distance of 24 to 30 inches.
   Bed linen should never be draped over a gooseneck lamp, since it may be a fire hazard.
4. A heat cradle is a heat source with a series of 25 watt light bulbs. It is used for treatment of large surface areas. The patient and heat cradle are covered with a bath blanket during the treatment. The temperature under the blanket should not exceed 51.6°C (125°F). Unscrew, but do not remove, one or more light bulbs to lower the temperature. The heat cradle should be placed 18 to 24 inches from the patient.
5. Warm pink skin indicates the desired effect. Skin that becomes red or uncomfortable is being burned.

6. Any patient undergoing light therapy must be assessed frequently.
7. Patients who are confused or uncooperative should not be left unattended during light therapy.

NURSING ACTION/RATIONALE
1. Assemble all equipment.
2. Verify the physician's order.
3. Identify the patient.
4. Explain the nature and purpose of the treatment.
5. Provide adequate lighting.
6. Provide privacy.
7. Wash your hands.
8. Position the patient so that the affected area is exposed. Drape the patient as necessary.
9. Put on exam gloves and remove any old dressings as appropriate and discard. Remove exam gloves.
10. Place the gooseneck lamp or cradle the recommended distance from the patient. If a heat cradle is being used, cover the cradle and the patient with a bath blanket.
11. Continue the light therapy for 20 minutes or as ordered.
12. Instruct the patient not to touch the bulb or move closer to the light.
13. Assess the patient every 5 minutes for redness at the treatment site or discomfort.
14. Instruct the patient to call the nurse regarding any discomfort at the treatment site. If complications develop, discontinue the treatment.

15. Apply sterile dressings to the area following the treatment, if appropriate.
16. Assist the patient to a comfortable position.
17. Discard equipment or return it to the appropriate area.

PATIENT AND/OR FAMILY TEACHING
1. Explain the procedure and its purpose to the patient.
2. Reinforce and clarify the physician's explanation of the disease process.
3. Explain any additional therapeutic orders.
4. Remind the patient not to touch or move closer to the light.
5. Instruct the patient to inform the nurse if any adverse symptoms develop.
6. Teach the patient how to continue light therapy at home, if ordered.

DOCUMENTATION
1. Site of treatment, strength of bulb used, distance from patient, and duration of treatment.
2. Assessment of site before and after therapy.
3. The patient's reaction to the treatment.
4. All patient teaching done and the patient's level of understanding.

Burn Care:
Semi Open Air Method

PURPOSE
1. Promote wound healing.
2. Prevent complications from infection or deformity.

REQUISITES
1. Sterile gloves—2 pairs
2. Sterile basins—2
3. Sterile forceps
4. Sterile scissors
5. Sterile 4 × 4 sponges
6. Sterile normal saline irrigating solution, warmed to 37°C (98.6°F)
7. Iodophor liquid soap
8. Antimicrobial topical medication as prescribed
9. Mesh gauze large enough to cover the burn area
10. Waste receptacle

GUIDELINES
1. The percentage of the body surface burned, the source of the burns, the location of the burns, and the degree of skin damage determine the method of burn care. These factors, as well as the patient's age and physical condition, determine the prognosis for recovery.
2. A first degree (superficial) burn involves only the epidermis. A second degree (partial thickness) burn involves the epidermis and part of the dermis. A third degree (full thickness) burn involves all layers of the skin.
3. After stabilization, severely burned patients are usually transferred to a regional burn center where specialized personnel and equipment are available to treat the victim.
4. There are various methods of caring for a burn, including the open air method, the semi open air method, and the occlusive method.
   a. The *open air method* is useful in treating burns of the trunk, face, neck, and perineum. The burn forms a hard crust (eschar) in 72 hours, which protects the burn area. Topical antimicrobial agents may be applied to reduce infection in the burn. This method of treatment may require protective isolation.

   b. The *semi open air method* is also useful for burns of the trunk, face, neck, and perineum. A mesh antimicrobial-impregnated gauze is placed over the burn area and is changed daily. Protective isolation may also be used for this type of treatment.
   c. The *occlusive method* is used for burns of the feet and hands. Antimicrobial ointment or impregnated gauze is placed over the burn and a sterile dressing is applied.
5. The major complications following a severe burn include infection, fluid and electrolyte imbalances, and respiratory injury.
6. In addition to topical applications of antimicrobial agents, burn areas are treated with bath therapy, preferably in a Hubbard tank. Debridement of the burned areas can be done much earlier if bath therapy is instituted.
7. Skin grafting is usually performed following third degree burns. A variety of skin grafting techniques may be used.
8. The physician's order will determine the type of treatment for a burn.

NURSING ACTION/RATIONALE
1. Assemble all equipment.
2. Verify the physician's orders for treatment.
3. Follow any isolation precautions necessary before going into the patient's room.
4. Identify the patient.
5. Explain the procedure to the patient.
6. Administer an analgesic prior to the procedure if appropriate.
7. Provide adequate lighting.
8. Provide privacy.
9. Wash your hands.
10. Position the patient so that the burned area is exposed.
11. Rewash your hands.
12. Open the sterile supplies.
13. Cleanse the burn area:
    a. Pour iodophor soap and warmed, sterile normal saline into a sterile basin.

b. Pour warmed, sterile normal saline into the second basin.

c. Put on the sterile gloves.

d. Place sterile 4 × 4 inch gauze sponges in each basin.

e. Remove the old mesh gauze dressings and discard.

f. Cleanse the burn area with the soapy solution, using the 4 × 4 inch gauze sponges. Remove any medication or dead tissue.

g. Rinse the burn area with the normal saline.

14. Remove your gloves and discard.

15. Put on the second pair of sterile gloves.

16. Remove any additional dead tissue with a sterile forceps and scissors.

17. Apply a layer of the prescribed medication with a sterile gloved finger, covering the entire burn area.

18. Cover the burn area with the mesh gauze.

19. Reassure the patient frequently during the procedure.

20. Remove the sterile gloves and discard.

21. Assist the patient to a comfortable position.

22. Discard equipment or return it to the appropriate area.

23. Wash your hands.

PATIENT AND/OR FAMILY TEACHING

1. Explain the burn care to the patient as well as what discomfort to expect.

2. Reinforce and clarify the physician's explanation of the extent of the trauma.

3. Instruct the patient regarding the action and side effects of the medications.

4. Explain any additional therapeutic orders such as planned skin grafting.

5. Explain any activity restrictions to the patient.

6. Instruct the patient regarding range-of-motion exercises that can be done to prevent contractures.

7. Instruct the patient regarding good nutrition for wound healing.

DOCUMENTATION

1. Date and time of procedure, method used for cleansing the burn, and medication used to treat the burn.

2. Any analgesics given.

3. An assessment of the burn.

4. The patient's reaction to the procedure.

5. All patient teaching done and the patient's level of understanding.

Treating Patients with Pediculosis

PURPOSE
1. Therapeutically treat a patient with pediculosis.
2. Prevent the spread of pediculosis.

REQUISITES
1. Pediculicide shampoo or lotion (type as ordered by the physician)
2. Water-soluble bags
3. Red plastic isolation bags
4. Exam gloves
5. Equipment for a bed bath or bed shampoo, if necessary

GUIDELINES
1. Three different types of lice are found on the human body: head lice, body lice, and pubic lice (crabs). Head lice and body lice have very similar morphological characteristics (Figure 9-6a), whereas pubic lice have a considerably different appearance (Figure 9-6b).
2. Identification of the type of louse is important because treatment and prevention measures vary. In general, the louse can be identified by the part of the body infested. Head lice are found on the scalp, usually behind the ears or at the nape of the neck. Body lice are usually found on clothing or on the skin where clothing has close contact, such as the beltline. Pubic lice are found in the pubic hair but can be found on the eyelashes, on mustaches, and in axillary hair.
3. Frequently, louse eggs are observed rather than the adult. Head and pubic lice attach their eggs to hair follicles. Body lice generally lay their eggs in the seams of clothing.
4. Lice are spread by direct contact with an infested person or by indirect contact with clothing, bed linen, or personal items such as combs and hairbrushes.

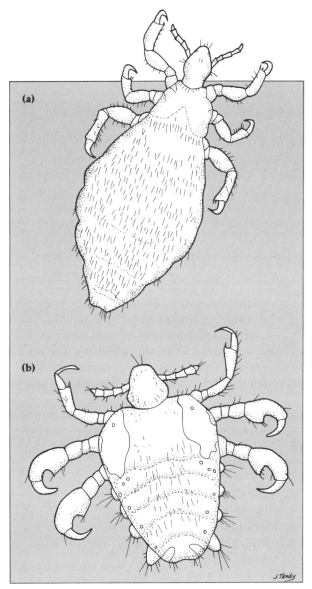

Figure 9-6. Types of lice. (**a**) Head or body louse. (**b**) Pubic louse ("crab").

5. The incubation period for louse eggs to hatch is one week under optimum conditions. Treatment with a pediculicide should be repeated after one week to ensure that any lice that were in the egg stage during the first treatment are destroyed.
6. Lice cannot survive 10 minutes of exposure to temperatures exceeding 52°C (125.6°F).
7. An assessment of lice on a patient should be reported to the physician and the nurse epidemiologist to initiate treatment and prevent transmission to other patients.
8. The patient with body lice does not need to be treated with a pediculicide. The infestation can be handled by treating clothing, linen, and bedding as described in the procedure.
9. Pediculicides vary as to their application, length of time for treatment, and time for removal. Follow the product manufacturer's directions and/or the physician's orders.
10. Infestation with lice does not necessarily mean that the patient has poor personal hygiene. Discretion should be used when discussing treatment with the patient and family. The patient and/or family may be very embarrassed about the situation. A well-informed supportive nurse can alleviate fears and misconceptions by sound patient teaching.
11. Adjunctive treatment with antihistamines and antipruretics may be indicated to eliminate the patient discomfort and scratching of the infested areas.

NURSING ACTION/RATIONALE
1. Assemble all equipment.
2. Identify the patient.
3. Explain the problem and the procedure for treatment.
4. Provide privacy.
5. Put on exam gloves.
6. Shampoo the patient's hair with pediculicide shampoo, if ordered. Assess the scalp for irritation.
7. Bathe the patient. Assess the patient's skin for irritation.
8. Shampoo the pubic hair with pediculicide shampoo, if ordered. Assess for skin irritation below the hair.

9. Comb the patient's scalp hair and/or pubic hair with a fine tooth comb to remove any lice or eggs attached to the hair.
10. Apply pediculicide lotion to the entire body, if ordered.
11. Assist the patient into a clean hospital gown.
12. Change the bed linen.
13. Bag the used bed linen, gown, towels, and washcloth in a water-soluble bag, then double-bag into a red plastic isolation bag.
14. Bag all the patient's personal clothing to be sent home for laundering.
15. Soak the patient's combs and brushes in pediculicide for 6 minutes or place them in 52°C (125.6°F) water for 10 minutes.
16. Remove the exam gloves.
17. Contact the housekeeping department to vacuum the patient's room and any upholstered furniture and to scrub the toilet seat.
18. Send the double-bagged linen to the laundry for washing.
19. Wash your hands.
20. Repeat the procedure in 1 week, or as ordered.
21. Follow up on removing the pediculicide after 24 hours if indicated by the product manufacturer.

PATIENT AND/OR FAMILY TEACHING
1. Explain the problem and the procedure to be used for treatment.
2. Answer any questions the patient may have and encourage questions.
3. Explain to the patient that a second treatment of pediculicide may be needed 7 days after the first treatment. Instruct the patient how to do the second treatment if the patient will be discharged.
4. Instruct the family or significant others to contact the public health department for a check to determine possible infestation and to obtain treatment, if necessary.

5. Instruct the family to launder the patient's personal clothing and bed linen in water 52°C (125.6°F) and to dry in a hot dryer for 20 minutes. If clothing cannot be laundered, dry cleaning will also eliminate the lice. An alternative is to keep all infested clothing in a plastic bag for 2 weeks, the life expectancy of the pubic and head louse. The body louse can remain dormant up to 30 days, so the plastic bag method is not recommended for body lice.

6. Instruct the patient and family not to share clothing, combs, brushes, and other personal items.

7. Instruct the patient to avoid scratching the areas of infestation.

8. Instruct the patient on the availability of antihistamines and antipruretics, if appropriate.

9. Instruct the patient and/or family regarding personal hygiene, if indicated.

DOCUMENTATION

1. Area of infestation and notification of physician.
2. Assessment of scalp or other skin areas.
3. Time, route, and dosage of all medications, including medicated shampoos and lotions.
4. Disposition of hospital linen.
5. Disposition of the patient's personal clothing.
6. Treatment of the patient's personal care items.
7. A follow-up assessment of the patient's skin and hair.
8. All patient and family teaching done and the level of understanding.

Teaching Manual Milk Expression to the Breastfeeding Mother

PURPOSE

1. Maintain a mother's milk supply when she must be hospitalized and separated from her nursing infant.
2. Obtain breast milk for infants unable to nurse.
3. Relieve breast engorgement.

REQUISITES

1. One of the following breast pumps may be used:
   a. Electric breast pump with sterile accessory kit (collection container, nipple shield)
   b. Breast milking/feeding unit with sterile collection bottle, cylinder, nipple shield, rubber ring
   c. "Bicycle horn" hand pump with collection container

GUIDELINES

1. A mother may need to be hospitalized for medical or surgical problems during lactation. Any separation of mother and baby should be as short as possible. If feasible, the baby should room in with the mother so that breastfeeding can continue.
2. If breastfeeding must be temporarily discontinued, breast milk can be adequately expressed either by hand or with a breast pump. However, this is no substitute for nursing the baby directly.
3. Mothers should express their milk regularly and frequently, about every 3 hours, to maintain their milk supply.
4. With adequate handwashing and sterile supplies, sterility of the milk can be maintained, if necessary. The nipples naturally secrete a cleansing oil and do not need to be cleaned off prior to hand expression.
5. Milk supply is related to fluid intake, rest, and nutrition. Fluids should be encouraged unless contraindicated.
6. Mothers on medication may have to discard their milk. The pharmacist is a good reference regarding the effect of drugs on breast milk.

7. When radioactive isotopes are used for diagnostic testing or general anesthesia is used for surgery, the mother may have to temporarily discontinue breastfeeding.
8. The degree of illness may affect the mother's ability to produce milk.
9. The "let-down" reflex, a hormonal response, causes milk to be released. This reflex can be assisted by providing privacy and encouraging the mother to look at a picture of or think about the baby.
10. When one breast is being emptied, the other breast may start to flow. Do not try to stop it.
11. The mother should be informed that practice and patience are needed to learn how to express milk. Praise the mother for her efforts and allow her to verbalize anxiety concerning her infant and any separation.
12. Milk to be fed to the infant should be collected in a sterile plastic container or bag. All parts of the pump need to be sterilized.
13. Collected milk should be refrigerated immediately. If it is not to be used within 48 hours, it must be frozen. Breast milk can be stored for up to 2 weeks in a refrigerator freezer and up to 6 months in a deep freezer.
14. Milk stored at the hospital should be labeled with the patient's name and the date collected.
15. In assisting the mother to select the best method of milk expression, several factors should be considered:
    a. *Availability*—how quickly can the pump be obtained? If the desired pump is not available at the hospital, contact the local chapter of La Leche League. Some pharmacies rent electric breast pumps. Hand expression is the most available method.

b. *Sterility*—how well does the method maintain sterility? Sterility can be easily maintained with the electric breast pump, since each mother receives her own accessory kit. The entire breast milking/feeding unit can be sterilized. Sterility can be maintained when using the hand pump with the attached bottle; however, the hand pump without the attached bottle cannot be adequately cleaned, since milk may enter the bulb. With proper handwashing, sterile technique can be maintained with hand expression.

c. *Collection capacity*—how much milk can be collected before it must be transferred to another container? Eight ounces can be collected with the electric breast pump without breaking the system. The maximum amount of milk collected with the breast milking/feeding unit is 3 ounces, but the infant can be fed directly from the collection container. The hand pump without the attached bottle holds less than $\frac{1}{2}$ ounce.

d. *Cost*—some insurance plans do not cover the cost of a pump. The electric breast pump may be expensive to rent. The hand pump is less expensive than the milking/feeding unit. However, hand expression is free.

e. *Effectiveness*—how well does the method of milk expression work? The electric breast pump provides a high level of breast stimulation. It is recommended for mothers who need to express milk on a long-term basis. The other methods are recommended for occasional or short-term use.

f. *Mobility of the mother*—the breast milking/feeding unit is contraindicated with women who have limited mobility of their arms.

NURSING ACTION/RATIONALE

1. Wash your hands.
2. Identify the patient. Instruct her to wash her hands.
3. Assemble the breast pump according to the manufacturer's directions.
4. Explain manual expression by the chosen method to the mother.
5. Provide privacy.
6. Assist the patient to a comfortable position.
7. Have the mother massage and stroke her breast toward the nipple to bring the milk from the milk ducts into the milk reservoirs.
8. Have the mother manually express the breast milk from one breast:
   a. Electric breast pump (Figure 9-7**a**):
   (1) Place the nipple shield over the nipple area. Ensure a good seal.
   (2) Adjust the lever for desired amount of suction.
   (3) Turn the machine on.
   (4) Allow the milk to flow into the collection chamber, keeping the container below the level of the nipple shield.

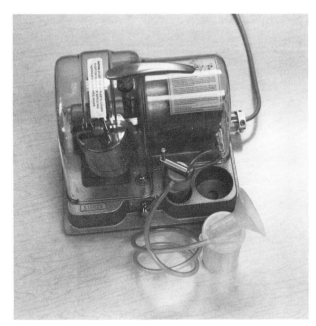

Figure 9-7a. Electric breast pump.

b. Breast milking/feeding unit (Figure 9-7**b**).
   (1) Place the nipple shield over the nipple area. Ensure a good seal.
   (2) Gently slide the collection container back and forth in a pistonlike manner to produce suction.
c. "Bicycle horn" hand pump (Figure 9-7**c**).
   (1) Depress the bulb halfway.
   (2) Place the nipple shield over the nipple area. Ensure a good seal.
   (3) Release the bulb partway, observing the suction on the nipple.
   (4) Continue compressing and releasing the bulb partway to produce gentle suction. Do not release or compress completely.

d. Hand expression (Figure 9-8).
   (1) Hold the container under the breast.
   (2) Place the thumb and the first two fingers about 1 to 1½ inches behind the nipple. Position the thumb above and the fingers below the nipple.
   (3) Push into the chest wall.
   (4) Roll the thumb and fingers toward the nipple, as if to make fingerprints.
   (5) Repeat this sequence around the nipple. Avoid squeezing, pulling, or sliding, which can hurt the breast tissue.

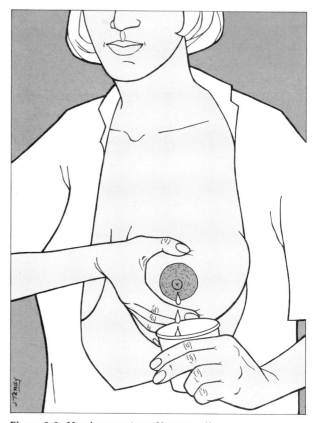

Figure 9-8. Hand expression of breast milk.

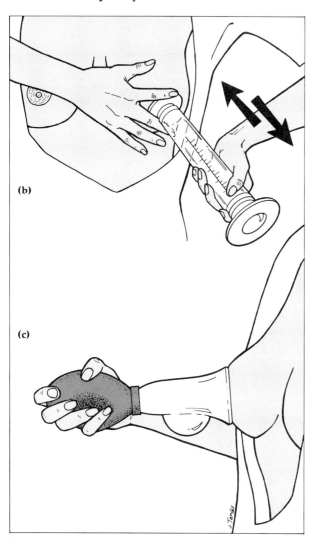

Figure 9-7 (continued). (**b**) Breast milking/feeding unit. (**c**) "Bicycle horn" hand pump.

9. After 5 minutes or when the collection container is full, have the mother break suction by inserting a finger underneath the nipple shield. Empty the collection container and store or discard milk as desired.
10. Repeat steps 7, 8, and 9 on the second breast.
11. Stay with the mother until her milk is flowing and she is comfortable with the procedure. Provide encouragement and reinforce the technique.
12. Have the mother continue to alternately massage and express each breast for the same amount of time that her infant would be nursing.
13. Return all equipment to the appropriate area.

PATIENT AND/OR FAMILY TEACHING

1. Explain breast milk expression methods available and their advantages and disadvantages.
2. Instruct the mother to massage the breasts before and during milk expression.
3. Teach and demonstrate the chosen method of milk expression to the mother.
4. Teach the mother the importance of good handwashing and reinforce the regulations for storing the milk.
5. Observe the return demonstration by the mother to evaluate her technique.

DOCUMENTATION

1. Method used to express milk.
2. An evaluation of the mother's expression technique.
3. Whether the mother is discarding or saving her milk.
4. All patient teaching done and the patient's level of understanding.

Vaginal Irrigation or Douche

PURPOSE

1. Cleanse the vaginal canal.
2. Treat a vaginal infection.
3. Reduce inflammation of vaginal tissues.

REQUISITES

1. Vaginal douche unit
2. Solution (amount and type as ordered by the physician)
3. Cotton balls
4. Clean basin with warm soapy water
5. Waterproof bed protector
6. Bath blanket
7. Sterile gloves
8. Water-soluble jelly
9. Bedpan
10. IV standard

GUIDELINES

1. A physician's order is required for this procedure.
2. The special nozzle on the tubing of the douche unit has holes on the side to minimize the risk of fluid passing through the cervical os into the uterus.
3. Normally, the nozzle is rotated during the irrigation. Never rotate the nozzle if the patient has had recent vaginal surgery or has a diagnosis of cervical cancer.
4. The patient should empty her bladder before the irrigation. A full bladder may be painful when irrigating.
5. Always observe clean techniques but wear sterile gloves for the procedure.
6. Solution for irrigation should be warmed to 38 to 40.5°C (100 to 105°F) unless otherwise specified by the doctor.
7. Assess the patient's perineum for excoriation before irrigating. Excoriation can be painful when in contact with some irrigating solutions; consult with the physician before proceeding.

NURSING ACTION/RATIONALE

1. Assemble all equipment.
2. Identify the patient.
3. Explain the procedure to the patient.
4. Instruct the patient to empty her bladder.
5. Assist the patient onto the bedpan and place the patient in a dorsal recumbent position with knees flexed and legs spread.
6. Drape the patient and place the bed protector under her buttocks.
7. Wash your hands.
8. Clamp the tubing on the bag and fill the bag with the warmed solution.
9. Unclamp the tubing and clear all air. Reclamp.
10. Put on sterile gloves.
11. Cleanse the patient's perineum with cotton balls soaked in warm water. Start cleansing from the outer edges of the labia in smooth downward strokes. Use each cotton ball once and discard.
12. Lubricate the nozzle with water-soluble lubricant.
13. Hang the irrigating bag on an IV standard, no more than 12 inches above the patient's vagina.
14. Separate the patient's labia with one hand. Gently insert the nozzle into the vagina, angling it upward and then downward toward the patient's back (Figure 9-9). Advance the nozzle about 2 inches into the vagina.

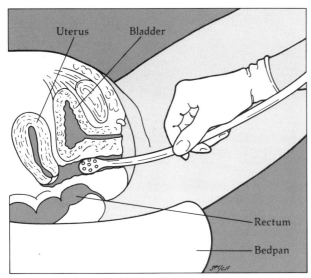

Figure 9-9. Placement of irrigation nozzle in the vagina.

15. Open the clamp and allow the solution to flow into the vagina by gravity. Gently rotate the nozzle during the irrigation.
16. Clamp the tubing when the irrigation is completed and gently remove the nozzle.

17. Allow the patient to remain on the bedpan for a few minutes to completely drain the vagina.
18. Remove the bedpan and wash the perineum with soap and water. Dry thoroughly.
19. Assess the perineal area.
20. Remove gloves.
21. Assist the patient to a comfortable position.
22. Discard equipment or return it to the appropriate area.

PATIENT AND/OR FAMILY TEACHING
1. Explain the procedure and rationale to the patient before starting.
2. Instruct the patient in the steps of the procedure for self-administration, if appropriate.

DOCUMENTATION
1. Procedure performed.
2. Amount of medication or solution used.
3. The patient's reaction to the procedure.
4. Assessment of the perineum.
5. All patient teaching done and the patient's level of understanding.

Index